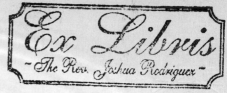
HEALING
THE
MIND
THROUGH
THE POWER OF
STORY

The Promise of
Narrative Psychiatry

LEWIS MEHL-MADRONA, M.D., Ph.D.

Bear & Company
Rochester, Vermont • Toronto, Canada

Bear & Company
One Park Street
Rochester, Vermont 05767
www.BearandCompanyBooks.com

Bear & Company is a division of Inner Traditions International

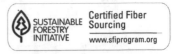

> *Note to the reader:* *This book is intended as an informational guide. The remedies, approaches, and techniques described herein are meant to supplement, and not to be a substitute for, professional medical care or treatment. They should not be used to treat a serious ailment without prior consultation with a qualified health care professional.* ***Anyone who is currently taking psychiatric drugs should not stop taking them without the support and guidance of a qualified health care professional as serious withdrawal symptoms can ensue.***

Library of Congress Cataloging-in-Publication Data
Mehl-Madrona, Lewis, 1954–
   Healing the mind through the power of story : the promise of narrative psychiatry / Lewis Mehl-Madrona.
      p. ; cm.
   Includes bibliographical references and index.
   Summary: "Psychiatry that recognizes the essential role of community in creating a new story of mental health"—Provided by publisher.
   ISBN 978-1-59143-095-7 (pbk.)
   1. Narrative therapy. I. Title.
   [DNLM: 1. Narration. 2. Psychotherapy—methods. 3. Indians, North American. WM 420 M498h 2010]
   RC489.S74M443 2010
   616.89'165—dc22

                                                                      2010007197

Printed and bound in the United States by Lake Book Manufacturing

10 9 8 7 6 5 4 3 2 1

Text design and layout by Priscilla Baker
This book was typeset in Garamond Premier Pro with Avant Garde

To send correspondence to the author of this book, mail a first-class letter to the author c/o Inner Traditions • Bear & Company, One Park Street, Rochester, VT 05767, and we will forward the communication, or contact the author at **www.mehl-madrona.com.**

This book is dedicated to my mother, Emily Bradley Mehl, who was not only crazy enough to bring me into the world, which I'm sure was not terribly easy in many ways, but who has been there to help me out many times, even though I'm supposed to be a grownup and not need help.

Contents

PART I
History and Foundations

PART II
Science and Mind

Acknowledgments

I want to thank my friends who helped me through the completion of this book, especially Magili Chapman-Quinn, Kitty Ketner, Skyler Madison, Peter Blum, Sheila and Sheldson Lewis, Thomas Vietoricz, Aiyana Stern, Lorna Chase, Gordon Pennycook, and Karin Mack. Each of these people read chapters and gave me invaluable feedback. A big thanks to my Mississippi catfish buddy, Rocky Crocker, for his wonderful support and assistance, and to Barbara Mainguy, with whom I discussed the ideas of this book and who helped me in innumerable ways with making my writing more clear and presenting these ideas that are not always so easy to articulate. Thanks to Andrei Vinogradov, who has been teaching me Russian in between some great conversations, and who taught me that Brezhnev was a minor political figure in the era of Alla Pugachova, the Russian pop star. Thanks to John Charles of Sturgeon Lake First Nation for his healing and support. And thanks to my students at the University of Saskatchewan, who gave me important feedback about the clarity of presentation and the plausibility of these ideas. Thanks to Tony Gee, for much of the editing of this book was completed in the back seat of his car as we drove around Australia, meeting with different aboriginal groups in hopes of inspiring further movement of culture into health care. The remainder of this book was edited on United Airlines, and I thank the flight attendants who took care of me while I completed this work, especially Ted Pizzino. Thanks to my editors at Inner Traditions: Jamaica Burns and Nancy Yeilding, whose help was invaluable.

Preface

This book was written during my four years of practicing psychiatry in rural and remote areas of Saskatchewan, Canada, and extends the concepts I developed in my previous work, *Narrative Medicine: The Use of History and Story in the Healing Process,* into the field of psychiatry.[1] In all of my books, I have struggled to follow the advice of Austrian philosopher Ludwig Wittgenstein (1889–1951), who urged us to write simply and plainly, without jargon. Wittgenstein believed that technical terms should never be used when plain language would suffice.

In keeping with Wittgenstein's vision, I have worked to create a new genre of writing, one that is simultaneously popular and academic, interesting to professionals but accessible to the general public. I disagree with the ideas that ordinary people cannot understand complex concepts and that complex concepts cannot be simply revealed without jargon or technical language.

Besides Wittgenstein, two other figures loom large as my guides for this work: His Crazy Horse and Ohiyesa. His Crazy Horse, which, translated from Lakota, literally means "His Horse is Crazy" (ca. 1842–1877), was a Lakota visionary who had an amazing vision. He saw great, gray ribbons stretching across the prairie, on which large bugs were traveling at incredibly fast speeds. People were looking out from many openings in these bugs. His Crazy Horse also saw great birds flying across the sky. Inside these birds were many people, looking out of holes that opened along the length of the bird. They were all coming to learn about healing from the Lakota people.

His Crazy Horse predicted that in seven generations, the children of the conquerors would come to learn Lakota spirituality and healing. They would pick up the ways of the Lakota, to the chagrin of their ancestors. We are now in that seventh generation, and the prophecy is coming true. People of all origins who live in North America are embracing traditional Native spirituality. His Crazy Horse was right, so I write in support of his vision.

Ohiyesa—Charles Eastman, M.D. (1858–1939)—was an Oglala physician. People have told me that we might be related. I hope so. Eastman lived a traditional Oglala hunter/gatherer lifestyle until his missing father resurfaced when Ohiyesa was fifteen years old. Given up for dead, his father had actually been in a U.S. government prison for the crime of insurgency. Upon his return, he announced that Charles must "learn the cunning of the white man." Charles did. He applied himself to the task and graduated from Dartmouth College. He proceeded to study medicine at Boston University. Following his internship, he returned to be the physician at Wounded Knee, South Dakota, and tended the injured at the Massacre of Wounded Knee in 1890. Eastman helped to found the Boy Scouts, blending Oglala cultural symbols into the organization, and inspired the creation of the Order of the Arrow, Scouting's National Honor Society.

Eastman wrote over ten books about Oglala culture and spirituality, some of which are still in print today. He truly tried to blend cultures and to enrich mainstream America with the wisdom of Native America. That has been my goal too. My mother was Cherokee and Scottish, while my father was Oglala Lakota and Quebecoise. So I have attempted to weave an indigenous perspective into all that I write so that the resulting narrative is applicable to both mainstream North America and the indigenous world. I hope Eastman would be proud of my efforts, for he is part of the audience to whom I write. Throughout the writing of this book, I have asked for his spiritual help, along with that of His Crazy Horse, Ludwig Wittgenstein, my grandfather Archie, and any others who could assist.

There's Nothing But Story

Telling stories is a human universal. It develops
spontaneously without training in childhood.
BRIAN BOYD, *ON THE ORIGINS OF STORIES:*
EVOLUTION, COGNITION, AND FICTION

Healing the Mind through the Power of Story furthers the renewal of interest in the importance of story and of individual human lives in medicine and in psychiatry. Stories are a very important source of medical knowledge and wisdom, perhaps even the basic unit of information gathering in medical diagnosis and research, and are the essential ingredient of human relationship and communication. In what has become an increasingly impersonal world, both medicine and society at large are beginning to realize and rediscover the importance of relationship and stories in healing.

At first the concept seems simplistic. Of course we all tell stories: for fun, for entertainment, for camaraderie, but facts are what matter, the results of scientific research, the *truth*. What I will try to show in this book is that the facts that we worship in our global, modern, industrialized culture are just the summary line of story. Having been a physician now for thirty-four years, I know that the stories science produces change every two years. It's hard to study for exams, for example, because it is often not clear which version of the story will be on the test. In 2005, we didn't think digoxin helped the kind of heart failure that is called diastolic dysfunction, meaning that the heart doesn't fill properly and the amount of blood pumped is below 40 percent of normal. In 2008, we learned that the problem was dosage. Low-dose digoxin did help, while the higher doses we were using didn't. This was a relief because we didn't have to keep checking blood levels with the lower doses that worked better anyway. But on my 2009 geriatrics exam, which would be the right answer to the question, Is digoxin useful for diastolic dysfunction heart failure? That depends on what year the test was written.

Much of contemporary science is like this, and all of it is based on a worldview that variables are independent and not interconnected, which most of my elders think is ludicrous. They can't believe any educated person would actually think in this way (have such a story about the world). Every "fact" that we state is the result of many stories. As one Lakota elder told me, "It's all story. There's nothing but story."

We would not survive without story, for story defines our meaning and purpose, our identity, our goals and values—everything that makes life worth living. Australian aboriginal people have four levels of meaning and interpretation of story, all of which are crucial for our lives.[1] There is the level of the text itself, as in explanations of the natural features of the world and animal behavior, so common in traditional, indigenous stories. Then there is a second level of relationships between people and within communities. On this level, stories tell us how to relate and behave and form a community with others. A third level shows us how to negotiate the relationships between our own community and the larger environment. A fourth level teaches us about spiritual action and psychic skills. This level includes the practices, ceremonies, and experiences that give access to the esoteric spiritual knowledge that lies within the story. Australian elders also teach that all stories and all versions of the same story are true, and that discernment comes in knowing when and how to use a story and for what purpose.

Stories teach us empathy. They help us understand another person's position. This is because stories contain so much more information than we can possibly convey in the statement of facts. Stories give us unique access to the inner lives and motivations of others. The twelfth-century Persian poet Nizama wrote, "While each warrior thought of nothing but to kill the enemy and to defend himself, the poet was sharing the sufferings of both sides."[2] History is written by the winners, but story allows everyone's perspectives to be told, even those who are conquered. In movies, even the stories of villains can be told—Hannibal, Al Capone, Adolf Hitler, and more. As University of Auckland Professor Brian Boyd puts it in *On the Origins of Stories: Evolution, Cognition, and Fiction,* "Stories come most alive when *all* the principal characters have their own vivid life."[3]

Stories assist us in developing empathy by helping us see the world from others' perspectives. When I want to know how someone came to believe what she believes, I ask her to tell me a story to illustrate her point. When I hear enough stories, I come to realize the experiences that led her to draw a particular conclusion. When I was in graduate school, a researcher put pro-choice and anti-choice advocates together in the same room. He didn't ask them to argue their beliefs. He asked them to go around the circular table and tell stories about the life experiences that led them to come to the beliefs about abortion that they held. No one changed their beliefs, but they left the room with a profoundly greater respect for the other side's position—that there might be reasons to think differently than we do.

Stories give cognitive and emotional significance to experience. Stories are amusing, memorable, and absorbing; they are also instructive, informative, and orienting. Through the hearing and telling of stories, children learn how to be a child and how to relate to their parents and other adults who populate the world around them. We construct and negotiate our social identity through the stories that we tell other people (and through the stories that then get repeated about us). Stories assist us in developing a moral sense, as they give moral weight and existential significance to actions and events.

Stories enhance our creativity and help us to think beyond the here and now. Just as yesterday's science fiction becomes today's reality, stories give us new vantage points from which to contemplate the possible and eventually create it. They stimulate our imagination and allow us to see alternatives. Without story, our lives and environments would be hideously drab and uninteresting. As Boyd puts it, "A mental architecture that processes only [facts] remains severely constricted. . . . Most discovery involves supposition."[4]

Stories keep us connected in social networks, which build and shape our brains. Just as our brain makes maps of our sensory body and of the outer physical world that it explores and interprets, it also maps our social world.[5] These social maps, which consist of stories that we have constructed about our experiences, guide our action in the world. By storing information about our social world in narrative form, we are able to quickly assess the motivations of others, their intent, how they make us feel, their status in our social hierarchy, their feelings about us, the context of the situation, and what behaviors would be considered normative. Recalling a story brings this knowledge to the fore of our awareness with a complexity and richness of information that is staggeringly greater and more complex than any series of statements of "beliefs."

According to Boyd, "Nature did not design us to think in the abstract. Minds evolved to respond to their immediate surroundings and could hardly do otherwise. Yet, nature *has* prepared minds to attend to and to act in response to other agents and actions and has shaped *human* minds for play, through their long childhood, with models and ideas of agents and actions and reactions. As we grow, we learn to dispense with physical props and to rely more and more readily on the cultural props of our narrative heritage, always on call in memory, in order to think in sustained ways beyond the here and now."[6]

Stories unlock the mysteries of psychophysical suffering that declarative facts cannot reveal. Social life is the performance of stories. Physiological life is the consequence of the performance of those stories. The enactment of story has deep physiological consequences for all involved. For example, my client with back pain told stories about people at work who wouldn't get off her back. She told stories about being unable to say no to others who then became "burdens around her neck." Language arises from the body, and story presents the meanings that are embedded within the body. We verify the truth of these stories when we act on them and the body changes. My client finally said no, quit her job, and ended her relationships with her "hangers-on;" and her back pain disappeared.

Another client with sciatic pain spontaneously told a story about being raped at age seven and being unable to tell anyone. Her pain had begun at that time, followed by intermittent flare-ups ever since. Immediately after the rape, she had come home sobbing inconsolably. Her mother had been insensitive to her pain. She related her frustration at her mother not even asking why she was crying and acting as if her pain was trivial and even annoying. Healing came when she told the story during somatic therapy (also called body work, massage therapy, osteopathic manipulation) on the sciatic area of her body. In telling the story, along with relating a recurrent dream that had plagued her since that time, she was able to grasp the meaning of her experience, her dream, and her pain. She practiced telling a new story about how she wished the postrape experience had gone with her mother and family. In that story, her mother was concerned and pried from her the story of what had happened to her. Her mother then confronted the boy and his family, and amends were made. My client felt supported, loved, and transformed. After that retelling, her long-term sciatic pain resolved and has not returned.

Such stories are common; they confirm our intuitive grasp of the relationships between our life events and our bodies. While they defy the usual type of medical research, they nevertheless form another kind of epistemology, different from that valued by medicine—that of narrative inquiry.

We can reinvent psychiatry as the art and science of story. We can draw on the wisdom of the narrative movement in philosophy and psychology for support in transforming our vision of brain and behavior from one of defective brains (genetically or structurally) to defective stories.

The global crisis in mind and mental health arises from the domination of a biomedical, clinical point of view over all others. It defines mind as brain and creates experts (psychiatrists) to medicate defective brains. What disturbs me is how much this approach erodes personal relationships. We cannot really care for chronic, long-term patients or incurable patients without appreciating the stories of their lives. It is only through these stories that these difficult patients come to be human for us and our relationships have meaning over and beyond the little interactions of caretaking.

Genetics fits within the narrative model. Brains that are very different, such as individuals with autism, can be understood in terms of story-environment mismatch. When the stories of these individuals match their environment, they can thrive. In a similar manner, the people who suffer from what we call "severe mental illnesses" are not so different from us. Mental illness is not a qualitatively different thing from being "normal," as contemporary psychology would have us believe, but rather, the extreme of a continuum in which we all live. For example, we all hear voices. Some of us think we are talking to ourselves. Some of us think the voices are outside of our heads. Some of us call these voices "self-talk." Some of us call these voices memories of conversations. When I work with a person, I start with his beliefs and I ask for stories to show me how he came to form those beliefs. Inevitably, we find that they are partly formed by people who made conclusions for him or interpreted the world for him. He is, like all of us, enacting stories shaped by his social networks (past, present, and future).

A person who has been hospitalized for hearing voices is not so different. She has simply lost (or never learned) the capacity to manage her voices. She might have fantastic stories to explain how these voices became associated with her. Sometimes her voices tell these stories. As we work together, most of her voices become ordinary people from her past. Her stories about her voices change. The voices are now attached to images. Over time she learns that such voices are the internal representations of people from her outer life and they are still saying the same things they said when those people were actually present in the past. Then the voices can be countered. With my support, along with that of a larger community of family and friends, she can "fight back" and make the voices go away (except for the kind or loving voices she may want to keep). She has learned to manage her voices in the same way the rest of us do.

Occasionally, people who were previously suffering miserably discover that some of the voices are actually beneficial and may have ontological status above and beyond mere internal representations. These voices become spirit guides or guardian angels, and the people who hear them emerge wiser and more comforted than those of us who have none. This awareness is part of what the psychiatrist Stanislav Grof called a spiritual awakening.

Consider Mary, a thirty-four-year-old woman living at home with her parents, tormented by voices for nine years. She refused to accept the standard psychiatric explanation that she is genetically defective and must be on medication for the rest of her life. She tried medication and found it a worse experience than hearing voices. "At least with my voices, I've got company and I have myself," she said. "The medication didn't stop the voices and I lost myself. No one was home anymore. All my creativity went away. Everything that I value about life disappeared. I'd rather keep the voices."

Mary needed a counter-narrative about voices. She loved the idea that everyone hears voices and that she could retrain her brain to manage her voices better. She preferred this interpretive story to the conventional one. She was able to work within it to manage her voices. Her voices resolved into one really bad one that assumed the appearance of many people from her past, changing its tonality, phrasing, and accent to match the person it was mimicking. Mary eventually decided that this voice was an evil spirit that had attached itself to her when she was homeless. Whether this is true is unimportant, since it worked. Stories slowly emerged of the ways she had been abused, including being raped when homeless. Over time the evil spirit voice differentiated into a concatenation of the voices of the people who had abused her on the streets and the demeaning and belittling stories they told her about herself. We were then able to rid her of the voices and their stories one at a time. She kept some of her comforting voices, relabeling them as angels. Over two years of working, Mary emerged as socially competent and able to manage herself in the world, feel better, and suffer less. That was a far better and more exciting outcome than the results of the prevailing biomedical story would have been.

I will tell similar stories about what we call schizophrenia, arguing that we all have schizophrenic experiences, but most of us call these
experiences dreams, daydreams, fantasies, and so on. The person labeled
schizophrenic is merely at the extreme of a continuum of being unable to
tell the difference between dream and ordinary waking life. He or she can
relearn that capacity. Similarly for autistic individuals, given a sufficiently
powerful motivating story, the person can learn (with the help of a supportive community) a theory of mind that includes other people.

**To do this kind of work and to see the world in this way, we need
strong supporting stories.** In this book, I will offer scientific stories, not
as fact, because fact will change, but as plausible stories about the world
that produce better outcomes and are more aesthetic than the stories they
are replacing. Stories about neuroplasticity, neurogenesis, epigenetics, and
social learning are more practical and desirable than stories about fixed
genetic defects that cannot be changed. These newer stories lead us to do
practical things that help people suffer less and to do them in more effective ways than we did before we heard them.

I have been especially impressed with Dr. Edward Taub at the University
of Alabama, who has developed what he calls constraint-induced movement
therapy for people who have had strokes and can't move a "paralyzed" limb.
From basic science research, Taub figured out that because they are unable
to move the limb in the acute phase immediately after the stroke, these
people "learn" that moving it is impossible. Once the acute phase of the
stroke is over, even though they are then capable of moving, they continue
to tell themselves the story (believe) that they can't move. Taub constrains
the movement of their working limbs, forcing them to move their other
limbs and reconfigure a brain map for those limbs. He forcibly counters
the story that they are paralyzed. The results are phenomenal.[7]

I have been doing something similar with those who hear voices and
are unable to reality test. I am challenging the story that these people
can't change, and I am placing their experiences in normative contexts and
giving them exercises and procedures to manage voices. I help patients
who have been diagnosed as bipolar learn how to manage their moods
in very similar ways. What will surprise most psychiatrists (and people

who live in the mainstream world) is that all of this is possible without medication if there is enough social support in place. I do occasionally prescribe medication, but mostly when it is necessary as a substitute for social support.

What I will argue in this book is that the split previously believed to exist between "functional" and "anatomic" brain changes is a bad story. In the past, we believed that if brain changes could be demonstrated, then the problem was "physical" and deserving of a "physical" solution (drugs, shock therapy, surgery) and if brain changes couldn't be demonstrated, then the problem deserved a psychological solution. Instead I am suggesting that we need different stories, stories that convince us that we can all change and relearn or learn for the first time how to better function in the world. In fact, all experience changes our brains.

In his *The Brain That Changes Itself: Stories of Personal Triumph from the Frontiers of Brain Science,* Norman Doidge wrote about another inspiring neuroscientist whose work underscores this point.[8] Michael Merzenich of the University of California, San Francisco, literally coined the term *neuroplasticity* through his experiments with cutting peripheral nerves and letting them grow back. To everyone's surprise and amazement, even though the regrown nerves were all jumbled up compared with the nerves before they were cut, the brain sorted this out and created a working map that entirely normalized the jumbled sensory input.[9] This is what I am arguing we can do for people with "severe mental illness." We can provide experiences for them that will enable their brains to unjumble their perceptions and reconfigure their brain maps. We can do this through teaching them better stories about themselves and the world.

Critical periods exist in which environmental stimulation is required for proper brain development. For example, the visual cortex of kittens will not develop if the eyes are kept shut during this critical time. If one eye is forcibly kept shut, the part of the brain that is supposed to map the shut eye gets recruited by the working eye and won't go back to serving the shut eye when that eye is opened.[10] A host of other brain areas have been found to have similar critical periods. I suspect that similar phenomena happen to people who are diagnosed as schizophrenic. Perhaps their lives are so miserable that it's more pleasurable or protective to pay attention to dreams or fantasy, and eventually the part of the brain that keeps track of waking life versus dream life gets recruited by the dreaming brain and loses its appropriate function. We can retrain that function!

Narrative approaches to psychiatry allow us to bridge from indigenous knowledge to scientific knowledge. Another focus in this book is based on my realization that most of what I am suggesting is already known by indigenous people. My inspiration for a narrative approach to psychiatry actually came from my studies of traditional North American healers for the past thirty-six years. I didn't initially know about narrative philosophy or psychology—even though I was practicing it—because I had learned it from traditional elders who didn't have those words. As one Lakota elder put it, "Isn't it exciting that neuroscience is finally catching up to the Lakota?" Indigenous medicine will live on because it contains the wisdom of healing through story. It appeals to those who cannot find a holistic understanding of their ailments in present Western medicine. It can transform our contemporary world and foster healing among all concerned.

As so many indigenous and other healers have pointed out, healing is unique and individual. How people change and transform cannot be predicted by knowing the allopathic diagnosis from which they suffer. How people can heal is implicit within the unique story of their lives and their illness. We must discover those stories through our interaction and we must cocreate a healing future, as I did with the three people presented so far—who suffered from low back pain, sciatica, and hearing voices. Through the appreciation of the power of story, we can build bridges between the indigenous and the modern worlds to create an integration that allows for more people to be healed.

No one heals without community. Another focus of this book is to keep in continual awareness that we are all neurons in a social brain. We need each other to grow and change and heal. We cannot do so alone. We must overthrow the primacy of the individual story, especially that of the "rugged individual." I think such stories were written by the ruling classes to keep people down. Barbara Ehrenreich said in a lecture I heard that "the establishment always hated the communal expression of art, as in tribal dancing or dancing in the streets." The establishment has also hated the communal practice of healing, as in ceremonies. European-derived cultures are low on community healers because so many were burned at the stake. Indigenous cultures have communal and community-based healers and ceremonies, but look at the lengths that the United States and the Canadian governments went to prohibit the practice of these ceremonies. Massacres like that at Wounded Knee in 1890 occurred when people gathered to peacefully conduct their ceremonies.

I suggest that everyone form a healing circle (*hocokah* in Lakota) to help each other with healing, and in this book I provide suggestions on how to do so. Traditionally these circles formed around elders, but we are in short supply of elders these days. Also, because of colonization and Christianization and intergenerational trauma, some elders are more restrictive than helpful. We have to come together to help each other even if genuine wisdomkeepers are not available. We can make community, create community art, create community ceremony and dance and ritual and music for our healing, even if faced with the lack of blueprints for how to do this. We can dance. We can keep rhythm. No other primate from capuchin monkeys to nonhuman apes can keep rhythm. This is uniquely human, and we must use it to our full advantage to entrain ourselves to coherence with each other for maximal healing and transformation.

It not only takes a village to raise a child, it also takes a village to heal a person with schizophrenia or a bipolar disorder or to make an autistic individual happy and functional. Putting people into institutions and out of sight only compounds the problem. Jail, which is the contemporary psychiatric hospital, is not where our mentally ill people should be. They should be with us, in our midst.

I won't spend much time on the impoverished state of mental health care today. I will simply say that everything gets degraded in a class society run by money. Our current system exists because it is profitable for those in charge. It is not helpful for most of the seriously mentally ill people we are supposed to serve. I will mention studies to demonstrate this, but convincing the reader of the failures of contemporary mental health care is not my focus. It is rather to demonstrate a solution that is labor intensive, human focused, and grounded in story.

Although this solution may be a minority perspective now, it is always possible that eventually minority voices can rise to become the dominant paradigm. The Russians discovered that you can't kill art. In Czechoslovakia, for example, after the Russian invasion, samizdat art was everywhere. Coyotes like me are always around to challenge the status quo. Coyote is the North American Native symbol for change and transformation, for flexibility and humor. She's always in the wings, howling at our dominant culture to change. Art today can emerge from homeless people, runaway kids, and gangs—the disenfranchised. Like these people standing at the margins of society, Coyote stands at the edge of biomedicine suggesting another story that could work better for helping the people who are suffering.

Narrative psychiatry is decidedly *not* antidrug. Whatever works is good. But it is decidedly against practice through dogma. If drugs worked as well as they were presented to do in my pharmacology class in medical school, I would never have followed my current life path. If drugs were a panacea, people would take them. I have spent forty years with people who have been diagnosed with serious mental illness, and I respect them. If something would stop their suffering without compounding it, they would certainly use it, in a majority of cases. People are natural optimizers within the constraints imposed on their world by the stories they tell and share with others of their community.

Truth is not "out there" waiting to be discovered and measured, leading to rules and regularities. Truth is a story that people create through their social interactions, always provisional and contingent on context. Plato was wrong. No pristine, raw material exists, independent of beliefs or persuasion. We arrive at the meaning of our lives through collaboratively negotiating our stories with all those around us.

The ideas of this book can be summarized as follows:

1. Everything is story, including our identities, our selves, our meanings and purposes, our theories about the world.

2. Brains are organs of story, changing to match the needs of their environment, and specialized to understand story, store story, recall story, and tell story. Brains use stories to make maps of the external world, which we can never fully know. Those maps work more or less effectively. Changing story changes those maps and allows us to function better.

3. Culture shapes brains and genetics through the transmission of story. Culture consists of all the stories ever told and remembered in a given locale coupled with all the results (buildings, art, ceremony, and so on) of enacting these stories, which may come from a multitude of sources and are certainly not limited to one or even two ethnic groups. Stories can cross ethnic groups, as in northern Saskatchewan among the Dene (Navajo) people, where Bible stories are well known by all, but the group's own traditional stories are not. Stories are traded and exchanged as commonly as pots, pans, and viruses.

4. Stories are social "neurotransmitters." Stories facilitate communication between humans in the same way that neurotransmitters facilitate transmission between neurons. People are neurons in a social brain.

5. The world is amazingly more complex than we can ever imagine. But through our construction of stories we synthesize its complexities into narratives that do explain the universe in more than just linear terms. Stories allow us to file extremely complex amounts of information effortlessly even from short encounters and to retain and recall that information accurately much longer than episodic memory. Story holds the richness of the interconnectedness and complexity of the world in a way we could never articulate otherwise.

6. The highly improbable is very likely to eventually happen. When it does, we will generate a story to explain it and give it meaning and purpose. Whether the story is true is less important than whether it comforts us and allows us to continue to maintain a sense of continuity and empowerment in our world. Healing and

improving function is more about improving those stories than proving them right or wrong.

7. <u>Treatment doesn't work, people do.</u> Our relationships and the dialogue among us are most important in facilitating change and transformation. We decidedly need each other. We need community, for it is dialogue within community that leads to healing, growth, transformation, and change.

8. Healing (or therapy, though I prefer the word *healing*) is an emergent process through dialogue that shifts the stories of all involved. Because of its dependence on dialogue, it can never be fixed and is forever somewhat mysterious. We learn best how to do therapy through reading novels, watching movies, writing stories, acting in plays, studying dancing, and living life large—talking, loving, laughing, and staying close behind the hero of change and transformation, the beloved trickster, my friend Coyote. Healing nurtures the intent to create wellness and transformation (and a little Divine Grace can't hurt).

Join me as I spin a new story, which weaves together threads of indigenous wisdom and modern medicine to create new possibilities of healing. Let us explore together the promise of narrative psychiatry and the power of story for healing minds and brains.

PART I

History and Foundations

1
Conventional Mental Health Today

Like play, art can reshape minds.
BRIAN BOYD, *ON THE ORIGINS OF STORIES:*
EVOLUTION, COGNITION, AND FICTION

We accept all guests in the hospital emergency department, turning no one away, although administration has devised a new scheme for seeking deposits from patients who are classified as nonurgent, a status that our psychiatric patients have found clever ways to avoid. Considering their pain always urgent, these patients have learned magic words to defeat nonurgency. Whenever they arrive at emergency rooms they simply say, "I'm suicidal."

Threats of suicide generate quick responses, especially in the context of nurses who are not particularly tolerant of psychiatric patients. They typically believe these people are taking up beds that could be used by others with "real diseases."

The nurses dread the ugliness of the battles at the triage desk over deposit requests. "I'm afraid you'll have to pay a deposit," I once heard a nurse saying. "You don't have an urgent condition because it's been going on for the past six months."

Other typical explanations given for requiring a financial deposit in our emergency department included:

"Because your doctor's office is open and they say that they can see you."

"Because you can go to the Health Department for your problem and they will treat you for free."

"You could go to the VA Clinic today, and we'd be happy to call over and get you an appointment."

"Would you be willing to see your own doctor, if we could get you an appointment there?"

But there are other ways to get classified as urgent besides suicide. Our psychiatric patients have also learned the value of chest pain: "That gets you seen right away, 'cause you might be having a heart attack," whispered one of our frequent patients in the hallway, as he counseled a neophyte to tell the triage nurse about chest pain.

There are other tricks to being seen quickly, although psychiatric patients have a tendency to be rushed in and then left sitting for hours since no one knows what to do with them. Perhaps our hospital should have a special room with walls decorated with art done by our patients, paintings emerging from their madness. Desperation brought them to our demesne, and desperation should be depicted on our walls.

Coming Home

A howling prairie wind was blowing dust and flecks of snow against the sliding glass doors of the emergency department entrance. Psychiatric patients altered the mood of the emergency department in the way that an orchestra changes the feel of a concert hall when it starts to tune. Their presence was discordant and even cacophonous, yet there was a familiarity to them as if they represented a part of all of our families, or even of us.

I thought of them like the proverbial wolf of older times. Despite almost never attacking people, the wolf was reviled and avoided. For centuries people feared the gaze of a wolf as evil and sinister, believing that the stare of a wolf could make one speechless. In the Middle Ages, people steered their horses clear of wolf tracks, as it was believed that any horse whose hoof landed in a print would be crippled. Since that time, humans have shot wolves and displayed or buried them at the edges of their property and at town gates in hopes that the hides would keep other wolves away. No one ate wolf meat, as it was thought to be poisonous. This is how psychiatric patients are treated in emergency departments. Perhaps similar considerations apply to them as to the maligned wolf.

That evening I overheard the nurse explaining to "Jane,"* a frail-appearing wisp of a woman who had visited us many times before, why she should leave the emergency department. "The Guidance Clinic will take care of this for you. You've been going there for as long as I've known you. They're much better equipped to handle your questions and concerns than we are."

"That's nice," Jane replied nervously. "Maybe I'll just sit in the waiting room. Would you like that?"

Esther, the nurse, grew quiet and said, "I guess you could do that. I guess you could sit there as long as you want." This was perhaps a desirable alternative to the way Jane usually visited us—in a diabetic coma or close to it. Jane regularly used her diabetes as a method of near suicide. When she felt depressed, she simply stopped taking her insulin. Rarely did she have to wait long. Her diabetes had become quite brittle, meaning that her glucose was all over the map, sometimes very low, sometimes very high, but unpredictably so. Jane hardly ever controlled her high blood glucose and was beginning to develop complications of the disease, including vision problems. The threat of becoming visually impaired made her even more miserable, which inevitably translated into another emergency room visit for ketoacidosis, the manifestation of out-of-control diabetes in which too much acid builds up in the blood and the person becomes unconscious.

Jane was often quietly weeping when the EMTs brought her to us on the stretcher, her glucose rarely less than seven hundred—seven times the normal value. She also could vomit on command and did so often. Lately, she had begun to dabble with heroin. One of our psychiatrists tried to have Jane committed to the state hospital because of her poor diabetes care. But a local judge threw the case out of court, even though Jane liked the state hospital.

---

*Names and other proper nouns have been changed to protect confidentiality.

"I'll paint a picture for your waiting room," Jane said. "I'll paint you a picture of the gates of the state hospital." She had been there enough times to memorize many facets of those run-down, rambling buildings in Las Vegas, New Mexico, that qualified as the state hospital. Jane told Esther that the bread was hard as rocks at the state hospital and you could burn yourself on the coffee when it first came out of the urns.

"But why do you want to wait here?" Esther asked, trying to explain that there wasn't anything we could do for her, so it was pointless to wait for nothing.

I knew that Esther's perception of what would help Jane was worlds apart from Jane's, for we were Jane's only family in a perverse sense of the word. We were among the few living beings on this earth who actually cared for her and ministered to her when she was sick. Jane's coming to sit in the waiting room was actually a great improvement, although Esther could not see it that way. If only we could have exploited Jane's search for more healthy contact with us by letting her stay in the waiting room or by giving her simple jobs to do around the emergency department, perhaps she might not have had to get sick in order to come see us.

When she replied, "Because this is home," Jane was speaking so honestly that she sounded crazy. Jane had spent her childhood aching to be normal. Diabetes hit Jane hard in seventh grade and took a tyrannical hold over her. She had come to Clovis, New Mexico, in junior high school and, being already strange, had been excluded from the usual cliques and groupings of her peers—making her as isolated at school as she had been at home. Her whole life had become a bizarre mimicry of what she perceived normal to be. She could not lose the twang of Brooklyn, where she had lived until fate flung her across the country to the oil fields of New Mexico. Hard as she tried, her efforts at imitation caused her to be ridiculed.

Late evenings, when we were not terribly busy, I learned these things from Jane as I talked to her about her diabetes and her life, although as often as not, she refused to talk, catatonically suffering the nausea and abdominal pain of diabetic ketoacidosis until our drugs drowsily snowed her and calmed the turbulent waves of her stomach.

"Jane," Esther almost scoffed, "we're not your home."

"Home is where the heart is," Jane argued. "I'll just stay here for a while, if you please. I'll visit with my friend at the desk."

Maybe the emergency department world was as off-kilter and bizarre as the atmosphere in her childhood home. Maybe it was the companionship Jane found with other patients in the waiting room that made her feel at home, as I have been told by other patients for whom the contact and humanity they found in the waiting room was more important than anything the doctor could tell them in the examining room. But there was something so deep and unsettlingly disturbed in Jane that she was excluded from much of the waiting room camaraderie. Occasionally someone befriended her, or more often than not, took advantage of her. Jane's pain and sadness were like a killing dust that precipitated onto the furniture around her, as if from a cloud over her head, a dust that fellow patients fled to avoid and that caused staff to shun her as well.

Jane was afraid of dogs and cats and even her own shadow. She would sometimes peek at us from behind closed curtains when she was feeling better after one of her skirmishes with a coma. She jumped whenever anyone appeared to be coming near her. Her hands trembled when anyone interviewed her. She could not walk to the bathroom without looking behind her for hidden enemies creeping up to ambush her. I don't know if she was even comfortable inside the bathroom with the door safely locked.

Jane told me her parents had grown darker, not older. She shared their trait of waking up screaming from nightmares in the middle of the night and sometimes in the middle of the emergency department. Once I had asked Jane what made her scream, and she told me I must have been dreaming, since she had not screamed. Another time she had screamed a man's name over and over, although it was not a name we recognized, and afterward she denied screaming or having ever heard that name. This was typical of Jane's response to our trying to comfort her. By denying doing what we wished to comfort, she made it difficult if not impossible for us to give her comfort. I wondered if she were truly dissociated from her experience, really not knowing it had happened, or if she was just afraid to share her inner processes with emergency department strangers.

Perhaps it was wise for her to refuse to share since we were not in a position to help her with that knowledge anyway. But the urge to share pain is strong; even strangers in bars discuss their marital problems, their hopes and dreams and aspirations, in ways that are decidedly intimate, perhaps because they will never see each other again. Often we are driven to share our pain with anyone who will listen, however inappropriate the setting, the context, or the person with whom we are sharing. Even so, we may speak in another language, one that hospital staff have no time or patience to learn. But this is what medicine must reclaim from indigenous traditions—stillness and a willingness to listen.

As Jane and Esther talked, I wondered how an indigenous healer would handle Jane. Perhaps the traditional healer would begin by following her, watching her movements carefully from the great oak tree outside her ramshackle, subsidized apartment, studying her as one might track game. Then, once he had really observed and understood her, he could offer healing.

In the years of my work in New Mexico, Jane's darkness and unhappiness only deepened. She became fanatically absorbed with her music and carried her boom box with her all over town, only to have it stolen sometimes. This would precipitate another diabetic "underdose" and a visit to the emergency department, where Jane would continue her reticent patterns, with her baleful glares, her seeming hatred of and hostility toward those of us who took the time to care for her. The pain must have been acute, for our caring was ultimately mechanical and not lifesaving. Jane would sometimes sit up in bed and sing a plaintive, alley-cat cry, more off-key than the worse country singer, an expression of her diabetic delirium and her anguished life pain.

That night I talked to the nurses about Jane. I told them I would have liked to have worked with Jane were we to be in another context, another place, another time. I told them that someone should try to help her. But I could barely see the many patients that came and get my charting done. We did not have time to care. And the hospital's corporate management was insisting that we see 20 percent more patients per day, even though we could barely handle the number of patients who were already coming through our entrance doors.

Esther's response was to say, "No matter," and to take command again by forcibly picking up the telephone and calling the Guidance Clinic. "Hello. One of your clients is sitting here at my triage desk. You better come get her right now. No, I don't care if it's not your job. She doesn't belong in my emergency room. You're responsible for her. You come get her right now. You're supposed to be looking after these people or hadn't you heard? I expect to see someone soon if you want to keep good relations here."

Jane took a worn and ragged appointment card out of her purse and read it quietly before handing it to Esther, saying, "I guess I already have an appointment there. Maybe it all happened because of you."

I looked up from my charting at the desk and saw Jane's small, fearful face. She waved at me and I waved back. Life was a kind of concentration camp for Jane, her very own Bergen-Belsen, or at least I think this was what she was trying to tell us by refusing to control her diabetes. She could not leave the country of her hideous past. She played loud music through her boom box as some tawdry tribute to the pained spirits circling around her. Sometimes I thought I could see a lost soul peering out from Jane's eyes. It was a look of tears and terror and uncontainable fury, so unlike the meek, downward gaze that Jane usually brokered.

Esther was trying to refuse to take credit for Jane's appointment, which had existed before Jane pulled the card out of her purse. Jane insisted that the appointment and the card had not existed before Esther had just now thought to call the Guidance Clinic. People diagnosed with schizophrenia often speak the plain truth of quantum physics. They suffer because everyday life tends to ignore these insights and proceed as if quantum physics had never been invented. Physicists, shamans, and people diagnosed with schizophrenia all know that our reality is created as we go and that no evidence can be brought forth to explain a continuous world. A medicine person would agree with Jane that Esther had created that appointment card, like pulling a rabbit out of a hat. Each day our dreams and our nightmares are assembled, seemingly from nowhere, remaking the world from its raw material, bringing it into existence as we awaken, ceasing to exist when we close our eyes.

People diagnosed with schizophrenia and other sufferers with insight often reel under the shock of the truth and fall deeper and deeper into the abyss of their pain. You have to be smart to be crazy. Traditional healers, however, can bear these insights and still empty the garbage and cook dinner.

I prayed that Jane could meet a healer who could plumb the depths of her pain, the black gold lying beneath the surface of physics and mysticism, who could strike oil because he didn't care to argue metaphysics; he already believed it and would dive straight for the pain. Healers see the tortured lives so many of us live hiding beneath our social pleasantries or, in Jane's case, behind bizarre behavior. Maybe even a traveling evangelist could help. I have no doubt that some of them are genuine healers, their powers wrapped in a cocoon of Christianity, hidden to all but a discerning few. Jane's spirituality bore fruit in darkness like a still-living moth whose silver, powdery wings are pinned as it is chloroformed and the lid of the collector's case is closed.

Esther was finally giving up and telling Jane it was all right for her to go paint in the waiting room and wait for someone from the Guidance Clinic to come, although I was sure they were never going to come, having not been impressed by Esther's pleas. Jane was telling Esther that they wouldn't come, that nobody wanted her there—that was why she came to the emergency room. Jane was clearly communicating that she felt loved by us, that our physical gestures in placing her IV or examining her lungs were meaningful to her, that what little caring we did give was so much better than the rest of her life, and it made me angry to think that the Guidance Clinic, our mental health system, had failed Jane so much. Meanwhile, Esther was getting sucked into arguing with Jane, playing the endless game of telling Jane she had talents and could make something of herself, forgetting the severe pain that inhibits all action, even as I have sometimes done for fear of the misery and despair that lies in its wake.

Esther was insisting that Jane had to have interests. Maybe she cared about other patients she had met, maybe she liked to cook, maybe she was a vegetarian, maybe she believed in animal rights, cared about desert turtles, and so on. Jane, warming to this game and seeming to thoroughly enjoy it, proudly announced to Esther that she had no interests whatsoever because they'd all been taken away from her. In her pleasure Jane was growing dreamier and more withdrawn. Esther was insisting that someone at the Guidance Clinic could find her an interest, and Jane was telling her that no one there cared enough to do that. I wondered why Esther couldn't accept that simple fact for Jane. If anyone had cared for Jane, the pain would have spilled out of her in a voracious and undiluted manner.

Esther said Jane needed something to take her mind off her misery, something she could do all day, while Jane countered that she could bleed all day and that bleeding returned power to the earth and that her menstrual blood was at the center of her anguish. Jane was telling how she shed her menstrual blood for the anguish of others, just like Jesus Christ. Maybe Jane was right, that she would have held her blood inside if not for the suffering of others, that she would have made a baby, become a mother, gotten married, if not for her preoccupation with her own suffering and the suffering of others. Jane was paying tribute to the untrustworthiness and unscrupulousness of humankind, to the fact that the world is dangerous. That is how she hooked Esther, for their feelings and thoughts were actually much alike. Esther, however, had the strength to maintain an exterior facade, a feat Jane could not do.

Finally, Jane let Esther win by changing the subject to Esther's nice hair, saying how appropriate the color was for her face, mentioning that she was glad Esther was not a nudist anymore, while Esther blushed and gave up her battle to reform Jane, content with being able to call a cab for her. Jane was telling Esther that she wanted to stay with her, but Esther was dialing City Cab, the number embedded in her mind from the many other times she'd called them to get someone, telling them to come get Jane when the dispatcher answered. Jane was like the holocaust survivor who looked for the Nazi within every Christian she met, mistakenly convinced that anyone who wasn't Jewish must be a Nazi. Esther had clearly met her match.

"You're treating me no better than a dog," Jane said in what sounded like genuine horror.

"Chilly weather we're having, isn't it?" Esther was finishing the write-up of her triage sheet.

"Yes, it's getting colder every day, isn't it," Jane said, looking wildly around the room, as if she were searching for something to grab when the taxi came. "Do you think it might snow again tomorrow?"

They continued like that until the battered white cab came. "I'll see you later," Jane hollered as she left with the cab driver. We would see Jane again.

We saw the cab driver frequently, too. She smoked too much and drank too many beers. She had emphysema and cirrhosis of the liver. Both were mild enough to permit her to still drive a cab, huffing for air and puffing on her cigarettes.

"I hope to God they help that girl," Esther said, her nerves obviously frayed by another encounter with Jane.

"You know they won't," I said. "They see her for fifteen minutes, once a month, if she's lucky. They give her medicine she won't take. She's right that we care more about her than the Guidance Clinic does."

"Don't they do psychotherapy anymore?" Esther asked. "I thought all those counselors over there talk to people."

"Budget cuts," I said. "Too many patients and not enough staff for them to spend time with one person, so they spend no time with many people. I think I'd prefer to really help a few people and turn the rest away, than to pretend to care for everyone and really help no one."

"What are these poor, mixed-up people going to do?" Esther wondered. "We can't be their therapist. You're a psychiatrist, aren't you? Why don't you fix her?" (I was not there as a psychiatrist, but in my other role, as an emergency room physician.)

"I can't do much in this setting," I replied. "It's all I can do to see the patients we have. I can't take the time to sit with someone like Jane, and besides, I'm not here to see her every week. Every day would be closer to what she needs."

I was saddened by how woefully inadequate our mental health system had become and by my inability to do anything more. "Why don't they just send her to the state hospital?" Esther was saying. "They could keep her there until she is well." A buzzing sound indicated the arrival of lab test results through the pneumatic tube.

"They don't do treatment anymore even at the state hospital," I said. "And they certainly don't keep people very long unless they're criminally insane, which Jane isn't." A light was flickering on and off on our shabby Christmas tree, which sat on a base of white cotton that poorly mimicked snow.

"What would you do with a person like this," Esther asked, "if you were going to work with her?"

"I'd see her every day, if I could. If she had any religion, I'd get her priest or minister or rabbi involved."

"Maybe we could send her to church," Esther reflected.

"If some congregation took her in and took an interest in her, it'd sure beat nothing," I said as Esther walked back to her computer to resume entering data on our trauma patients for a state survey in which we were required to participate.

"Maybe my church could adopt her," she was saying. "Give some of the people who want to meddle in other people's lives a life that needs some meddling." She was framed by a calendar on the wall with pictures of New York City, where another nurse had spent a holiday.

"Something like that is probably her only hope," I said. I was thinking this was like Native American healers who took in patients who were unable to care for themselves.

The Odor of Trauma and Scandal

After-hours in the emergency department, you get used to the iodine-like smell. It's only when you leave that you suddenly realize that outside smells funny, because the disinfectant odor is gone. Hospitals must cultivate that odor, like haunted houses.

Our command central was a long desk located in the center of the bay of beds, where, at any given time, several people were usually lying in various stages of being processed.

"Harriet" was my next patient of the weekend. She had passed out at her home, where she lived alone at age sixty-eight. Even a quick inspection revealed that she was delirious as she moaned about a war that had long ago ended and mistook Esther and me for her children. She looked too white to possibly live in New Mexico, and her blue eyes were suspicious and fearful. We could tell she had pneumonia from the wispy absence of breath sounds in her right lower lung, from her shallow, rapid breathing, and from her cough. I imagined that Miss Harriet had moved here years ago from someplace in the East and that she lived behind thick curtains to keep the sun away from her too-pale skin. I thought she would have complained bitterly if she'd had the strength to make a scene. She awoke fitfully when Esther started the IV in her arm, but otherwise she dozed. Cranky as Esther was when she worked, she cared for the Miss Harriets of Clovis with grace and good cheer.

Esther's children spanned two generations, with her daughter Rachel's two children playing with Esther's four-year-old daughter. Esther's marriages were deep wounds from pasts that still actively bled on those occasions when her ex-husband, Jackson, came drunk to the emergency room, found passed out somewhere in town. A month before this evening, severe tragedy had hit; he had run into a telephone pole guide wire while drunkenly riding his motorcycle, going so fast that his speed carried him up the wire to the pole itself. The wire had stripped the flesh from the bone of his leg in one of the nastiest injuries we had seen anyone in Clovis survive.

Each of us had our family secrets and hidden scandals that could show up in the emergency department to embarrass anyone who worked there, for the emergency room is where everyone comes—the drunks, the psychotic, the depressed, the drug addicted. I was lucky that my family scandals could not appear in Clovis, since I did not live there.

A month earlier, when Jackson had been brought to the ER by the ambulance crew, his leg had been bleeding profusely. Miraculously, he had missed severing any of the major vessels that could have instantly killed him, and the artery in his thigh that he had cut was holding together with a fine clot. People still came to look at the pictures that the fire department had taken of Jackson's leg with the skin peeled back to reveal dull white bones. We covered those bones as best we could, while Esther sat at the desk and cried, her young daughter clinging to her leg and Rachel standing behind her, one hand on her mother's shoulder, the other holding her baby, who seemed dazed and confused by the whole affair, wanting to play peek-a-boo with the firemen who stood around the desk drinking coffee, their role in the whole business finished.

Esther said she was crying for her four-year-old daughter, who ran the risk of losing her father, but we all knew the tears came from someplace deeper. She cried for herself as well, perhaps for the loss of marriage and family life that this man meant for her.

Despite the severity of his wounds, Jackson was too drunk to feel much pain. We packaged him as best we could while calling for the helicopter from Lubbock. He survived the trip, but after multiple surgeries and days in the intensive care unit, he eventually lost his lower leg. Esther bravely and angrily tried to do what she perceived to be the right thing for her daughter, hardly working during a month of vigils at the hospital in Lubbock. Much as she hated this man who had tormented her with his alcoholism, she kept watch by his side. One more injury, one more drunken evening when he shouldn't have been riding his motorcycle, but this time had been the worst ride of his life. We heard that, with shame and apology, he tolerated her often-hostile vigils at his bedside.

For that entire month we called for progress reports on Jackson, pretending to be the referring physician so we could learn more than they would tell Esther. Rightly, I suppose, we were the "referring physician," since Jackson's only health care was the emergency department, where he was brought when he was too drunk to make it home.

The Misery of Life

Emergency departments are full of the misery of life; the beds are full of schizophrenia, depression, drug abuse, and life's other maladies. The police bring us drunks as if our antisepsis could transfigure them to sobriety and make them walk home. Drunks are particularly frustrating because they can be so uncooperative in their care. "Lucy" was our first drunk of the Friday night, an in-home drunk, perhaps a younger, wetter version of our Miss Harriet, living in her large turn-of-the-century banker's house, where she tended to her garden and roses with a birdwatcher's compulsiveness, but always with a glass of gin at hand. Typically Lucy was found passed out around her rose bushes. Someone would call the ambulance, which would bring Lucy to us.

This evening, when things were quiet, I talked to Lucy about her life. She was less drunk than usual, loquaciously drunk instead of her usual passed-out drunk, her blood alcohol content having been "only" 0.27 when she arrived, instead of her usual 0.39. She told me about the tragic death of her one true love when she was only twenty-seven years old.

Although she would never admit it, I suspected that Lucy's misery predated the death of her love, who had died on the rough pine-board floor of the frontier home of her parents, original settlers of Clovis, both of whom had long since died of emphysema. Lucy accentuated her speech with pointed jabs of her tobacco-stained fingers, and I suspected that, before long, she too would be coming to the ER for shortness of breath in addition to her usual drunkenness.

"His parents never liked me," she slurred. "And when my Jack died, they took my children away from me, one by one, until all four were gone." Her life ended with the departure of her last child. I would never know if she had been drinking then, if she had been a good mother or a neglectful one.

The loss of her children had been her final blow, as it often is for even the most drug-hardened addicts, reminding me of similar stories from overdosed women lying semicomatose on hospital gurneys, still shedding bitter tears over the loss of their children. When I hear these stories, I marvel at the incredible suffering a person must feel to need such numbing from drugs or alcohol. But sometimes not even the threat of losing children can stop some women's tumultuous downward spiral toward drug- and alcohol-induced oblivion. It's out of all control.

Like the burned-out remnants lying in the wake of Sherman's prodigious march across Georgia to the sea, they lie in ruins on the bed. Such patients are tributes to our lack of caring or our inability to change the misery of people's lives, which is only worsening in these days of managed care. The time doctors have to spend with patients shrinks smaller and smaller, until five minutes seems like a lot in some offices.

"Did you talk to anyone or get any help after your husband died?" I asked Lucy. She had shaken her head and smiled wistfully at me. "Who would have talked to me, who would have cared, where would I have gone? Not even the minister," she sighed. "And I didn't have any family nearby."

I sat on the stool beside her, thinking that she could have been quite beautiful at age twenty-seven, long before the alcohol and tobacco had dried and cracked her skin. I found myself drifting away from her story of lawsuits from the grandparents and no money to defend herself. As she droned on with her long tale, I wondered how people could be so cruel to each other.

Meanwhile, I was hearing another casualty of family life on the police scanner in the background. A man was holed up with a gun outside of town, surrounded by sheriff's cars. The police were bringing us his five-year-old niece for a rape exam even as Lucy continued to speak. She had told her mother that her uncle had put his "pee-pee" inside her and that he had made her cry, prompting a hysterical call to 911. Lucy continued to ramble, oblivious to my departure from her bedside. I needed to know what we could expect about the standoff. Luckily I would not be called on to do the rape exam. Those of us who did not live in Clovis were not expected to see cases that would definitely require legal testimony.

The city attorney had made a deal with the medical staff that only the doctors who lived and practiced in town would deal with such cases. This was fine, since there was little I hated more than inflicting the trauma of a rape exam on an already brutalized person, especially a five-year-old. The sheriff's deputy who had brought the girl told me that the uncle would probably shoot himself. "They either deny everything or they kill themselves, and the fact that he's holed up with a gun tells me he's not going to deny the charges. So we'll probably have to bring him in to see you, dead or dying, once he gets the courage to shoot himself, which could take most of the day," the deputy muttered, shaking his head.

As if to mark his words, we suddenly heard a flurry of shouting on the radio. "I heard a shot!" someone yelled.

"It came from inside," came another voice. A third person shouted, "Call the ambulance. Call the ambulance." We could already hear its siren in the background noise of the radio, getting louder and louder. The drivers would park far enough from the range of the guns to keep the EMTs safe, but close enough to bring us casualties in a hurry.

"He's shot hisself in the chest," came a new, very Texan voice. Then we heard the voice of Ernie Toutousis, our fire captain and head of the EMTs, on the special ambulance radio. His voice was calm as he announced an open, sucking chest wound that they were transporting code three (sirens blasting), attempting to place an IV en route. We heard the sounds of the ambulance's siren receding on the police radio. Then the EMT driving called to tell us that their attempt at placing an IV had been successful, and they were turning the corner onto the truck bypass that would lead them to the hospital.

"How far out are they?" I asked Esther. We knew they were coming from somewhere near the state line. I wasn't sure how long it would take an ambulance traveling code three to go that short distance to us, but I knew it was time to get things ready, including checking the code cart and breaking out the basic equipment we would need, such as laryngoscopes, endotracheal tubes, and central line kits. I had heard most of the story in snatches as I chatted with Lucy and later while frequently being interrupted by the many other questions that come up in the emergency department, such as what dose of children's ibuprofen to give for a fever, whether to use a tepid bath, and requests to look at a wound to see if it could be steri-stripped or would need stitches. I could hear Esther talking over the noise of many voices and radio calls, but could not make out her words. I saw others appearing to help us, so I knew Esther had called people from the respiratory therapy, lab, and x-ray departments.

We were about to hide behind what we do best—resuscitate the dying—but we were never able to address the terrible social conditions breeding child abuse and other social ills, and always too late to help the people involved.

I clipped the laryngoscope blade onto its handle and flipped it open to make sure the light would work. Then I inflated the balloon on the endotracheal tube with 10 ccs of air to make sure it worked and drew back the air into the syringe to deflate the cuff so that the tube could be inserted.

"Don't you dare try to save this sorry, no-good . . ."

"You know we have to try," I replied to Esther, wondering how serious she was.

It was cold enough outside for a thin film of ice to have formed on standing puddles, and the oil rigs surrounding the town stood like bizarre dunking birds blanketed by a rare coating of snow. Esther was identifying with mother and child, but still I was surprised by her fervor in wanting this child molester to die.

"What do you want me to do?" I asked Esther.

"I want you to pronounce him dead even if his heart's still beating, because he will be dead sooner or later, and you'll save the county a lot of money." She looked at me with piercing eyes, as the sheriff's deputy vigorously nodded his affirmation.

"Think how much money you'd save the county by doing that." This was the deputy talking, but Esther was nodding her head too.

"Someone like that doesn't deserve help." Esther sometimes talked too loudly when patients were around and was accused of an error of taste. But she had been a nurse for seventeen years and was a good one, and her "errors of taste" were usually just her version of the plain-spoken truth.

"You guys are making me nervous," I said. "You know what our duty is." Esther's view on life was simple, never disingenuous, and always aimed at ridding the world of filth and pollution. She meant to make Clovis a safer, more Christian place to live. Perhaps, through oversight or ignorance, she had not grasped that her means did not always seem terribly Christian. Esther typically kept her mouth shut around administration and had learned to cover her mistakes well, but this time she was not to be silenced yet. "They should have just let him bleed to death in that house," she hissed.

"Is this your plan for all would-be criminals?" I teased her. "You're now going to decide who lives and who dies?"

"Just child molesters. I'd do different terrible things to the other kinds of criminals," she said. But she winked, tipping me that she was not entirely serious. "And that deputy would let me get away with it." She winked at the sheriff's deputy.

I put my finger to my lips to bid them quiet because Eleanor, the triage nurse, was bringing back a child whose mother thought he had an ear infection. "To Serve and Protect" was the motto emblazoned on all Clovis police cars, but the police had been getting bad publicity lately after a three-hundred-person riot during one of the high school football games. That night we had seen fifteen people with minimal injuries, who were all there for documentation so they could file lawsuits against the police. One of the parents had screamed at us about being honkie racists. He wanted more x-rays than I thought his son needed. Four family members were parked around the bed, all muttering about the lousy health care provided at the hospital. Yet that family seemed to spend part of every weekend in our emergency room.

Just then the ambulance radio crackled loudly: "This is IV Tech Charleston in Med Unit Two calling." The radio broke his urgent-sounding voice into barely understandable staccato bursts.

"This is base," Esther answered, holding down the button on the microphone by the radio. "Go ahead Med Unit Two. We copy you." The static was heavy on the radio.

"We are traveling code three with a man about thirty years old," the reedy, high-pitched voice was saying, "self-inflicted gunshot wound to the chest, sucking chest wound. Vital signs are as follows . . ." We left the trauma room to gather around the radio, to listen to the drama unfolding so near our doors, as if we were in an earlier time, perhaps like the first people to hear Orson Welles' *War of the Worlds,* though this was real.

"What's their ETA?" I asked again. "Five minutes," Ken, another nurse, was telling us, for he had heard the entire radio transmission. Our team was assembled. We watched in motionless silence as the ambulance pulled up at our front door.

"Here she blows," Esther shouted.

"Inform us of any changes in condition," Ken was saying, belatedly. "LY445 clear." All that remained was the static.

"Let's roll," I said. Soon I was holding the endotracheal tube and the laryngoscope, standing at the head of the bed ready to intubate. We use the laryngoscope to press down the tongue and create a passageway to reveal the vocal cords through the mouth. Once I see the cords, I can then pass the endotracheal tube through them so that we can ventilate the patient. The voices of the EMTs were shrill and excited, growing more distinct as they got closer to us. They rushed their gurney to the bed at the center of the trauma room and pulled the patient onto the bed, where we were waiting to work on him.

I was poised with the endotracheal tube, Esther was poised to start another IV, and Jay was ready to cut off the man's clothes. Medical "codes" always have an other-worldly quality to them, and when we're working well, there's a calmness that settles over everyone, though by all rights we should be anxious. I lifted up the patient's tongue and passed the tube between his vocal cords. In the distance, we could hear someone wailing, could hear the eerie call of a woman's shrieking grief traveling through a kind of sound tunnel that our intense concentration formed, making it seem as far away and plaintive as the cry of a heron or an egret on a midnight marsh.

"Do we have to do this?" Esther whined under her breath, all the while preparing her IV setup, since we needed two large-bore IVs to replace the volume in fluid that he would be losing in blood, lying motionless beneath us, the room in constant motion around him. The respiratory therapist was operating the ambubag, an apparatus that ventilated the patient through the endotracheal tube. Two women from the lab were taking the blood we had just drawn to the lab, while Michael rolled the portable x-ray machine into our trauma room. He was an ex-hippie x-ray technician, his long blonde hair turned gray, taller than anyone in the room. I was getting out the chest tube kit because it was clear we would need to drain blood from the chest cavity.

I was proud to be a part of the excellent care we gave in the midst of the desolate, high-plains mesa country in southeast New Mexico, even better sometimes than what I had seen in the great medical centers where I had trained, hospitals with hundreds more beds than ours. We were all autodidacts, training ourselves to a standard of excellence required of the only hospital for 110 miles in any direction. I never felt that same pride working in New York, California, or Arizona as I did here. Already, Esther was taking charge of the body before us, as it oozed its life blood onto the floor. While she worked to get our blood pressure cuff onto the man's arm, I was examining the wound.

"Is that his heart beating in the bottom of that hole?" Michael asked incredulously, his height enabling him to look down at the wound from high above the table. "That's the biggest chest hole I've ever seen in someone who's still alive."

"That is his heart," I confirmed.

"How did he miss it?" Michael wondered. "Not that it matters all that much. I can't imagine how anyone could survive that wound. Could anyone survive that wound? Can he survive that wound? Do you think?"

Donna, the respiratory therapist, was ventilating the man. I was trying to figure out how to manage his chest wound, which he had made with a shotgun. I had never seen a person still alive with such a large hole in his chest, but the reality was that we had to seal it, and it was too big for me to know how. As a stopgap measure I decided to lay sterile plastic over the wound, the kind that could create an air seal. I found the spot on his side where I wanted to place the chest tube and made an incision with the scalpel. I spread apart the tissue between the ribs, first with a clamp and then with my finger, until the hole was large enough to pass the chest tube through. I was fairly happy with the resulting gush of blood and air into the collection chamber, which bubbled through water to create a vacuum seal. Nevertheless, the man was going downhill fast, and despite the fluid pouring into him, his blood pressure was slowly dropping.

I grabbed the central line kit, took out a long needle attached to a syringe, and probed his neck until I drew back blood. That was the internal jugular vein, which provided a direct and large passageway for fluid and drugs to reach the heart. Soon I had threaded a metal wire through the inside of the needle. I pulled out the needle, threaded the wire through the large catheter called a percutaneous sheath, and shoved it through the hole alongside the wire until it was completely inside.

Blood poured back, and we connected the line to fluid, letting it go as fast as possible into the heart. Nevertheless, the blood pressure continued to fall, and the pulse got faster and faster. I asked Esther to start a dopamine drip to raise the blood pressure at least temporarily, and she rushed to start it up. Her prior comments had certainly not affected her efficiency as she rapidly started the dopamine.

Although it was temporarily effective, the dopamine was also failing. I had already called our chest surgeon. The man's pulse was getting weaker and weaker, even though his EKG still looked strong. His pulse was failing as the surgeon walked into the trauma room, and I was trying to imagine the best way to do chest compressions. That surgeon walked up to the table and stuck his gloved hand into the wound, grabbing swabs to absorb the blood that splattered on the tattoos covering the patient's arms. He was muttering to himself. The dopamine was running as fast as possible and the fluid was flowing through the three IVs, while the lab had still not delivered the blood we had requested.

"I can't help him," the surgeon said. Then he asked for clamps that could be found only in the operating room, cursing when we did not have them. What we had was his own special pack that he had prepared himself and that sat in a cupboard in the trauma room until he asked for it. But even the surgeon's own prepared kit did not contain what he needed. He himself looked like a bushy-eyebrowed, Eastern European pianist, throwing his head back as he pounded the piano keys.

After his concert, he stepped backward off the stool he had been standing on, since he was too short to stand on the floor and still see well into the wound. Esther wore a bewildered expression that could have been disbelief or fear, her face looking as it had been flash-frozen. We all knew what was coming, but felt helpless to interfere with the course of events.

"I can't help him," the surgeon said simply, "so you might as well stop. His arteries are too badly damaged to reconstruct, he has lost too much blood, and what you are doing is hopelessly prolonging the inevitable. So I am going to make it easy on you and call this code, unless anyone objects, which no one should."

The surgeon's accent had remained thick throughout his life, although he was actually Italian and not Eastern European. Esther was crying now. She had apparently forgotten her sentiments about what this man had done and was grieving the tragic loss of life that we saw all too often and that had almost befallen her ex.

We stopped and watched the EKG slowly deteriorate to a single flat line. Someone mercifully pulled the sheet over the body, though the blood still dripped steadily onto the floor even as did Esther's tears, much as she tried to hide them, quickly rubbing her cheeks and taking on the tough air that she often carried. But I had seen her sorrow, her sadness, and her pain. We had shared those emotions of loss that we feel when we lose a young person no matter what their circumstances, whether rapist or drug addict or All-American teenage drowning victim, and those were the emotions that had driven us to health care. How rare that we could show these feelings! How sad that American health care had driven these feelings out of our day-to-day work most of the time. How important and necessary that we find ways to create something different and better!

If only our society had better means of preventing and addressing its social and emotional ills—its mental health—perhaps none of these tragedies that I just related would ever have happened. That is what the rest of this book is about.

The Failure of a Promise

The stories I have just told are typical and representative of how the system of care that has evolved doesn't work for patients. Psychiatric disorders remain among the most important contributors to worldwide health burdens.[1] The promise of relief from suffering via drugs has largely not been realized. Related controversies—such as questions about the withdrawal syndrome from antidepressants and the increased risk of suicide, along with metabolic syndromes created by antipsychotic drugs—spark widespread concern.

The Clinical Antipsychotic Trials of Intervention Effectiveness (CATIE) studies, funded by the National Institute for Mental Health and coordinated by the University of North Carolina at Chapel Hill, showed low efficacy of antipsychotic medication for schizophrenia. The World Health Organization confirmed, over the course of thirty years and with thousands of patients, that people with psychosis did better and had higher recovery rates in third-world countries where drugs were not generally available than in developed countries with medication.[2] A 2008 meta-analysis on antidepressants showed no difference from placebo when all reported trials (to the U.S. Food and Drug Administration) were considered instead of just the trials published in journals.[3] Bipolar depression is associated with substantial disability, with up to 80 percent of patients remaining symptomatic despite conventional treatment.[4] In the twenty-first century, 0.4 percent of people diagnosed with bipolar disorder commit suicide each year, a rate that is twenty times greater than the general population.[5]

I am suggesting that we need a new course, a human approach, an approach to caring and compassion that reconnects to the world's indigenous healing systems and explores their use and integration. The counterclaim of the conventional biomedical system is that people just don't take their medications and are noncompliant; if people took their medications, everyone would be fine. The CATIE studies have refuted that claim. Many of the participants stopped taking their medications because they didn't work or because the side effects were too burdensome. That's certainly been my clinical experience. People stop medication, largely, because it isn't working.

Others have made these same points. As early as 1996, psychiatrist David Kaiser wrote, "As a practicing psychiatrist, I have watched with growing dismay and outrage the rise and triumph of the hegemony known as biologic psychiatry. Within . . . modern psychiatry, biologism now completely dominates the discourse on the causes and treatment of mental illness, and in my view this has been a catastrophe with far-reaching effects on individual patients and the cultural psyche at large."[6] He saw "patients [being] . . . reduced to something less than fully human, as they become an abstract collection of symptoms without meaning to be 'managed' by technicians called psychiatrists."[7] The end result of this process for the patients was to "reify in them an identity as a chronic patient with a bad brain. This identification as a biologically impaired patient is one of the most destructive effects of biologic psychiatry.[8]

Kaiser had observed a fundamental change in his patients: "Now when a person becomes depressed, for example, they are less able to read it as a sign that there may be a problem in their life that needs to be looked at or addressed. . . . Instead, they identify themselves as ill and submit to the correction of a psychiatrist who promises to take away the depression so they can get back to their lives as they are."[9]

American psychiatrist Phillip Sinaikin wrote in 2003 that the field appeared to be evolving from "an eclectic discipline of many perspectives to a self-certain and self-validating, reductionistic medical 'science,' which some of us find disheartening and frightening."[10] A narrative critique of conventional medicine finds it based on a preference for the general over the specific, objective over subjective, quantitative over qualitative, and it threatens to become a story to end all stories. It lacks a way of measuring inner hurt, despair, hope, grief, and moral pain, which frequently accompany the illnesses from which people suffer.

Changes similar to what Kaiser described have also been happening in indigenous communities. Whereas historically, cultural beliefs about emotions and their vicissitudes identified them as springing from relationships and their disturbances, a modern Cree family I recently saw sprang to the position that the disturbances in their relationships were due to their private mental illnesses. The father argued that he shoved his daughter "because of his bipolar." The daughter argued that she was irritable around her mother and wanted to spend her time with her friends "because [she] was bipolar." The mother said perhaps the family was having problems because her "depression made [her] withdraw." This perspective was so uncharacteristically Cree as to stand out for me. I wondered who were these "spirit beings"—bipolar and depression—who ordered people around and made them do things. The traditional Cree notion of emotional accountability had been replaced by making "clinical entities" responsible for people's difficulties with one another. The implication here was that my job was to find the right medication for each family member so the family could relate well again and be happy. When asked explicitly if this was their expectation, they agreed.

Disciplines find their own ways of deciding what constitutes "good evidence" to support current practice. Disciplines also regulate what is considered "serious" research and what is not. For current psychiatry, pharmaceutical research is considered more serious and valuable than social research or micronutrient research. Rhetoric and social negotiations allow us to arrive at definitions for what types of studies are considered "most valid" or "most effective." My most recent experience with this came when I submitted a paper to the *Journal of Biological Psychiatry* about the equivalence of high-dose, high-potency micronutrients (vitamins and minerals) to risperidone (brand name Risperdal) for eighty-eight children diagnosed with autism. The editor rejected the paper in less than twenty-four hours, saying it would be of no interest to their readers.

This told me that changing psychiatry and mental health will have to be a grassroots movement. Psychiatry will not readily change. The impetus for reform must come from outside it, aided by those within psychiatry who will support such change (currently a minority). Now we will turn to what we need to understand in order to be adequate workers for paradigm change.

2

Good Stories and Mental Health

Poetry is capable of saving us.
I. A. RICHARDS, *CAMBRIDGE MINDS*

Dr. Rita Charon, a physician at Columbia University in New York City, first coined the term *narrative medicine,* defining it as medicine practiced with narrative competence, which is the ability to acknowledge, absorb, interpret, and act on the stories and plights of others. She wrote, "With narrative competence, physicians can reach and join their patients in illness, recognize their own personal journeys through medicine, acknowledge kinship with and duties toward other health care professionals, and inaugurate consequential discourse with the public about health care. By bridging the divides that separate physicians from patients, themselves, colleagues, and society, narrative medicine offers fresh opportunities for respectful, empathic, and nourishing medical care."[1]

In *Narrative Medicine: The Use of History and Story in the Healing Process,* I built on this narrative framework to suggest that all theories are narratives—explanations of how the world works.[2] Not only that, but we can use people's stories about their illnesses to come to understandings about how illnesses and lives interact, and even how illnesses arise from the performance of stories. The way we live has physiological consequences, and we live by enacting the stories we believe to be true.

Story-Making: Our "Default" Mode

We are narrative creatures, consummate storytellers. For thousands of years, we have been telling stories to each other. We "have told stories around the campfire . . . have traveled from town to town telling stories to relate the news of the day . . . have told stories transmitted by electronic means to passive audiences incapable of doing anything but listening (and watching). Whatever the means, and whatever the venue, story telling seems to play a major role in human interaction."[3] Whenever we encounter something new, surprising, different, or interesting, we tell a story about it.

Once upon a time, only those interested in literature studied stories and how they worked.[4] The ideas of narrative were lost within literature departments. Among the most active early contributors to narrative thought were Russian literary theorists. Rather than focus on the meaning of stories, they focused on how good stories were told.[5] They asked what gave stories their familiar structure. They were concerned with heroes (main characters) and what happened to those heroes.[6]

More recently, however, the study of storytelling has entered many fields. Within psychology and psychiatry, neural imaging studies are showing that brains are designed to function most efficiently in creating, recalling, storing, and telling story.[7] A developing body of evidence suggests that a default state of the brain is one of making up stories (part of what is called the theory of narrative generation). Midline activity in the brain's frontal cortex underlies both story-generating activity in which the mind wanders along a narrative trail[8] and the default mode of brain activity associated with resting attention.[9] When the brain is in story-generating mode, it is focused on elaborating a story that links memories of past events with present activities and imagined future possibilities, involving ourselves and other characters, and reducing our immediate sensory awareness of the world around us. In contrast, in what has been called mindful awareness or mindfulness, we inhibit the making of stories in favor of a broad, free-floating awareness of sensations and mental events that is storyless.[10]

When not much else is going on, we fall into default mode and begin to imagine and create vignettes. This has the positive aspect of enabling us to practice how we will act in a social situation. Repetitions of such stories give us the opportunity to practice until we get it right, simulating life by using the capacity of this circuitry, which also involves memory regions in the hippocampus. The down side of this mode is that we can be sitting on a beautiful beach under a blue sky on vacation, feeling warm and comfortable as we listen to the sound of the waves rolling toward the beach, but not even notice, for we are so engaged in our simulation of our interactions with people back home or at work. Narrative mode can lead to distressing ruminations, while mindfulness mode can stop these ruminations or obsessional simulations by returning our attention to the beauty around us. Suddenly we notice the beach and the waves again. Mindfulness mode disengages those narrative circuits that also keep track of the story about who we think we are, which creates a historical, continuous self.[11]

A 2007 study by Dr. Norman Farb and colleagues at the University of Toronto observed that during story-making a particular area of the brain was activated. This area includes parts of the middle frontal lobe (the ventral and dorsomedial prefrontal cortex) and a network of brain areas in the left frontal lobe that deal with language production and how we make meaning through language (the inferior lateral prefrontal cortex, the angulate gyrus of the temporal lobe, the middle area of the temporal lobe), and the hippocampus, which is involved in memory. The individuals in the study who were taught mindfulness meditation through an eight-week intensive course learned to make a pronounced shift away from these parts of the brain toward a very different right-brain network (the right ventral and dorsolateral prefrontal cortex, the right insular cortex— a region related to perceiving bodily experience, the right secondary somatosensory cortex of the parietal lobe, and the right inferior parietal lobe). In doing this, they turned off the story-making part of the brain. The anterior cingulate gyrus is involved in this, for it is the area of the brain activated when we switch our attention.* Our brains apparently default

---

*The functioning of the anterior cingulate gyrus is also related to what is called obsessive-compulsive disorder. In these situations, people have difficulty switching their attention and perseverate on one thing over and over.

to idling in story-making mode.[12] Active effort is required to transfer to another mode.

Story and Our Sense of Self

This default brain activity also provides a sense of self. Neuroscientist Marcus Raichle of Washington University in St. Louis and others saw that every time a person engaged in a mental activity, such as memorizing a list of words, a collection of brain regions consistently *decreased* activity compared with their "resting levels." Only when people recalled autobiographical memories or imagined different simulations of possible futures or alternate pasts did this brain network become more active. Raichle hypothesized that this network has to step into the background to facilitate our being able to fully concentrate on specific tasks.

The parts of the brain that coordinate these activities are the medial prefrontal cortex, posterior cingulate cortex, retrosplenial cortex, precuneus, inferior parietal lobe, and hippocampus. They are primarily located along the crevice separating the brain's hemispheres, and on each lobe behind and above the ears. Consensus is growing that this circuit has two major hubs: the posterior cingulate cortex (PCC) with the precuneus, and the medial prefrontal cortex.

The medial prefrontal cortex is involved in imagining, thinking about yourself, and the "theory of mind," which encompasses the ability to figure out what others think, feel, or believe, and to recognize that other people have different thoughts, feelings, and beliefs from you. The precuneus and PCC are involved in pulling personal memories from the brain's archives, visualizing yourself doing various activities, and describing yourself. Both of these areas are necessary for creating good stories about the world.

Health requires our ability to create good stories about the world in this "default mode," or baseline condition. This mode is not properly coordinated in patients with schizophrenia, related to poor connectivity between brain networks.[13] The regions of the brain known previously to be abnormal in patients diagnosed with schizophrenia also function abnormally in the default mode network. The extent of the default mode abnormalities correlates with the severity of auditory hallucinations, delusional thoughts, and attention deficits. What this suggests is that schizophrenia arises out of a difficulty in forming good stories, which is supporting by clinical experience. People with schizophrenia are not able to tell strong, coherent narratives about their experience.

Unstructured mental activity—be it remembering your homecoming football game in high school, thinking about an anticipated unpleasant meeting with your boss at work and what your coworkers might say afterward, debating whether to take that new job you were just offered or keep the one you have, or recalling your adolescent attempt at being a rock star—is all part of this default narrative mode, being what the brain does when it is doing nothing in particular. It's the brain's core, both physically and mentally. It recalls stories because that's how we best store memory.

We replay a vignette from homecoming, especially as it involved our interactions with others, as opposed to recalling a chronological list of what happened that night. We replay the events that have emotional significance and meaning for us, often wondering what would have happened if things had gone otherwise. We play many "what-if" games in our mental simulations. This is one of the amazing values of story—that we get to experience "what if," "what might have been," "what could have been," and thereby learn from experience.

Stories Store Memories

A story is the most efficient way to save memory. Stories contain items of sensory description. They have emotional coloring. They hold our interest and activate our attention. Stories clump information together into packages. Our nervous system typically is limited to holding seven bits of information in consciousness at any one moment (some gifted individuals can go as high as ten). Stories clump information into larger chunks so that much more information is available to consciousness at any one moment. The affective, or emotional, tags that are attached to a story make it very easy to recall, much easier than isolated bits of information.

Stories facilitate learning since they're so much easier to store and recall.

Roger Schank of Northwestern University and Robert Abelson of Yale University "argue that stories about one's experiences, and the experiences of others, are the fundamental constituents of human memory, knowledge, and social communication." They state three propositions: "1) Virtually all human knowledge is based on stories constructed around past experiences; 2) New experiences are interpreted in terms of old stories; 3) The content of story memories depends on whether and how they are told to others, and these reconstituted memories form the basis of the individual's 'remembered' self."[14]

When I want to teach about all the four directions and their associated values, emotions, animals, and colors, I tell the story of how the four directions were formed (see my book *Coyote Medicine*[15]). It communicates everything a person needs to know to participate in a Lakota sweatlodge ceremony in an informed manner, but in the form of a story about how the four sons of the wind walked around the world on a mission from the Creator to set the four directions so people would never feel lost. They had epic adventures, encountered supernatural creatures, and overcame vast obstacles. It's hard to forget this epic tale that can take up to two hours to tell. Then when anyone asks me a question, such as what the color of the west is, I ask him or her to recall the story and figure it out. That virtually always works.

Any student can tell you that what psychologist Theodore Sarbin called paradigmatic memories, or isolated facts, are much harder to recall. This is because they have no context, no emotional coloring, no meaning or purpose, or no arousal/activation value. They don't hold our interest. They don't motivate or inspire us to action. A number of developmental psychologists have determined that you have to engage children's interests first before you can teach them anything. This was the logic behind the popular children's show *Sesame Street*.

When we have an "event" that stands out in our lives, we tell others about it in the form of a story. It's those stories that get stored in memory to be recalled and told again and again (changing each time we recall and tell the story, since we are constantly modifying our stories to match the interests of the audience to whom we are telling them). Through recall of stories, we can quickly assess a new situation in comparison with past experiences that seem similar. "We remember not words but our inferences about sequences, causes, and goals. This is their power for negotiating the minefields of human social life."[16]

Stories Live Us

Here's the part that gets really interesting. Psychologist and educator Jerome Bruner wrote that stories live us, not the other way around.[17] We act out the stories we have internalized about how we are supposed to be in any given situation. Russian developmental psychologist Lev Vygotsky (1896–1934) wrote beautifully about this.[18] He described young children repeating simple stories to themselves that they heard from their mothers and other caregivers. Slowly but surely these stories became more and more elaborate until well-formed narratives emerged around age four.

Those of us who have children and grandchildren are well aware of this. My two-year-old grandson tells elaborate stories, but in a language that's difficult for me to understand. He clearly doesn't grasp that his language doesn't communicate his ideas yet, because if I show any signs of being inattentive, he becomes irate and demands the return of my full attention to what he is saying. His storytelling abilities are far ahead of his language constructional abilities. But he is rehearsing. His frontal lobe will catch up. The rest of his language circuitry will mature. The words will eventually emerge in a way that I can understand. But he has the tonality now. He has the expressiveness and the prosody of a master storyteller, because we are all master storytellers.

By age four, the story starts to form, and a six-year-old can "talk story" at length on many topics, sometimes to the exasperation of parents who must accomplish tasks (clean floors, wash dishes, pay bills) but who don't wish to hurt the feelings of their child who is so excited by his story and wants the full attention of the audience.

The stories we hear as children are captured forever within our nervous systems. These stories contain information about the meaning of our lives, what values we should hold, what is respectable and what is not, what is ethical and what is not, and how to behave in the situations we encounter.

Even though I had the privilege of an upbringing rich in stories, I am not so different from anyone else. Comparing my childhood with that of others, however, I realized I was primed to see the importance of story. My grandmother was a storyteller. My mother was an English teacher who eventually worked as a children's librarian. I was encouraged to read widely. Our house was full of story, including traditional stories of our Cherokee ancestors.

Stories and Social Relationships

Stories are our primary means of relating; at all gatherings, people talk story, telling the most interesting or revealing vignettes about their lives since the last meeting. At weddings and funerals, what do we do but tell stories? Wedding stories are more cheerful and funny, often about unusual members of both families, or about funny deeds of the bride or groom from their childhood, often to the embarrassment of both. I was recently a part of such a situation.

My stepson and his wife and child had joined me for a ceremony in Woodstock, New York, and a number of us went out to dinner afterward. We were telling stories as people do. I was asked to tell the funniest story I remembered about Ben from childhood. He cringed with anticipated embarrassment and told me to tell it anyway. I told the story about how he and his friends took his mother's car for a ride around 2 a.m. one Friday night. What made this funny is that his mother's license plate said "MIDWIFE" and all the police in our little town knew her and her car. They quickly surmised that six young people at 2 a.m. in what we called "the midwife-mobile" was out of the ordinary, so they proceeded to stop the car. No one in the car was over fourteen. Ben was thirteen. He jumped out of the car and ran away, dashing into the nearby woods and eventually making his way back to the house, where, of course, the police had already come, knowing full well who he was and where he lived. The story is funny because it happened in Vermont, where a certain tolerance and peacefulness exists. Had Ben done this in Arizona, the police would have certainly shot him, and it would not have been a funny story. Then the rest of us proceeded to tell funny stories of silly things each of us had done as children.

What was the point of this? Of course, it was interesting and entertaining. But I think it also had the effect of welcoming Ben as an equal with us. Most of us were twenty or more years older than he. The first story acknowledged his being younger. Then our successive stories informed him that we had all been just as silly as he and invited him to consider himself an equal in our group. The functions of stories at weddings are to bond the two families and to facilitate everyone's "getting along." The functions of stories at funerals are to set the memories that will persist of the departed and to comfort those left behind. Funeral stories can also be funny, but in a way that honors the memory of the departed and makes everyone feel a bit uplifted.

Stories Shape Our Brains

Human lives are organized through stories or narratives. Stories—and the social milieu in which they are told—shape our brains. I have met children who sat in cribs in orphanages until they were six years old. I particularly remember one young child from Bulgaria whose American parents had adopted her at age six. When I saw her at age ten, she was far from normal in her social interactions. She could readily have received several psychiatric diagnoses. Her story was that she had had virtually no human care until age six, and her brain reflected that lack of development. By age twelve, she was still biting herself, having dangerous tantrums and experiencing difficulty in modulating the extremes of her emotions, overreacting to situations, and barely able to interact with much younger children. She and other similar children highlighted for me the degree to which our social environment shapes the circuits of brain that regulate emotion and mood and mediate our relationships to each other. On the individual level, environment shapes brain more than brain shapes environment.

Having written this, I suddenly hear the voices of my students at the

University of Saskatchewan, for this is how the mind works. I can recall our conversations about these topics. My memories consist of dispersed conversational vignettes about the various topics. I can see images of the students who are speaking. I remember when the room was too hot or cold. I can become so absorbed in these recollections that I lose track of what is going on around me. Sometimes this is called daydreaming.

I don't necessarily remember the conversations accurately. Memory doesn't work that way. I may have invented much of it, but it feels real to me. What is extremely accurate is the gist of the conversations, the big picture, the social emotions that flowed through the room, the sense of the students' characters. We store our really important memories in story form, recalling them as a story in much the same way that we remember a piece of fiction: more in terms of characters and their emotions, the gist of what happened, the biggest picture, and the meaning that we attributed to the story, rather than what actually happened detail by detail. Our brains fill in (some would say confabulate) the detail to match the present situation.

My students would be clamoring to be heard. They would be saying, "Wait, isn't mental illness genetic? Doesn't it come from chemical imbalances? What do you mean we learn how to be mentally ill?"

They are lost in the nature-versus-nurture argument. Is behavior the result of life experience, or is it hardwired in the brain? Here's what those theorists didn't know. The brain (nature) is shaped by experience and interacts with the environment to change itself to match its experience. In chapter 7 we will discuss epigenetics ("over the gene"), the new science of how social experience modifies our genes. This new realization by molecular geneticists that life experience reshapes our DNA moment by moment is exciting to those of us who tell stories about healing. The structure of the gene may be as important as the sequence of the genetic code with which we are born. This structure can be completely reshaped by life experience. How this is done has been the subject of numerous *Scientific American* magazine articles. For our purposes it is enough to say that it is done through chemical alterations (methylation and acetylation) of the DNA and of the histone molecules (protein chains) that support and maintain its structure.

The shape of a molecule is incredibly important in biology. Shape emerges from the interaction of the component groups of the molecule. A methyl group consists of one carbon atom and three hydrogen atoms. An acetyl group is only slightly larger, with an oxygen atom added. When these molecular fragments are added to the DNA or the histone that surrounds it, the structure of the gene shifts, causing the messenger RNA to copy it differently and change its expression. Life experience can be transmitted by this form of structural change to at least three successive generations. We really do benefit (or suffer) from the experiences of our parents, first genetically at conception, and then in reshaping our DNA after conception through the life experiences they give us and the stories they tell us.

On the whole, social relationships and experience are perhaps more powerful in changing our brains than drugs.* This has certainly been my experience working as a psychiatrist. In the World Health Organization's long-term studies of schizophrenia in third-world countries where drugs were minimal (reviewed in *Narrative Medicine*), the people with schizophrenia had much better outcomes when they were kept within their families and communities, were given jobs that conferred meaning and purpose, and were still honored as members of those families and communities.

This is crucial for the sustainability of human life on the planet. Drugs are expensive and require large factories and distribution systems. They require natural resources to produce. They contaminate the environment. (The concentration of psychoactive medications in the water supply and in marine animals is alarmingly high.) Human care and compassion

---

*I do acknowledge, however, that there are circumstances, particularly for people who are chronically psychotic, in which psychiatric medications are useful, both to relieve suffering and to ensure safety. My approach is to use the lowest possible doses of antipsychotic drugs to reduce acute suffering and psychosis while we work with the person and the family to change perception, to restore a healthy story-making capacity, and to build and change social relationships. The drugs may be a temporary but practical bridge to keep the patient (and others) safe and enable the person to gradually enter the relationship-building process. **Another important note: People taking psychiatric medications should never stop taking them abruptly, as serious withdrawal symptoms can occur.**

is much less expensive, and in the future, people will be in much greater supply than natural resources. They need jobs. Imagine a mental health system in which we rely on one another to help families and communities to become whole again and to take better care of their members. I can envision a world in which drugs become largely unnecessary because we have the social knowledge and capital to heal one another through our relationships.

Experience Changes Biology

What is crucial about my vision is its inclusion of brain and biology. When I began to study narrative psychology and philosophy, I was uncomfortable with their general avoidance of discussing the body and biology. I realized this was because their proponents were largely coming from humanities backgrounds—comparative literature, literary criticism, creative writing, feminism, ethnic studies, philosophy, and so on. I was happy to bring my biophysics and medical background to the table. I wanted a narratology that included the body and the brain.

Traditional elders from multiple tribes have told me for years that experience changes biology. The essence of their social and spiritual healing practices relies on their acceptance and enactment of that story. They don't need a biochemical or mechanistic physiological explanation to accept the story arising from their observations. They know that changing the relationships among people in families and communities changes their biology. They know that changing our relationships to animals, plants, rocks, and spirits changes biology. They know that life-threatening illnesses can disappear given sufficient change.

My Cherokee ancestors had an ultimate ceremony that embodies this. If at least two teams of seven healers had not facilitated a cure for a very sick person and death seemed imminent, then drastic measures were taken. The person's name was changed. That seems absurd to our conventionally, academically trained minds. What we don't appreciate is how the name, in Cherokee culture, referred to all of the stories ever told about the person. With a new name, that person now had different parents, children, spouse, work, and status in the community. Cures were documented from this procedure. The early anthropologists who described it were astounded that it could happen, because they associated the identity with the visual body (European practice), while the Cherokee associated the identity with the symbolic body (the name). The Cherokee could do what the Europeans could not. They could completely change how they interacted with the person when that person had a new name.

I've often dreamed of doing this, but identity is more fixed today. It's the downside of driver's licenses, passports, social security, photography, videography, and the increasing documentation of all that we do. Changes in identity can no longer be accomplished by simply changing a name, though I have known people who have disappeared from their old life and reinvented themselves in a new place with a new name and a new situation and have gotten well. But the ability to do this is extremely rare.

We return to my students and their objections to social relationships powerfully reshaping biology. Their objections are philosophical, not data driven. Their objections come from their incorporation of the dominant story of contemporary North American society—that biology is biology and must be treated biologically. According to this story, even psychology is biology and should be treated biologically. This story tells us that pharmacology is the solution to our woes. To appreciate this, all one has to do is watch television. In the United States, commercials are available for most categories of drugs. The promises are enormous. A quickly and more quietly spoken mention of risks and side effects comes at the end of the commercial when we are too enraptured by the imagined benefits to listen or care. I call this story "better living through chemistry," an actual phrase from my childhood in the 1950s.

My students' objection (and perhaps yours) comes from growing up in a world saturated by the "better living through chemistry" story. We have been taught to seek help from a pill for every woe, every ache or pain. Of course that story has tremendous commercial appeal for the pharmaceutical industry and for those who own stock in it or are employed by it. Why do physicians continue to rely almost exclusively on pills, if they don't work so well? Drug companies have an obvious agenda—profit. Physicians, on the other hand, have different motivations—often being more concerned with status and feeling socially acceptable than with income. Physicians also want to give their patients what they want. They have accepted the "magic potion" story also and think, as their patients do, that drugs will solve the problem if they just give the right one. Too bad pharmaceuticals don't work as well as presented.

Without digressing too far from the flow of this chapter to present pertinent data, I will say that my experience in treating with psychiatric medication has been largely dismal for all types of psychiatric disorders: with a handful of exceptions, psychiatric medication for schizophrenia generally helps about 20 percent of the people, leaving another 80 percent to suffer. The CATIE studies funded by the National Institutes of Health for many millions of dollars similarly found that only "one-quarter of all the participants were satisfied with the level of symptom relief they experienced from [the initially prescribed] antipsychotic medication, were able to tolerate its side effects, and stayed on it for the entire 18 months of the study."[19] The study focused on primarily chronic patients. Of those who discontinued, a significant percentage did so due to lack of effectiveness and another significant percentage due to unacceptable side effects.[20]

What's more important is that the effectiveness of the drugs eventually wears off because medications do not change the social relationships that have shaped and continue to maintain the person's brain. Drugs can override this for a time, but not forever. Then the conditions of our lives overcome the drugs and force us back to where we were before the medications. This is because the brain is a socially maintained organ. It is created through our experiences and changes through our experiences. For the patients willing to continue in the CATIE study, a different drug was prescribed. This is in accordance with the biological model, which says correct the pharmacology, correct the imbalance, and all will be fine.

Drugs Can't Solve Everything

Despite the public's perception, my experience is that most psychiatrists do not offer any interventions besides medications. They work in accordance with what complexity theorists call a simple, closed-system model. But the reality of modern life is that there are few closed systems. Rather, behavior, symptoms, and suffering arise from multiple interrelated, inter-acting forces that drive brains (and people) to do what they do. Simply relying on drugs is rarely effective long-term because these forces bring things back to where they were (called homeostasis).

What my observations (and those of the traditional elders who have informed and taught me) have confirmed is that the brain is not a closed system. It is connected to a world of other brains. We are nodes in a social network. One elder told me that our world is modeled after a spider web. Each of us is an intersection in a web woven by Grandmother Spider to contain us all. Just as the motion of an intersection or a node in a web is constrained by the rest of the web, so our freedom to act, our actual human agency, is constrained by the web of our social relationships. These social relationships generate our health and disease. Change the relation-ships and you change the biology.

What happens when a brain is medicated and the social relationships in which that brain is engaged remain unaltered is that the environment slowly reshapes the brain back to its former state, but slightly different, because the drug is still on board. The person is now potentially worse, because higher neuro-hormonal levels are required to produce the same symptoms and overwhelm the effects of the drug. Sometimes this has been called biological tolerance, but I think it is more than that. I think toler-ance to drugs develops because our social relationships have not changed and thus eventually force us back to how we used to be.

How does this work in the body? Take the experience of fear as an example. Fear starts with the perception of danger, which may or may not be an accurate apprisal of the environment. In either case, the perception of danger activates the sympathetic nervous system, with the production of norepinephrine and many other molecules. Chronic fear leads to chronic activation, with associated higher levels of cortisol (the so-called stress hormone), which leads to the breakdown of our bodies—catabolism—as opposed to anabolism, the state in which our bodies are repaired.

Let's assume a drug called a beta-blocker is given to a person in a state of chronic fear. The beta-blocker prevents the sympathetic nervous system from responding. But the person's perception of danger hasn't been changed. And the environment in which the person lives may actually be dangerous (such as that of some of my clients who are regularly beaten when their spouse goes on a drinking binge). The need for the outpouring of catecholamines—hormones and neurotransmitters—still exists, and the body finds a way to produce them. It's just that now the set point is higher. In such a situation, short-term benefit has been achieved at long-term costs.

A substantial disability remains among people undergoing conventional psychiatric treatment.[21] A variety of stories define mental health and tell people how to be well and how to reduce suffering. People from different cultures define mind and mental health differently or not at all. The biological model is incomplete. It ignores a wealth of knowledge, both European and indigenous, about what really happens. As mentioned earlier, I am *not* against psychiatric medications. I am appalled, however, by our current model, which assumes that drugs will solve everything. Short-term use of drugs can sometimes reduce suffering sufficiently to allow the longer-term work to take place. I often use low doses of antipsychotic drugs to reduce acute suffering while I work with the person and the family to change perception, to restore the capacity to story, and to change social relationships.

What is necessary for avoiding medication is intense social support, which few people have these days. Once a person has become a chronic patient, the social support is minimal because so many families want no contact with their relatives who have been diagnosed with schizophrenia. They depend on the "mental health system" for care that it largely doesn't give except for some case management and medication visits. The intense social support that exists in India or that I have seen on reservations in Canada is largely lacking in urban America. Therefore, drugs in doses low enough that they don't cause side effects and scare the person may help reduce unbearable suffering enough to enable the person to begin the relationship-building process. And yes, sometimes vitamins, herbs, acupuncture, and any number of other modalities can provide short-term as well as long-term suffering reduction. The fallacy of the biological psychiatry argument is that only drugs can change brain function. Everything changes brain function. The question is how to do it with the least side effects.

Changing the "Inner Family"

Our waking and dreaming moments are full of countless others. Psychologist Richard Schwartz at the University of Wisconsin in Milwaukee describes the internal world of our brains as populated by people we have incorporated and given ontological status as people living within our skulls. He believes that we have created representations for all of our family members within our brains and that our emotions arise from the speech of these internal representations and also as reactions to what they say.[22]

The dialogue with our internal characters contains story and feeling. For example, I once said to a girlfriend, "I remember the time you got drunk and beat me up and threatened to have your gangster friends kill me, even though you don't remember it." That sentence continues as part of my internal dialogue. When I repeat that sentence, she is still there listening, regardless of how long ago it was. She still has her same puzzled reaction of not remembering what she did when she drank. I still have my same hopeless reaction to that situation, even though it has been years. The conversation and the story about that conversation remain present for the telling, which evokes in me the same reactions or feelings that I had initially. The story is stored with affect attached. Psychologist Gordon Bower of Stanford University called this "affect-dependent storage and retrieval of memory."[23]

The inner voices of people who are diagnosed with schizophrenia are largely critical, negative, and persistent, sometimes urging the person to commit suicide, saying that he or she is worthless and not deserving to live. Often these voices are imagined "outside" the person as disembodied beings tormenting the individual. Schwartz found that it wasn't enough for family relationships to change via external family therapy. He argues that we must also do internal family therapy to change these internal constructions of the outer world.[24] Another way to say this is that we must manage our inner voices, regardless of what ontological status we give them. For people suffering from psychosis, this often reduces their rage and anger. For sad people, managing the voices can mean eliminating self-deprecation. For worried people, it means erasing the voice that warns of impending doom. This concept of managing voices is catching hold. In Ireland, the Hearing Voices Network evolved to assist people with managing their voices. It is now spreading over the entire world.

Parts therapy was developed to help people manage their various parts, an idea presaged by ordinary language, such as when we say, "A part of me wants to go, but a part of me doesn't," or "I left my heart in San Francisco." A "part" can be seen as a "voice." This amounts to a modern interpretation of Siberian and Mongolian soul retrieval, which gathers parts of a person that have been left behind or lost, or have wandered off. The narrative perspective offers some fresh understandings: these parts are the tellers of the stories that guide our lives, they are formed from the original tellers of the stories that determined our fate as children, and they can be changed.

In Schwartz's perspective or in parts therapy, these parts or voices are more independent than assumed by self-talk, which assumes a unified self as the source of a monologue. Some have well-developed ontological status; they are beings in their own right, speaking to us independently. Rather than an integrated self delivering an integrated monologue, a cacophony of independent voices are competing to be heard.

I think these internal characters arise because we continue telling the stories we hear; the internal storyteller takes the form of the person who originally told the story. Just as the brain makes maps of our physical environment and our sensory environment, I imagine that we have an inner map of the outer social world that contains our representations of the people in that environment. We have the capacity to imagine dialogue, to create fictional scenarios that could happen or could have happened, to continue relationships and discussions for years after they are over. For us to really change, we have to change these inner voices and dialogues as well as change the outer world relationships. We need to change the stories that we repeat over and over about ourselves. We can learn how to tell a different story to others about who we think we are and to find ways for the people in our lives to tell different stories about us.

Boyd believes that we use our memory to evaluate new situations against what we have experienced in the past.[25] When faced with a new experience, we check it against previous related stories. If our past stories are challenged and appear inaccurate, we must revise them to facilitate our understanding of the present.

Holding Space for Nancy

"Nancy" is a good example of a person who was healed by a change in story. She had a psychotic episode during college and was admitted to a hospital, overmedicated for two months, eventually discharged, and—to her amazing credit and that of her family—gradually worked her way off medications and into a normal life within a year. She was able to go back to college, complete her degree, and earn a graduate degree in—what else?—clinical psychology. Of course, I believed that Nancy was a natural to be a psychologist: she was a wounded healer who had successfully recovered.

How did her recovery happen? Nancy's mother refused to believe that there was anything permanently or perpetually wrong with Nancy. She insisted that Nancy would "get over it" eventually and find her way. She refused to accept the dire pronouncements of the psychiatrists that Nancy was schizophrenic, doomed to a marginal life of low functionality and misery, and would require medication for the rest of her life. Unfortunately, psychiatrists often present diagnoses of mental illness as life sentences, stipulating that the patients will require medication to treat their conditions for the rest of their lifetimes. This relationship process—this type of storying—is very damaging to a patient, perpetuating in the person a very negative and likely untrue story about himself or herself. But "mental illness" is often not a life sentence, as we shall soon see.

Nancy saw her experience as part of a spiritual awakening and resented being medicated because the medication made her less able to think or experience what was happening to her. She had an unshakable belief that she would go through these experiences and emerge on the other side, changed for the better as a result of having taken the journey. She was also aware that she felt unsafe and lost even as she was having powerful spiritual experiences. She couldn't understand why the doctors and nurses in the hospital were not at all, even vaguely, interested in her personal spiritual transformation.

My favorite Nancy story comes from the height of her psychosis, when she believed she could drive along a winding road with a mountain on one side and a lake on the other without looking. Nancy closed her eyes and let go of the steering wheel, letting the car do whatever it wanted. Miraculously, she ended up in a ditch beside the road after going a full mile with her eyes closed. Apparently the car wanted to navigate several hairpin turns and did so very well. A friend of mine has a similar story about doing this with a lake on either side of the road for almost the same distance. She miraculously survived as well.

I don't have any trouble believing these stories. Many of my students have trouble with my beliefs in the supernatural realm, but as I tell them, I have evidence from the context of indigenous knowledge. Within that framework, spirits (angels) exist and help us in some of our most dire circumstances. They have saved my life several times.

Nevertheless, we will not go there. A person can be a dialectical materialist, even a good Marxist, and still work within a narrative psychiatry framework. You and I can agree that spirituality is a collection of stories. We can agree on the power of a story without agreeing on the "truth value" of the story. You can believe it's just a story and I can believe it's true, and that will be fine, because in the end, as philosopher Karl Popper proposed, we can never prove truth but can only possibly prove the falsity of something. For him, science is not the process of finding truths, but the process of making, refuting, and then revising claims. These claims, as Popper describes, are just our interpretive stories about what we think is going on.

So whether an angel saved Nancy, as I believe, or whether she hallucinated her drive on the mountain, as you may believe, what is important is that Nancy was able to taper off and then stop all her medications and find a normal life. She did this primarily through yoga, which aided her recovery enormously. She did yoga for hours every day, and slowly but surely found her way back to health.

Could Nancy have recovered if her family had believed the psychiatrists? I don't think so. I credit the faith and love and power of belief (also known as story) of Nancy's mother for creating and "holding space" to make healing possible.

Holding space is an important and rarely discussed concept. When we hold space for someone, we bear witness to them, their stories, and their pain. We serve as a supportive audience member, sometimes a coach, sometimes a warm shoulder for comfort. We hold the vision of the person being well, being happy, having recovered. The more people who hold that vision, the more possible recovery becomes. Having a good story to describe the person's travails helps us all to hold hands and look in the same direction. It gives us a sense of coherence, of being on the same page with each other. These are powerful feelings that make us feel that we belong to something greater than our single bodies, thereby creating the expectation that a miracle is about to happen.

After Nancy's recovery, she was forever changed for the better. Her life had a spiritual component never before present. Her other family members were at most agnostics, perhaps atheists. They weren't concerned about the spiritual. But Nancy had entered into a world of Hindu spirituality that worked well for her, stabilizing her situation so that she could return to college. Regardless of their different viewpoints, her family members were among the most supportive people on earth. During her recovery, Nancy was continually surrounded by loving sisters, brothers, father, mother, grandparents, uncles, aunts, nieces, and nephews. She was almost never alone unless she requested to be so (and not at the beginning at all lest she try "blind driving" again).

Finding the Words to a New Story

In our mainstream American culture, psychosis is more likely because of the lack of context for intense spiritual transformation. My Huichol and Yaqui friends from Arizona and northern Mexico tell me it is common for white Americans not to be supported in such spiritual processes because they have no familiar stories for understanding sudden, spontaneous spiritual awakenings. They believe such transformations are more common than we realize and are often misinterpreted as psychotic breaks.

Hindu cultures call these experiences "kundalini awakenings." Edgar Cayce (1877–1945), America's "sleeping prophet," called this a "kundalini crisis," occurring when a spontaneous spiritual awakening happens in the context of a body/mind/social environment that has not been properly prepared. Cayce, as well as Stan Grof, the American psychiatrist who lived and worked at Esalen Institute for many years, recognized that we need to be put into the correct context to receive and integrate intense spiritual awakenings, or we might go mad. Mainstream America lacks stories that contain the necessary instructions for contextualizing these experiences.

The late San Francisco psychiatrist John Weir Perry wrote:

All of us who have touched the deep, inner spaces of psychic life, whether in psychotic, psychedelic, or deeply meditative states, have experienced the convincing realness of these inner regions. Even while we know at first hand how overwhelming they are in their visual and feeling terms, we often sense how incapable we are of giving them words. For the beauty, the terror, and the love; for the visions and meaning and the flashes of insight, the words of our conscious instrumentation are found too small and cramped, too constrictive, and our modes of expression too encased in old structures of familiar experience.[26]

Part of my work with Nancy, and part of my work with all people who suffer from psychosis, is to help them give words to their experiences, to be able to tell a story about what they have experienced. It took some time, but Nancy now has many stories to tell about her psychotic experiences. She's actually become quite articulate in her descriptions, though she's still careful to whom she tells these stories. Working in the mental health field, she knows the biases toward anyone who has been psychotic.

I want to end my reference to Nancy with a story about an exacerbation of illness that occurred to her when she was thirty years old and had just married. Her husband had a son from a previous marriage. His ex-wife was chronically depressed and misusing substances—alcohol, marijuana, occasionally cocaine, and even heroin. Nancy lost some of her balance and poise when she invested herself in the story that she could create a corrective emotional experience for her husband's fourteen-year-old. The harder she tried, the more frustrated she became, and the angrier her stepson became. He got so enraged that he got really drunk and attempted suicide. (His storyline was, "I'll show you how hurt and angry I am by killing myself; then you'll really feel bad.") At the hospital, family members pointed at Nancy and said she was the problem; if she would only go away, all would be fine. Nancy experienced this as a hard blow to the chest and dropped into psychosis again. Enough of her awareness remained for her to come to me for a retreat into recovery.

Ten retreat days later, Nancy was feeling a bit fragile but was not psychotic anymore. She wasn't ready to return to her new family and its dynamics, but we had reimplemented her practices that worked—yoga, meditation, movement. Medication wasn't necessary. The safe structure took care of that. While it may seem to be part of "alternative" medicine, the stabilizing effect of Nancy's retreat can also be seen in more mainstream settings. I have a colleague at West Virginia University who never changes medication when a psychotic patient is admitted. He waits to see how the structure, protection, and stress-reducing aspects of the hospital will affect the symptoms. He finds, as I do, that life's exigencies often overwhelm the person's capacity to cope and that ten days of safety and structure is usually sufficient to bring things back to normal. Changing medications or raising doses is not necessary. If we were visionary, we would create much less expensive alternatives to hospitals that could still provide safety and structure; they would save the health care system enormous costs.

After she calmed down, we were able to look at the destabilizing story that had brought Nancy down—that she could fix her stepson, or that she could be the good mother to his bad mother, or that she could heal her loved ones. "You've bitten off too much," I said. "You should leave this work to Krishna, Jesus, Buddha, or the angels. Let your new family members all be who they are and don't play the stepmom from heaven, because that'll turn you into the stepmom from hell."

Nancy saw the wisdom of this, and we worked to help her construct a new story about equanimity and letting people be whatever they want to be without her feeling responsible for their healing and pain. "You have enough work in your practice to occupy your healing side without having to bring it home," I said. "Leave healing at the office."

Once Nancy became ready, I began having meetings with everyone involved. The finger-pointing was intense, but Nancy now had a story to protect her from accepting that energy directed at her. (My Cree friend John would call that energy a curse. He would have given her protection and asked her to pray for all those who were cursing her. He would have done ceremony with her, with the end result being the same—that she would have a new story that would protect her from taking on the wicked stepmother role.)

We eventually worked at the various family relationships. The stepson has his new story—that he doesn't give a damn about his stepmother; in fact, he can completely ignore her. (This actually allows him to have fun with her.) The boy's mother is still doing what she did and hating Nancy for replacing her, even though the woman hadn't been with her ex-husband for five years. The husband has given up his *Brady Bunch* fantasies of everyone getting along and being happy and somehow curing his son's pain and making his ex-wife happy. As I pointed out to Nancy, he couldn't make his wife happy when they were married, so how should adding Nancy to the picture improve that? It could only make the ex-wife less happy. Was the husband willing to get rid of Nancy to make his ex-wife happy? He wasn't. Gradually Nancy, her husband, and his son realized that they needed to see things as they were and to stop trying to change them. (Buddha said much suffering comes from imagining that things are different from how they actually are.)

Stories that Heal

Psychiatry is the science of stories and storytelling, because our social interaction is fully storied.[27] Most of what goes on in psychotherapy is an exchange of narratives, which seem to be illustrative and inclusive of basically all processes of meaning constructions: about awake and dream states; about the self, others, or the therapist; and about both the present and the past. The fundamental therapeutic functions that narrative has been shown to accomplish—emotional experiencing and relief as ways of working through thought and feelings—justify the pervasiveness of narrative.[28]

In fact, whenever we use language (and language is necessary for all things human), we enter the domain of story, for story is what language produces. British anthropologist and neuroscientist Charles Whitehead believes that language was the cultural big bang that turned an ancient primate social order on its head. Language helped create the nonbiological features of human culture, leading to the explosion of creative art and technology of the Upper Paleolithic era, transforming our precultural ancestors into people who could speak, share their dreams, and create fantastic systems of belief and social order.[29] With that explosion began story, or narrative, in the form we know today.

Therapy outcome is significantly related to changes in narratives about relationships from the negative to the positive.[30] Poor-outcome groups in therapy have a greater overall percentage of time spent discussing the actions of others or events or issues as opposed to reflexive stories about life experiences.[31] The good-outcome groups have a higher percentage of the reflexive mode (interpretation of either external events or subjective experiences) compared to the poor-outcome groups. An increase of reflexive narrative sequences seems to be related with a better outcome.

Written language has also been shown to have great healing power. Experimental subjects who write about deep personal topics have highly significant changes in clinically relevant measures.[32] They have significantly fewer health center visits for periods of up to six months, demonstrate improvements in their immune systems,[33] have fewer absences from work, have improved enzyme function for up to two months,[34] and have experienced improvements in physical health and grade-point averages.[35] Improvements in physical health experienced by research subjects are not due to dramatic changes in their behavior (including their drinking, sleeping, smoking, and exercise patterns).[36]

The narrative movement in psychiatry is concerned with understanding the stories of pain and suffering told by people within context. These stories have plot, costars, villains, and audiences of accountability. Suffering is not eliminated through the expert gaze of the law or of medicine. Putting something under the microscope for inspection does not change it. It reifies it and keeps it the same. It makes a changing story (verb) into a noun (object, no change). Equal partnerships are required for real change to occur. People must have a forum in which they can trust and believe in each other and simply talk about what troubles them and what they desire.

The narrative movement provides a bridge between European philosophy and concepts and the indigenous worldview and indigenous concepts of story, and how story becomes us and we become story and story is all there is. Our work is to render all people nondefective; to celebrate each person's unique resources, talents, and skills. Indigenous views of worth revolve around what we do within the relationships that we have. Dominant culture constructions of social relationships render some people inferior and ashamed. Our dominant culture thrives on large classes of people feeling that way (ethnic minorities, women, gays and lesbians, and so on). Lack of skill in negotiating within the dominant culture is turned into feelings of personal inferiority and self-defectiveness.

I remember my young male clients in Saskatchewan who joined Indian gangs. Tony, for example, had nothing. He lived in a two-bedroom house on a rural reserve with eighteen other people, who slept in shifts to accommodate the low ratio of beds per person. His parents were alcoholics, as had been his grandparents. Being in the gang gave him a sense of pride. He described it like being part of a war party in a more ancient time. The "braves" could raid "enemy camps" (other gangs) and count coup on those gang members as a way of gaining status. The sense of trust that his gang members would protect his back was incredibly comforting to Tony, for no one had ever protected him before.

Only through traditional healing could Tony find that same sense of community and camaraderie that he had found in the gang. It also provided him with a healing counter-narrative—a story that could undermine the assumptions of a particular story. Within society, counter-narratives that rebel against destructive conventional concepts or constructions like racism or the oppression of women (and I would add conventional concepts of anxiety and depression) are agents of social evolution. For Tony, the counter-narrative was that a sense of belongingness, meaning, and purpose was better found in traditional spirituality and ceremony than in a gang, especially because the risks of dying were so much less.

The transformative role of the counter-narrative can be better understood in light of quantum physics. Princeton University physicist John Wheeler (1911–2008) believed that the future shaped the past through the quantum reciprocal wave. In this idea, the future makes an observation and the observation sends an inquiry backward to reorganize the past to conform to that observation. Physicist and author Fred Alan Wolf, in writing about Wheeler's idea, thought of it as the future "pinging" the past with a message. Those pasts that can receive the message from the future (and are therefore reasonably compatible with the future) then respond by reorganizing themselves in such a way as to send back the "message received" response, thereby restructuring the past to conform to the observation made.

Wolf wondered if stories, each time they are told, alter the past in which they originated. If we apply this same principle to the retelling and reliving of our stories and realize the importance of reframing our stories—if we reconstruct and retell our stories in the future—we can actually change and heal the past. In doing so, we improve the healing relationship between all of us, eliminating the destructive constructs of "mental illness" and "depressives," and thus direct our improvement for the future.

What if we learn from the future? What if the future informs us about what we need to know and then we learn how to create the future based on information that the future provides? What if evolution is always goal directed, based on observations that have been made in the future and then reflected back to us in the past?

Kenneth J. Gergen, psychology professor at Swarthmore College, wrote, "Constructionist thought is not toward the enunciation of a new truth, [but toward] relationship. [T]his turn in sensibility opens a space for innovation and transformation."[37] We are moving away from the idea that there is one truth to discover about depression or anxiety, that these are explicit disorders or diseases, and toward the idea of human experience and its vicissitudes. Through relationship and dialogue, we make space to consider each other's sadness, fear, and pain. Innovation and transformation arise in that space between people and are, by definition, unpredictable. From this point of view, the so-called psychiatric disorders are not disorders, but rather conversations that can be redirected, explored, and transformed.

3

How Do We Learn to Be Who We Are?

My intention is to tell
of bodies changed
to different forms.
The heavens and all below them,
Earth and her creatures,
All change.
And we, part of creation,
Also must suffer change.

OVID, *METAMORPHOSES*

Learning involves the construction of new ideas or concepts based on a history or story that defines and describes those ideas.[1] We learn "who we are supposed to be" from other people. The Lakota believe that all learning (and especially learning about emotions) occurs in the context of a relationship. We are the result of all the relationships that construct us. All those relationships tell stories about who we are in them. As we learn, we incorporate those stories, select and transform them in ways that are more effective for us in the contexts and relationships in which we find ourselves, and construct a story that we continually revise about "who we are." This story is in the form of what are called cognitive structures in the terminology of cognitive behavior therapy (CBT). As we form new relationships in new contexts, our cognitive structures expand beyond the information given and we modify our story to provide meaning and organization to our ongoing and new experiences.

Development is not a smooth, continual process. We progress in a step-wise fashion, suddenly leaping ahead like jumping frogs. Qualitatively new psychological phenomena arise over the course of a life, consisting of novel operations, content, and relationships that are not continuous with previous ones. Consequently, perspectives and methods that are suitable for explaining early behaviors are not necessarily suitable for explaining later behaviors. Different concepts and methods must be devised to apprehend and integrate the different psychological stages.[2] New and developing relationships give us more stories (information), so our repertoire of stories expands, which changes our master story about who we are.

Lev Vygotsky's Social Development Theory

I have been most influenced in my thinking about development by Russian psychologist Lev Vygotsky. He believed that social interaction played a key role in human development (of the brain, of cognition, of imagination, of all mental functions that humans perform and animals cannot).[3] In contrast to French psychologist Jean Piaget (1896–1980), who believed that development is intrinsic and staged and precedes learning, Vygotsky believed that social learning (which occurs through social interaction) precedes development. He wrote, "Every function in the child's cultural development appears twice: first, on the social level, and later, on the individual level; first, between people (inter-psychologically) and then inside the child (intra-psychologically). This applies equally to voluntary attention, to logical memory, and to the formation of concepts. All the higher functions originate as actual relationships between individuals."[4]

Vygotsky believed that children begin with needs—for food, water, love, security, and safety—and use the available communication tools to attain those needs. Through gradual correlation of the mother's pointing at food with the state of being hungry, the child learns to point to food when hungry. Similar kinds of communication can involve crying when feeling afraid or alone, smiling when comforted, and so on. Initially, pointing or even crying had no meaning for the infant. Over time, through the intervention of a social other—such as when the mother or caregiver interprets the infant's desires or needs and fulfills them—the infant learns that crying or pointing has meaning.

In these shaping/learning situations, Vygotsky said the mother or caregiver is working within the infant's "zone of proximal development."[5] The zone of proximal development concept is crucial to Vygotsky's thought and is often described as a scaffold. Inside this zone are those things that the infant or person cannot do alone but can do with the help of a more experienced other (caregiver, teacher, mentor). Vygotsky believed that learning and development take place in this zone: we try things that we couldn't do on our own and master them with the help of a teacher, transcending our limitations to become more capable, competent, and skillful. Infants quickly develop a repertoire of communication skills for managing their parents and other significant caretakers. Through a similar shaping process, the child learns language. Vygotsky believed that the internalization of these communication tools led to the development of those uniquely human psychological processes and that full cognitive development requires social interaction.[6]

This learning in the zone of proximal development separates us from higher primates, who cannot do this. Vygotsky was impressed by the findings of animal psychologist Wolfgang Köhler, who determined that primates are able to use imitation to solve only those problems that are of the same degree of difficulty as those they can solve alone. Humans, on the other hand, can use imitation to solve problems beyond their current capacity to solve problems alone.

> Primates cannot be taught (in the human sense of the word) through imitation, nor can their intellect be developed, because they have no zone of proximal development. A primate can learn a great deal through training by using its mechanical and mental skills, but it cannot be made more intelligent, that is, it cannot be taught to solve

a variety of more advanced problems independently. For this reason, animals are incapable of learning in the human sense of the term; human learning presupposes a specific social nature and a process by which children grow into the intellectual life of those around them. Children can imitate a variety of actions that go well beyond the limits of their own capabilities. Using imitation, children are capable of doing much more in collective activity or under the guidance of adults. This fact . . . is of fundamental importance in that it demands a radical alteration of the entire doctrine concerning the relation between learning and development in children.[7]

Vygotsky's teaching paradigm provides a refreshing break from the usual instructional approach in which the teacher gives the student information to absorb. In Vygotsky's approach, the teacher collaborates with the student to bring the student into the zone of proximal development. In this zone, the student can do things with the teacher and through the support of the teacher that the student could not do alone.

This provides a model for collaborative healing relationships that can supplant the usual hierarchical therapist–client approach. In Vygotsky's model, one person who has a skill provides support for another to learn that skill. Thus, if I have the skill of knowing how to relax and knowing how to train others to relax and you need to learn how to relax, then together with me you can relax more than you can alone. If we spend enough time together in your zone of proximal development, you will learn how to relax and your skill will become equal to mine or eventually surpass mine. Then you will no longer need the scaffolding I have provided. Just as a scaffold is removed from a building when construction is completed, so is the scaffolding relationship unnecessary once the client learns what is being taught. One can readily see how different this approach is from that of psychodynamic psychotherapy or even rational emotive therapy or cognitive behavioral therapy, in which the therapist has the authoritative role.

Being a Marxist-Leninist, but with the transcendentalism and implicit spirituality that is inherent in the Russian language and culture, Vygotsky sought to explain consciousness as the end product of socialization.[8] I don't follow Vygotsky that far, however, having been taught by my elders that we enter the world with conscious awareness. However, that awareness must operate through a body and a brain (with the exceptions of intuition, spirit communication, and knowingness, which are not discussed in this chapter) and in a social world, from the moment we need to communicate, which happens at birth. Vygotsky believed that once we master language for the purpose of getting what we want, we internalize it and it becomes "inner speech," probably initially as the memory of speech we have heard, even if poorly understood, graduating as development progresses to well-developed auditory memory in which we can accurately reproduce what another has said. This is the origin of our inner voices, parts, self-talk, internal representations, or whatever we call our inner dialogues.

This capacity to memorize develops over the life of a child and can be followed by how well a child is able to repeat a story he or she has heard or tell a story about an event that has happened. Vygotsky and other neuroscientists would say that it is the attempt to reproduce or imitate speech, along with its many accompanying gestures, intonations, and tonalities, that activates mirror neurons within our brains; they then help us to activate the brain areas used for speech. A mirror neuron is one that fires both when an animal (including a human) acts and when that animal observes the same action being performed by another animal, especially those of the same species. Imitation leads to mastery.

The more we reproduce what another has said, the more we practice, at first verbally, reproducing speech, the more we build capacity to speak quietly, to speak without moving our lips. Eventually we learn to speak internally, using the same neurons as if we were speaking out loud, but suppressing the production of actual speech so that we can "talk to ourselves" silently. Vygotsky has marvelous descriptions of children talking to themselves until they realize at around age four that they can disengage the motor cortex and "think" a dialogue without actually speaking it. At first, they are still silently moving their lips, and eventually, not even that.

I associate this time in human development with our incorporation of others' voices within us. We begin to speak their speech and hear them without actually verbalizing. This is the beginning of the inner mind, the inner world, or the private world, as it has variously been described. These speeches and voices we internalize become the substrate for our adult lives.

Becoming Aware

Vygotsky also believed that the most fundamental qualitative change we could make over the course of a life was to become consciously aware, this awareness arising over and above our reflexive, biological processes. University of Massachusetts economist Nassim Nicholas Taleb distinguishes these as system 1 and system 2 processes.[9] System 1 is mediated faster than thought, using biological reflexes and stories we have stored and rehearsed about how to interpret the world. These stories have been used so often that they constitute a kind of automatic, or default, mode of response. The activities of the neurons and synapses that support these stories are virtually below the threshold for conscious awareness. System 2 processes require conscious reflection. In Vygotsky's words, this transition from "direct, innate, natural forms and methods of behavior to mediated, artificial, mental functions . . . parallel[s] the process of cultural development."[10]

Vygotsky believed that our lower, elementary processes are biologically programmed, natural behaviors that are immediate responses to stimuli, such as the sucking and rooting reflexes. "Higher mental functions are not simply a continuation of elementary functions and are not their mechanical combination, but are a qualitatively new mental formation that develops according to completely special laws and is subject to completely different patterns."[11]

We need to distinguish here the difference between psychological processes and consciousness. Consciousness intervenes, or mediates, between a stimulus and the response. Consciousness consists of psychological phenomena such as perception, emotions, memory, thinking, motivation, self, language, and accumulated learned information. Psychological processes involve awareness; they are humanly created mental phenomena. They are not natural biological "objects," although they require things like brains. Multiple metaphors have been derived to explain the difference between consciousness and psychological processes, but these explanations are largely conjectural.

For Vygotsky, there are no stages. Unlike Piaget, Vygotsky believed that the course of development was somewhat arbitrary, depending on the available resources at hand. A child develops the capacity to be conscious, cognitive, and conceptual based on successful exposure to adults or others who can help him or her to learn the necessary skills. Development occurs piecemeal, as adults or others happen to be around to help the child master particular tasks. In due time, the child develops into an adolescent, an "almost adult" who still needs certain scaffolding and assistance due to the immaturity of the frontal lobe, which keeps track of the consequences of our actions.

> Development of thinking has a central, key, decisive significance for all the other functions and processes. We cannot express more clearly or tersely the leading role of intellectual development in relation to the whole personality of the adolescent and to all of his mental functions other than to say that acquiring the function of forming concepts is the principal and central link in all the changes that occur in the psychology of the adolescent. All other links in this chain, all other special functions, are intellectualized, reformed, and reconstructed under the influence of these crucial successes that the thinking of the adolescent achieves. . . . Lower or elementary functions, being processes that are more primitive, earlier, simpler, and independent of concepts in genetic, functional, and structural relations, are reconstructed on a new basis when influenced by thinking in concepts and they are included as component parts, as subordinate stages, into new, complex combinations created by thinking on the basis of concepts, and finally under the influence of thinking, foundations of the personality and world view of the adolescent are laid down.[12]

Coming from a materialist perspective that regarded the human species, unlike other animals, as fashioning its own nature through productive activities, Vygotsky believed that human nature changes as socially organized activities change in history.[13] He further believed that historical changes in social activities have a directionality, and are therefore developmental. Thus, higher mental processes are rooted in the general history of humanity. Each individual also has his or her own developmental history, which consists of two lines: biological and cultural. "Natural processes regulate the growth of elementary psychological functions in the child— forms of memory, perception, and practical tool-using intelligence, those that are continuous with the mental life of apes and other species. Social and cultural processes regulate the child's acquisition of speech and other sign systems, and the development of 'special higher psychological functions,' such as voluntary attention and logical memory."[14]

Becoming a Competent Member of a Society

Research on neuroplasticity shows that the neurons in our brain grow and change in response to new experience and to learning, which causes the synaptic connections to reshape themselves and, in some areas, to form new connections.[15] The more we rehearse, the stronger and more reliable new synaptic connections become. Over time we rehearse (perform) certain stories so many times that they become virtually automatic responses—what is called second nature. Our recall of these stories is a path so well trodden that we no longer are consciously aware of these stories that we once had to struggle to grasp during a particular stage in our development. They have become automatic.

We become competent members of a society when we are able to sense or know directly—without the need to stop and reflect, nor to gather any evidence relevant to the matter—what should appropriately be said or done in most of the mundane circumstances we confront in our particular culture.[16] We do this by absorbing stories from this culture to a point that our brains can recall them faster than we can "figure out" a story to guide our behavior and actions. People who share the same well-rehearsed, automatic stories feel most comfortable around one another since they all behave in expectable, predictable ways. These people identify one another as belonging to the same group, regardless of what term they use to describe that group.

When Automatic Stories Conflict

Without shared stories, we would be aliens to one another—barely human, as in the past when the people who did not share our language and stories were subhuman, to be killed, used, enslaved, or discarded. Racism happens when people who have power do not share or appreciate the stories of those who lack power. Here is an example. In the summer of 2008, a young Cree woman who was a student of mine came to work with me at the family medicine clinic at which I was stationed. On her second day of work, she had missed an e-mail from me telling her that I would be late. She entered the building, wondered where I was, and was overwhelmed by what she perceived as hostility and aggressiveness from the clinic staff. They had not greeted her or addressed her in a friendly manner. Clinic nurses had been abrupt and dismissive. As a result of her interaction with them, she felt that they wanted her to disappear. She did not have stories to explain this. She had spent most of her life sheltered within the aboriginal community. She expected people to be friendly and welcoming, and was unprepared for the hostility she encountered. By the time I arrived, she was in tears.

How do we make sense of this? First, we must understand that those whom she encountered had stories connected with how she looked (like an Indian). I had the opportunity to observe that the staff behaved quite differently in a similar situation when an unknown white student came to the clinic. They did not realize that their way of interacting was intrinsic to their culture and its stories, which were about distance, detachment, and noninvolvement. They believed their way was the "right," or "correct," way to interact. They called it "being professional." I would have called it "being arrogant and patronizing," but they could not see this.

My Cree student's stories about how people are supposed to treat each other involved being warm, accepting, and welcoming. The contrast was devastating to her. We solved the problem by as quickly as possible getting her out into the field to collect stories and other information from aboriginal people.

University of New Hampshire professor John Shotter, who has written extensively about interpersonal relations, would describe this young Cree woman as lacking the knowledge needed to interpret the clinic staff's behavior because she did not participate with them in their activities. She had entered their world as a mere outside observer, which was extremely distressing and alienating to her. Shotter says that possessing a body provides us with immediate access to the *intentional* nature of human action: "With such an access we find that human action, in its very nature of always 'pointing to,' or of 'containing' or 'specifying' something beyond or other than itself . . . posits a world."[17] My Cree student could understand that the clinic staff were pointing and specifying, but her experience was that they were pointing her out as inferior or undesirable. Some of this was because she was my student and the mainstream, white, Canadian staff predictably regarded my pursuit of an aboriginal agenda in a conventional family medicine clinic setting as undesirable. This example illustrates what happens when the automatic stories of a dominant group mix with very different automatic stories of another person or minority group.

Our sense of who we are and what we believe is correct behavior becomes automatic as a result of the personal and cultural stories shaping our lives. Those who are labeled "mentally ill" are often people whose stories do not match those of the dominant group in power at the time. However, the stories of most psychiatric clients who arrive seeking help have also become so automatic that, to them, they do not feel like stories but like truth or fact. The results to these people can be devastating, because what they see as their own truth contrasts so sharply with, and feels overwhelmed by, the dominant party's truth. As a result many of them are not recognized as competent members of society. They lack many of the essential stories needed to negotiate a social world, especially one that is occasionally hostile. It then becomes my task to help these clients reframe their lives into narratives with which they can reintegrate themselves into the world.

From Vygotsky's point of view, we would say that these clients missed out on some key areas of social learning. Their social environment was lacking or not sufficiently rich to overcome whatever innate brain limitations they brought to the world. Vygotsky's views—the importance of teaching abstract thought—have been largely adopted by those serving and teaching people with mental retardation. While it was widely recognized that most mentally retarded clients were limited to concrete thinking, when all teaching was done in those terms, no improvement and even deterioration occurred. But when competent adults began teaching and challenging and supporting those with mental retardation to step out of their comfort level and into their zone of proximal discovery, their clients' capacity to engage in abstract thought and reasoning greatly improved.

According to Paul Ballantyne, historian of psychology, "Precisely because retarded children, when left alone, will never achieve well-elaborated forms of abstract thought, the school should make every effort to push them in that direction and to develop in them what is intrinsically lacking in their own development."[18] This is also what we must do for all mental health clients—engage with them in a dialogue in which they can transcend what is possible for them to do on their own.

We have to learn stories in order to organize and guide our behavior and to help us interpret one another in ways that work. Temple Grandin, Ph.D., an author who was diagnosed with autism, has described this process marvelously in the book she coauthored with Sean Barron titled *Unwritten Rules of Social Relationships: Decoding Social Mysteries Through the Unique Perspectives of Autism*.[19] What most of us take for granted, she had to painfully work out through trial and error, eventually culminating in a rule book for how to behave. Grandin is a wonderful example of someone who is different and has turned her difference into an asset, even a source of income through her writing and lectures. Dr. Grandin has authored or coauthored several additional books; see www.templegrandin.com.

Embracing Who We Have Become

I want to finish this chapter with another kind of story about development. Much of development is learning to appreciate who we have become through forces acting on us that are far from being in our control. In this traditional story we learn how Rabbit came to be how he is today, and we learn some important lessons about desirable behavior and about embracing what we are instead of wishing to be something else. We also learn about the helpful role that a therapist can play in helping a person who is suffering to alter his perceptions or interpretations.

I tell this story often to people who feel disabled or disfigured or changed in some negative way, with the goal of planting the seed that perhaps the changes are beneficial, or at least more so than they think. The idea behind the story for me is we can transform in ways that may at first be shocking and undesirable, but that turn out to be for our highest good.

This story comes from Vermont and was told to me by an Abenaki elder. It features Glooscap in the background and Rabbit in the foreground. Glooscap is the Abenaki trickster, just as Coyote is the trickster for the people of the plains and southwestern deserts, and Raven is for the Pacific Northwest. In Abenaki lore, Glooscap ruled over the people in a kind of loose, friendly way. He made many of the animals, and some worked out, but others were treacherous and dangerous. In time, however, he culled out the bad ones and gave posts of honor to those whom he could trust and who were proud to help him. Because Rabbit had the kindest heart of all of the animals, Glooscap made him his forest guide.

In those days Rabbit looked very different from the way he looks today. His body was large and round, his legs were straight and even, and he even had a long bushy tail. He did not hop-hop-hop as he does today, but ran like a dog.

One day in springtime, when fiddler ferns were breaking forth in the marshes and lilacs were blooming, Rabbit was resting beside a fallen log. He could smell the fresh mint. Perhaps he had even fallen asleep, when he was startled by a sudden wailing. When he raised himself from his resting place, he saw Fisher coming down the trail toward him, weeping and wailing. For those of you who don't know Fisher, he is one of the larger animals of the weasel tribe.

Inquisitive Rabbit wondered what was upsetting Fisher. Rabbit's soft heart went out to Fisher, whom he wanted to help. When Rabbit popped his head up over the log, Fisher nearly jumped out of his fur with surprise. "Rabbit!" yelped Fisher. "You nearly killed me from fright."

Rabbit went straight to the point. "Why are you crying, Fisher?"

Fisher sighed. "I'm going to my wedding."

Rabbit was surprised. "Turn around and run the other way if getting married makes you feel like that," he said.

"It's not that I don't want to get married," said Fisher. "I do. But I've lost my way, and I'll never make it in time."

Rabbit was not used to time deadlines. Time had only recently been invented, and no one took it too seriously. Rabbit preferred to tell time by whatever was blooming in any given moment and to mark the changes of the seasons by what was currently best for eating. "Just take your time," Rabbit said. "Use your nose and you'll soon find your way again." Rabbit was always eminently practical about guiding people through the forest. He preferred to let them figure it out on their own unless Glooscap called or a serious crisis was at hand.

"I have no time to use my nose," shrieked Fisher. "My future father-in-law has sworn that if I do not arrive for the wedding by sunset, he will marry his daughter to Crow. And look, the sun is already nearing its sleeping place!" Fisher began wailing again. Rabbit covered his big, sensitive ears. Rabbit's desire to nap wrestled with his good nature to help a friend in distress, but his mouth took over to save the day.

"In that case," Mouth said, "Rabbit will show you the way. Where are you going?"

"I am going to that village near where the river doubles back on itself," said Fisher. "Do you know it?"

"I know it well," said Rabbit. "Follow me."

"Thank you so much, Rabbit," said the happy Fisher. "Now I will surely arrive in time."

Rabbit led the way, but Fisher was not as fast as Rabbit. Fisher was used to traveling in trees, and he moved more slowly on the ground. Rabbit was not entirely virtuous and was getting impatient with Fisher. If not for Rabbit's long, bobbing, bushy tail, Fisher would have lost him amid the grasses and the bush. So maybe you could say that what happened next was Rabbit's fault, for it might not have happened had he been more patient. Fisher could barely afford to look where he was going, lest he lose sight of Rabbit's tail, and in one fateful moment, he went tumbling headlong into a deep pit. His pitiful cries soon brought Rabbit back to see what had befallen Fisher.

Rabbit was at least cheerful, if not patient. "Never mind," Rabbit said, "I'll get you out." He tossed his long tail down into the pit, telling Fisher to catch hold of the end and to hang on tight.

Fisher desperately clutched Rabbit's tail while Rabbit strained with all his might to haul Fisher up. Rabbit's tail was long, but not so strong as Possum's. Fisher had put on weight, what with all the wedding feasting, and just before Fisher reached the top of the pit, Rabbit's tail broke off with a loud snap. To Rabbit's horror, his tail and Fisher fell back down into the pit. Poor Rabbit's tail had broken off right at its root, leaving him with just a tiny nubbin!

Lesser animals would have given up in pain and bitter despair. They would have forgotten about Fisher and gone home to nurse their wounds and damaged pride, slinking home in that time when the shadows begin to cover the sun. Not so with Rabbit. Glooscap had chosen well. Once Rabbit had committed to a task, nothing would deter him. There would be time later to mourn the lost tail or to see if Glooscap or Grandmother Woodchuck could reattach it; now the business at hand demanded his full attention. Fisher needed to make his wedding lest Crow run off with the beautiful bride.

Rabbit had another idea. He grabbed a stout tree with his front paws and lowered his hind legs into the pit. "Take hold of my legs," he told Fisher, "and hang on tight. My arms and my legs are stronger and tougher than my tail was. With any luck at all, I'll soon have you out."

Rabbit pulled and pulled until his waist was made thin. To his horror, the back of his mind could feel his hind legs stretching and stretching. Soon he feared they might break off like his tail had. But just as he thought they would surely give way, Fisher's head rose above the edge of the pit and his front claws grabbed hold of the earth, allowing him to scramble to safety. As they toppled over backward, Rabbit noticed that the moon was full.

Exhausted, Rabbit sat down to catch his breath and assay the damage. "Well," he said in dismay, "my waist isn't so round as it was, and my hind legs are much longer. I don't know how I will be able to walk." When Rabbit tried to walk, he just tumbled head over heels. He struggled to find a way to move ahead with legs longer than his arms, and finally, he came to hop. To his surprise, hopping worked and was certainly better than rolling on the ground. After some practice, he found he could hop rather quickly through the forest. Soon Fisher was having just as much trouble keeping up with Rabbit as before. Instead of a bushy tail to guide him, Fisher kept his eyes on Rabbit's ears, bouncing above the full grass on this almost August eve.

At last, just before the sun touched the door to his sleeping place, Rabbit and Fisher arrived at the bride's village. Tall maple trees surrounded the clearing and their dwellings. All the relatives and members of Fisher's tribe were gathered, waiting. Fisher's appearance broke the tension and all cheered except Crow, who was far from glad! Everyone else was so happy that they tactfully failed to notice the dramatic change in Rabbit's appearance. "There'll be enough time for questions after the wedding," most thought. They didn't even notice Crow fly angrily out of the village.

Despite the dramatic transformations in Rabbit's appearance, which no one knew how to discuss, he was a most welcome guest at the wedding. After the ceremony, Fisher explained to the other guests how Rabbit had come to look as he did, and that made Rabbit ever so much more the hero. Rabbit filled the four corners of the night. Everyone feasted and made merry, and Rabbit danced so hard with the bride that she fell into a bramble bush and tore her gown. This put her in a dreadful state; she believed she was not fit to be seen in company and ran to hide behind a tree. Rabbit felt so contrite for what he had done, wanting so much to help her and make amends. So he hopped away to get a caribou skin he had seen drying in the sun, and made a new dress out of it for the bride.

"You must have a fine belt to accompany this dress," said Rabbit, and he cut a thin strip off the end of the skin. He put one end of the strip in his mouth and held the other end with his front paws, twisting the strip into a fancy cord.

He twisted and twisted, and he twisted it so hard that the cord snapped out of his teeth and split his upper lip right up to his nose! And that is how rabbits came to be harelipped!

Fisher's bride was shocked and wept at Rabbit's wound and misfortune. Being Rabbit, he urged her to stop. "It's all right," he said, "it couldn't be helped. Now run off and enjoy your wedding." Rabbit gave her the belt to tie around her waist, satisfied that he had paid his debt for her mishap.

"Wait right here," said the bride as she ran off. Shortly afterward she returned, carrying a lovely white fur coat. "This is for you," she said shyly. "It is the color of the snow, so if you wear it in winter, your enemies will not be able to see you."

Rabbit was touched and delighted with his present and promised not to wear it until the ground was as white as the coat, since his brown coat would hide him better in summer. When the wedding celebration ended, he said his good-byes to Fisher and the bride, and started for home.

Before he had gone far, he came to a small pool in the woods, so smooth it was like a mirror. Looking into it, Rabbit saw himself for the first time since his accidents and was aghast. Who was this creature staring back at him with the split lip, the hind legs stretched out of shape, and a tail resembling a small white mouse?

"Oh dear, oh dear," he sobbed. "How can I face my friends looking like this?" In his misery, he called out for Glooscap. "O Glooscap! Look what has happened to me! I'm not fit to be seen anymore, except to be laughed at. Please put me back to my former shape."

High up on his sacred mountain, Glooscap heard Rabbit and came striding down from his lodge to see what was wrong. When he saw poor Rabbit's new shape, it was all he could do not to laugh, though he kept a sober face so as not to hurt Rabbit's feelings.

"Rabbit," he said, "things may not be as bad as you think. Remember how fond you are of clover?" Rabbit nodded wretchedly. "And you know how hard it is to find. With that long cleft in your lip, you will be able to smell clover even when it is miles away!"

"That's good," said Rabbit, cheering up a little, "but it's very uncomfortable having to hop everywhere I go."

"Perhaps, for a time," said Glooscap, "but have you noticed how much faster you hop than you used to run?" Rabbit did a little hop, and a jump or two, just to see.

"Why, I believe you're right!" Rabbit exclaimed, but then the discouragement returned. "But my tail! I mind that most of all. I was so proud of it," he said.

"It was certainly a fine-looking tail," admitted Glooscap, "but bear in mind how it used to catch in thorns and brambles."

"That's true!" cried Rabbit, eagerly, "and it was very difficult to maneuver when Fox was chasing me! Now I can slip through the narrowest places with no snag at all!"

And he laughed with glee. "With my new legs, my cleft lip, and without my long irksome tail, I'm a better rabbit than I was before!"

"So you are!" said Glooscap, and at last he could laugh. When Glooscap laughs with gusto, the land shakes and the trees bend over, so Rabbit had to hold on tightly to a tree to keep from being knocked over. "So you are indeed!" laughed Glooscap.

And that is why Rabbit and Rabbit's children and his children's children have had, ever since that day, a little white nib of a tail, a cleft lip, and long hind legs on which they can hop all day and never tire. And since then, too, in winter, rabbits wear white coats.

What are the values implicit in this story, and what can we learn from it? What are your wounds, and how do you make the most of them? What stories did people tell you to help you see your wounds as advantages? How did your traumas become gifts?

4

How Do We Learn to Feel What We Feel?

Our thinking and language has a deeply metaphorical structure that gradually takes its shape from the way our physical bodies interact with the environment from the earliest moments of our existence.

BRIAN BROOM, *MEANING-FULL DISEASE*

According to the most prevalently held view in psychiatry today, emotions, language, and personality primarily arise from the biology within the organism moving outward. Disturbances of emotion come from disturbances in biological mechanisms that must be treated biologically. Language then mirrors reality as a representational device. The Hungarian developmental psychologist Pyotr Bodor captures this type of scientific view of emotions: "When they move us, the dirty animal moves. Its moral is straightforward: Let's repress it."[1] In other words, "Tame the beast."

The common psychiatric reductionist model says emotions are evolutionarily evolved moving forces executed by physiological mediation and accompanied by special display patterns.[2] This is a complicated way of saying they are brain generated and essentially out of our control. Bodor summarized all these approaches as sharing a simple assumption: "Emotions are casually produced by molar (ethological) and/or molecular (physiologic-biochemical) biological mechanisms."[3] Social interaction is given a secondary, constraining, or repressing role in the formation of emotions, language, and personality.

Some figures in biological psychiatry attempt to be more social by embracing the James-Lange theory of emotions, in which emotion is the subjectively felt sensation or physiological state of the body in its process of making biological responses. From this perspective the behavioral response to danger or injury is so fast that we become aware of pain only after we have withdrawn our hand from the flame; we perceive danger only after we are already running away.[4] Harvard psychologist William James observed, "Bodily changes follow directly the perception of the exciting fact, and . . . our feeling of the same changes as they occur IS the described emotion. . . . We feel fear because we flee, and grief because we weep."[5]

In the 1930s, however, Harvard physiologist Walter Cannon criticized this theory as lacking biological validity, although psychology generally ignored him.[6] Schachter and Singer summarized the account of this theory—which continues to prevail today—as emotion being "cognitively labeled felt arousal, whereas the underlying original emotional process was an emotion-specific state of physiological arousal, subsumed under the broader term of 'emotional arousal.'"[7] Despite the tremendous volume of research these ideas have generated since the early 1960s, evidential support for these concepts is still lacking.[8]

Changing Perspectives on Emotions

The most interesting criticisms of these approaches have been posed by historical studies of emotions. Stearns and Stearns studied five hundred years of diaries and noted major changes in how people perceived their worlds and in how emotions were defined and expressed.[9] They discovered that the definitions, expressions, and descriptions of emotions have evolved over that time. Many of the feelings we have today were not possible three hundred years ago, for no words existed to define them. This lends support to the idea that some psychiatric diagnoses could not have existed in 1680 because the emotions were not there to support them.[10]

The word *emotion* is derived from the Latin word *exmovere*, meaning "to move something." Until the mid-eighteenth century the word itself merely meant movement. The root, *motion*, remains. Not until the late eighteenth century did the word *emotion* come to mean "a sense of strong feeling" as its primary definition. At that time, powerful, visceral feelings were seen as sharply contrasting to the then-desired norm of controlled, rational, calculating thought.[11] People began to perceive that we are moved to act by passions or strong feelings instead of a sense of duty, vengeance, or similar, earlier concepts of motivators.

At this time, Europeans developed the view that emotions and thoughts were two different phenomena. Emotions were thought to be natural and governed by biological mechanisms beyond conscious control. Thought was assumed to be voluntary, learned, controlled, and dependent on cultural symbols and concepts. Emotions were associated with art, beauty, poetry, and music. Thought was associated with logic, science, and calculation. Emotions were said to interfere with thought; clear thought supposedly required eliminating emotions from it. Indigenous people of other lands did not share this view, nor did Europeans before the 1800s.

Unfortunately, these ideas persist in common usage today when people talk about left-brain and right-brain people and tasks. The "split brain" studies from which these differentiations arose don't actually apply to people, since our brains are connected across the hemispheres, and the concept has been abandoned by neuroscience long ago. Thought and emotion both require the entire brain. The richest, most wonderful experiences we can imagine are full-brain experiences. The left-brain versus right-brain metaphor has persisted in common usage, however, just because it reflects what Europeans already believed about differences between thought and emotion. Probably it was originally proposed because it was already the assumption.

In fact, thinking and feeling are inextricably intertwined.[12] For example, thinking about going to court entails feelings of displeasure, while thinking about going on vacation entails pleasurable feelings. Thinking about chronic pain entails feelings of frustration, despair, and anger. On the other hand, scientists can be passionate about their "thoughtful" work. They can feel a sense of intrigue, frustration, satisfaction, and even elation and aesthetic appreciation at discovering a new phenomena or formulating an elegant theory. The thoughts that are felt may be implicit and difficult to fathom, but they are ultimately knowable.[13] Feelings and thoughts are two sides of the same coin, different aspects of one thing, so the term *emotion* must be reconceptualized to denote the feeling side of thought or its coloration rather than being postulated to be a distinctly separate entity.[14]

Emotions and thought are part of the same whole-brain phenomenon of responding to the world. It was with this insight that University of Pennsylvania psychologist Aaron Beck invented cognitive therapy. He realized that changing our habits or thinking changed our emotions and vice versa.[15]

Emotion, Self, and Society

The critique of biological reductionist theories of emotion, such as that provided by University of Massachusetts psychology professor James Averill, emphasizes two points: (1) that emotions are intimately related to a person's sense of self, both in terms of eliciting conditions and consequences; and (2) that emotions can be understood only in the context of broader social and interpersonal relationships.[16] For years, Lakota elders had been making the same point to me—that we would have no emotions without relationships, that relationships teach us to feel and how to feel. This view is implicit in many indigenous knowledge systems about mind, emotion, and mental health, although it is largely ignored by science and psychiatry as quaint and ethnic.

American psychologist Martha C. Nussbaum believes that emotions are not feelings that well up in some natural and untutored way from our natural selves; they are contrived, social constructs.[17] We learn how and what to feel. Tom Lutz has proposed a theory and examples of emotion as aspects of cultural meaning systems that people use in attempting to understand the situations in which they find themselves.[18] Thus, emotions are socially negotiated. The social context surrounding the person gives meaning to feeling and to behavior, and provides criteria for judging one's own emotions and the emotions of others.

How could we develop compassion unless pain hurts and we had a means for appreciating pain in another person? Why should we read a novel or watch a movie unless we feel the grief or joy experienced by others—even when these others are fictitious? How wonderful that neuroscience is catching up to indigenous people to explain how we do this: through the activity of mirror neurons. Monkeys[19] and humans[20] have brain areas that operate during both execution and observation of instrumental, goal-directed action, such as pulling the skin off a banana to eat it. Giacomo Rizzolatti and his research group at the University of Parma (Italy) Department of Neurosciences found that when we observe another person smelling a foul odor, the same neuron population is activated in us as though we ourselves had smelled a foul odor.[21] Tanya Singer's research group at University College London showed that observing others in pain and feeling pain ourselves activated the same brain areas.[22]

University College London anthropologist and neuroscientist Charles Whitehead points out that emotions and affect-laden sensations such as pleasure and pain are associated with largely involuntary signals.[23] He notes that it requires a self-conscious effort of will (and conscious awareness of the presence of others) to suppress emotional expression. He argues that spontaneously occurring autonomic states are mapped onto (defined as) emotions not only by the individuals experiencing them but also by those who observe the accompanying displays of spontaneous autonomic activity and interpret these displays as emotion. This supports the idea that emotions are social acts. Even the words we use for emotions are derived from embodied social experiences. Broom, for example, describes how the commonplace metaphorical phrase "they greeted me warmly" can be linked to the early experience of feeling warm while being held affectionately.[24]

Emotions appear to be part of our inborn system for intersubjectivity.[25] We enter the world with some basic ways of recognizing pleasure and pain, and desirable and undesirable states and experiences. I think psychologist Paul Ekman (1934–) at the University of California, San Francisco, is correct that we come wired to quickly learn the specific emotions of sadness, fear, and anger. Clearly animals and young children have emotions that are expressed nonverbally. I came upon a baby rabbit trembling near the path on which I was running. It was afraid of me. I suppose its best strategy was to freeze. We have seen an angry dog snarling at another dog. We have seen a mother bear grooming and loving her cubs.

Ekman postulated universal facial expressions: anger, disgust, contempt, fear, sadness/anguish, surprise, and enjoyment. He described more than ten thousand different possible facial expressions related to three thousand emotions. However, he reported never seeing more than a few hundred in any conversation he studied. In fact, he found that two or three expressions dominate most interactions.[26]

Emotion, Language, and Culture

Tremendous cultural variability of emotional life and emotional vocabularies has been demonstrated,[27] even though Ekman's group found correlated physiological responses to posed facial displays among indigenous people in West Sumatra.[28] He himself described culture-specific attitudes about each emotion, including rules for its display, rules for what can properly trigger it, and so on. For example, at a beauty contest in the United States, it is "proper" only for the winner to cry, not the losers. At a middle-aged man's funeral, it is not appropriate for a secretary to show more grief than the wife.

A study was done in Japan in which male and female students were left alone in a room to watch a video, without knowing that a concealed camera was photographing them.[29] As they reacted without awareness of an audience, American students and Japanese students showed a correlation of facial muscle movements of 0.9, meaning that their muscle movements were 90 percent the same. When a researcher (an audience) entered, that correlation dropped precipitously. An American student from Berkeley, California, for example, then magnified his disgust response while a Japanese student masked it with a smile.

Ekman believes that the purpose for emotions—the reason they originally developed—was so that we could solve problems quickly without our consciousness interfering. He notes that the defining characteristics of emotions arise unbidden, resulting in fast appraisal that is often opaque, with triggers being evident only afterward.[30] Naturally, physiological responses play a role in the emotions since the brain perceives and interprets situations and reflects on our role in these situations. We are designed to compare new situations with our memories of previous situations. In some circumstances, this comparison results in dramatic responses, as in running away from a dangerous animal. That emotion is called fear. It is a performance act that includes the autonomic nervous system, the voluntary muscles of running, sounds and cries that we might make, and more. Ekman thinks that anger has a universal trigger—interference with goal attainment—and that most specifics around anger are culturally learned, such as how to stop the interference, how to eliminate the threat to the goal.

Ekman also identifies multiple enjoyable emotions, some of which are culturally affected. Cultures have developed their own language terms to describe specific emotions, such as the German word *schadenfreude,* which refers to pleasure derived from another's misfortune. In Yiddish, *nachas* refers to the distinct pleasure you feel in the accomplishments of your offspring. In Italian, *fiero* is the pleasure you get from stretching yourself to the maximum and accomplishing what you set out to do. In his study, all Ekman could see in the faces of his subjects was that one of the enjoyable emotions was occurring. People must speak in order for us to know specifically which one it is.

As soon as we use language to label our responses, the emotions begin to come under social control. For small children, emotions and their expression are mediated through adults who teach children the appropriate way to perceive and express emotions for their culture. Then social learning refines that basic learning into the complexities of human emotion that we encounter as older children and adults and that psychiatry purports to study and treat. As language skills develop, they are used in the service of recognizing and modifying emotional experience to conform with the expectations of the larger group for how emotions should be performed.

Emotions are "interdependent and interpenetrating" with all other cultural phenomena, including language.[31] Emotions and their triggers, their modes of expression, and their function in discussion are shaped by social activities and cultural concepts as we learn language and communication skills. Biological processes—including hormones, neurotransmitters, peptides, autonomic reactions—underlie (mediate) but do not determine emotional qualities and expressions. Rather, emotional qualities and expressions are determined by the evaluation we learn to make of the social context in which we find ourselves. Emotions are the colorations or valuations we make of the narratives in which we live. They arise from our sense of how desirable and undesirable our situations are compared with what we have learned to expect or desire. Biology provides the means by which culture operates within the individual but does not determine what will happen.

Language complicates emotions. Unlike animals, we begin to have feelings about abstractions. The basic fears and rages are quickly overwhelmed by a plethora of complex meanings and valuations of those meanings. Our participation in language and the culture that produces that language modifies these basic emotions to fit the stories being told in that locale. By naming or directly articulating an emotion with language, we inherently limit it or reduce it from the full richness that it deserves. We separate it from the complexity of its entirety. Story is powerful because it hints, teases out, and exposes the complexities of the emotions and meanings attached to the events of our lives. The really important stuff can only be told, understood, and communicated through story.

Very early in life, we internalize stories that tell us how to react to others. We humans get passionately angry about things that animals don't know to care about. We fear abstractions that animals lack the mental capacity to consider. We love invented concepts that cannot be touched—an alien concept to animals. An example comes from religious wars and persecutions. The Spanish Inquisition sought to punish people (and often kill them) for errors of thought, a concept that an animal could never grasp. In the year 346 CE, more Christians killed each other over the question of whether God was three beings in one or one being with three parts than were killed by the Roman Empire before it was Christianized. In 2009, the Iranian government continues to persecute and kill members of the Baha'i faith. The Chinese government continues to persecute practitioners of Falon Gong, a spiritual form of chi gong. Further examples abound. Humans punish "bad" thoughts, while animals apparently respond and react only to behavior.

Many types of situations are linked to the emotions they afford *by convention*. The link is neither biological nor deterministic, but sociocultural.[32] From the perspective of the sociocultural environment, emotions contribute to the maintenance and ratification of the local value systems and moral order by members.[33] As cognitive schema, the emotions contain an internal representation of social rules; they consist of an internalization of the local social mores.[34] Of course, we can all agree on universal extremes of emotions and their expression, such as those evoked by being chased by a raging bull or bitten by a snake, but powerful as these emotions are, they are trivial to our discussion exactly because they are so obvious and relatively rare. More interesting to our discussion are the bulk of ordinary feelings and transactions about feelings and the diagnoses of "pathological feeling states," such as anxiety and depression.

Similarly, we become upset at people who are not upset by events we believe to be cultural universals (although evidence is accumulating that they are not as universal as we believe). Examples include people who fail to be upset by the death of a child, by suicide bombings, or by murders of innocent people. We say there is something wrong with these people. For example, in a famous case from Australia, a woman named Lindy Chamberlain was convicted of killing her baby. She maintained throughout that a dingo ate her baby. She was not believed because the performance of her story in court was not sufficiently grief stricken and distraught. Later, she was released from prison when a climber's accident on Ayer's Rock resulted in the discovery of the baby's clothes with dingo teeth marks riddled throughout. One could say that her problem was poor coaching in how to perform her role for the judge and jury.

Upon review, we often find evidence that people who do not perform their emotions as we expect they should have had very different training about emotions and their expression in their childhoods than we did. This evidence, however, arises from a careful elicitation of the stories about the person's past. Especially in the case of heinous criminals, these stories often become biographies, since people want to explain such acts and seek explanations (probably to assure ourselves that we are morally superior and could never do what they did). Fundamentally, we seek explanations in the reading of life narratives. We compare ourselves to the other person and find relief as we argue that we could never be like this, that our experiences are too different. As an example, Lindy Chamberlain's dingo story is being made into a television show, a mini-series, a documentary, a movie, and an opera.

Cultural Psychology and the Wolakota Perspective

In psychiatry, culture enters into our definitions of emotion. We are more concerned about emotions within relationships and the stories that describe those relationships than we generally are about imminent danger to life and limb. Vygotsky believed that cultural phenomena are humanly constructed artifacts rather than natural products, and that cultural phenomena are social facts in the sense of being emergent products of social interactions rather than individual creations.[35] This matches the Lakota perspective. The cultural phenomena are the stories. They emerge through social interaction. We do not create stories except for audiences. Even in rehearsal before the first telling, stories are meant to be heard. The elders also taught me that emotion is inseparable from story. Stories have affective components. A movie, for example, uses music to set the affective tone and to make some reactions within the viewers more likely than others. They taught that we begin our lives by absorbing all the stories told around us.

Vygotsky believed that we collectively devise activities, such as producing goods, raising children, educating the populace, or treating disease, and that we survive and even thrive through these socially organized activities, which are basic to the ways in which we interact with any aspect of the world we can perceive.[36] Our solitary pursuits are modeled on these collective activities and often feed back to social activities when they are completed. Even our thoughts and meditations are often about our social activities.

Practical, socially organized activities stimulate people to collectively construct concepts about things and people. Therefore, socially constructed and shared conceptual representations, or meanings, of things reflect the way things and people are treated in social activity. For example, the activity of worship changes dramatically over time and from culture to culture. Similarly, the project of defining and "treating" "abnormal" emotions has changed from one of none at all to what now constitutes the enormous "mental health system," a system that rarely considers health and usually focuses on "disease."

Ratner explains Vygotsky's views on the way that culture affects emotion as what Vygotsky called cultural historical psychology.[37] Cultural psychology explains the basis, character, and function of emotions as grounded in macrocultural factors. Similarly, within Lakota traditional thought (*Wolakota*), as taught to me by elders, emotions exist because of relationship. One elder said that if we had no relationships, we would have no feelings. All feeling is brought about through relationship. Taking this further, he said that emotions are not within an individual, but between beings who are relating. The effect of the relationship on the individual can be seen in his or her body, but this effect is not the emotion. Similarly, what is generally called mind would be considered in Wolakota to reside between relating beings.

This is so different from the typical mainstream American perspective, in which emotion and thought are considered as separate, even if intertwined. Mind is associated with thought and feeling with heart. Contemporary neuroscience does not, however, support this perspective. In brain imaging studies, we see that thoughts are emotional and storied and that the entire brain is involved in experiencing. Of course, heart is connected to brain through the vagus nerve and other neural inputs, but the association of heart with feeling is a more metaphorical level of explanation than a biological one. Thoughts do not happen independent of emotions. They are a unified, whole-brain phenomenon.

Within Wolakota, life could not exist without relationship, which comes first and is primary. We begin through the relationship of our mother and father. We grow through the relationship with our mother. We are born and develop relationships with those who take care of us. Without relationship, we could not exist. Relationship creates and maintains the individual. Wolakota says emotion arises from our participation in relationship as a valuation of what is happening within that relationship. We experience that relationship as pleasant or unpleasant. We feel hurt or anger; we feel sad or fearful. What the other does matters, and emotion is our response. Of course, these relationships can also be with elements of nature, with spirits, and with the Great Mystery.

Within Wolakota, we have awareness, but the moment we communicate, we have entered into the relational sphere. From a Wolakota perspective, no human could have ever learned language without the assistance of another person. Our thoughts can always be traced to one relationship or another. As we develop, we learn to speak silently, as rehearsed statements that may not be uttered. We learn to be aware of saying something silently, repeating it, and monitoring our own responses to it as if we were saying it to another. We have internalized the other as a character with whom we can have "practice conversations." We develop a community of voices who speak the stories of our past. And occasionally, through transformative practices, we again become able to experience a world without language. This is often called trance.

To integrate Vygotsky and Wolakota, we could say that:

1. Humans only exist in social networks, which provide for their basic survival and fulfillment. Each relationship within a network generates affect-laden stories that explain "how things work" and "what must be done." Culture is the collection of all stories being told within a particular social network. This is how we can speak of a family culture, a kinship culture, a village's culture, and even the culture of a country. A social network is more powerful, supportive, knowledgeable, stimulating, and enriching than separate

individuals who may physically coexist together, because the interactions within the network generate new stories that have never existed before and evolve the culture.

2. The stories within social networks call forth special behaviors that serve the group over the individual (altruism, self-sacrifice, placing survival of the group over survival of the individual). The stories contained within social networks serve to place the needs of the group above the instinctual needs of the individual.

3. Social interactions shape human psychological phenomena within limits determined by biological capability.

4. Our social networks are also embedded in meta-narratives—larger stories that live us and live through us that come from social institutions (government, corporations, educational and health care systems, religious organizations). Many of us are not even aware of these larger stories as they are so "taken for granted as being true."

5. These narratives and meta-narratives inform us what to feel, how to feel, and how to express our feelings from a very young age. Parents, for example, can frequently be overheard telling their child not to cry, not to hit others, not to pout. Or they can be seen labeling their child's behavior as indicative of "sadness," "anger," or "rage." We learn to link behavior, internal sensations, and a cultural label.

Enhancing Emotional Awareness

The Dalai Lama believes that most of us are at the behavioral and emotional awareness levels of kindergarten students, far from the Ph.D. level to which we aspire.[38] Emotional skills include impulse awareness, behavior awareness, awareness of others' emotions, using information constructively, and identifying our own emotional profile. Typically, it's only after we have experienced emotions that we become aware of what they were. When we act emotionally, we often first learn about it when another person asks, What are you upset about? We don't readily observe ourselves or reflect on the story we are enacting. For example, I'm reading a book. I'm turning the pages, I'm thinking about a talk that happened earlier in the day. My conscious awareness is not monitoring what I'm doing. Suddenly I realize I have no memory of the last few pages I was reading. I have been lost in the earlier conversation, replaying it, reacting to it, and perhaps playing out alternate scenarios of how the conversation could have gone or how it will resume the next time I see the person. If it is my most recent boss, who humiliated me at every opportunity, I will have emotions that surpass my capacity to read the material.

The stories related to what we feel are so overrehearsed as to become automatic, even habitual. Achieving conscious awareness requires slowing down the activation of the story and its memory in order to reflect on it and change it. That may be easier to do in relationship with other people rather than alone.

Emotional awareness of others occurs as we monitor the sensations in our own bodies. When we monitor the sensations of our body, we can become more aware. Ekman showed that voluntarily making the appropriate facial movements for an emotion actually generates the physiological changes of that emotion.[39] The face muscles are caught up in a circuitry of emotion management. The theater director and teacher Constantin Stanislavsky (1863–1938) said, "Make the movement, and the feeling will follow." If someone wants you to know how they feel, you will. If someone doesn't want you to know what they feel, you probably won't.

Ekman believes that people do not distinguish between emotion, mood, trait, and disorder, even though they are different. Moods include being irritable, apprehensive, blue, or euphoric. Ekman believes that moods—in contrast to emotions—are nonadaptive and distort reality. We almost always know afterward what triggered an *emotion,* but we rarely know what triggered a *mood.* Emotions act as filters, but only for seconds or minutes. Moods, on the other hand, filter out anything that doesn't fit them. Traits include hostility, shyness, melancholy, and risk taking. For him, enduring characteristics include optimism, cheerfulness, well-being, and *sukha* (outlook). While happiness comes and goes in a moment or two, well-being is a much better evaluation of how you are doing in comparison with your peers. The Buddhist concept of *sukha* is the platform from which you greet life.

Narrative Psychiatry and Emotions

In psychiatry, we primarily treat *communications* about feelings—both mood and emotions. We may make our own observations such as describing a person as tearful, as looking sad, as distressed, as anxious, but primarily we ask people questions to determine which category of diagnosis should be applied to them. To diagnose depression, we inquire about whether there is sadness more of the time than not, poor concentration, poor memory, loss of appetite and libido, disturbed sleep, lack of interest in pleasurable activities, and the like. We ask about thoughts of death or suicide. We mainly rely on what people tell us. When we measure improvement, we again rely on what people tell us.

There is no absolute, concrete internal state that is being described. What we get is a language act that purports to present to us an internal state, but does far more than that by virtue of our participation in the interaction and the questioning. Some of our more enlightened colleagues include work performance evaluations, other independent assessments, and the participation of family members in the discussion about the patient's depression, but this is far from the rule. Primarily we diagnose and treat language acts.

When these language acts are too far from the norm, we may compel treatment through legal means. We do this to prevent people from harming themselves or others. But even then, the threat to harm becomes a language act. When I worked in a locked inpatient psychiatry unit in Arizona, I met many drug dealers in the ward who had arrived at the emergency room claiming to be suicidal. What was actually happening was that a drug deal had gone bad. Their goal was to be safe from those who wished to kill them for a few days until things blew over. Remarkably, we couldn't tell the difference between those who claimed to be suicidal but were hiding out and those who actually were suicidal and later made attempts after leaving the hospital. I was fortunate to be running a narrative group in which people were invited to tell their stories in confidence. The dealers believed me when I assured them of confidentiality and proudly boasted of their ability to "snow psychiatrists." I suspect anyone could "snow us," because everyone knows the language acts that we use to diagnose, to commit, and to treat. We learn them at the movies and sometimes, unfortunately, in our own families.

We psychiatrists are terribly poor at inferring motivation or internal states from watching people perform. We cannot predict who will be violent or who will be suicidal. We are stuck with responding to what people tell us, and unfortunately, the truly suicidal person may perform the role of a happy, contented person. A friend's ex-wife in Baltimore did just this. My friend had arranged for her to be admitted to the hospital, convinced she was serious about killing herself. She was discharged two days later after a stellar performance in which she convinced the staff that her ex-husband was just harassing her and that she had no intention whatsoever of killing herself, that she had everything to live for, including her children, and that she failed to meet the diagnostic criteria for depression. She left the hospital, drove straight to a bridge, and jumped. Lucky for us, in psychiatry, people often perform a role of feeling suicidal or homicidal *and wanting to be stopped*. Lucky for us, these people are not as hard to recognize, and occasionally we do stop them.

From the standpoint of people, emotions serve the evaluation of situations and the organization of responses to them. This definition readily includes the brain pathways involved in evaluating and organizing responses. It has the advantage of connecting brain to an environment. Pierre Bleau, a psychiatrist at McGill University's Health Centre in Montreal, says, "There are no defective brains; only mismatches between brains and environments.[40] Thus, I am suggesting that what psychiatry primarily treats is a social construction and not the brain itself, as many assume. We are treating the stories made and used by the brain, which is why social experience and relationship are so important. The advantage of a social constructionist approach (intrinsic to narrative psychiatry) is its ease of incorporating biological research and contextualizing that research in a sociocultural environment.

Some research on emotions ignores neurophysiology and concentrates on sequences of infant-caregiver communications to observe how infants learn to make appropriate emotional responses from their mothers. Other studies focus on the neurobiology of fear and finding which brain pathways mediate fear responses. All are interesting. All are valid. Someday we may connect these different arenas of research, but for now, we can feel confident that we are addressing an important phenomenon, one that manifests in our clinical world as complex language acts to be understood in context.

The separation of emotion from language goes against what we know about brain function, in which both left and right hemispheres participate simultaneously in decoding and storing our experiences. Well-formed and well-stored narratives involve both hemispheres. Poorly formed and stored experiences, such as those without words that only involve emotion, are hard to manage—for example, trauma that is beyond words or trauma that occurred before language developed.

Communication, whether verbal or not, is inherently emotional for it is associated with values, desires, interests, and motivations—the creation and maintenance of desirable states and the avoidance or termination of undesirable ones. At least, this appears to be how communication begins with infants, both from my observations and from those of Vygotsky and others.

Emotions arise from the values we have learned to apply to our experience and are intrinsic to the stories we tell ourselves to make sense of what is happening.[41] Without the story there would be no emotion, for we would have no way to interpret our experience. We need a context and a set of values. We need a frame.

The stories we carry about why we feel what we feel are central to our well-being and quality of life. Psychiatry gives us contemporary stories of emotions being controlled by genes or genetic biochemistry. But if emotions *were* controlled by genes, it would render people powerless and helpless, with little ability to make a difference in their quality of life without the services of expert biologists who can manipulate biochemistry.

Much of psychiatry is about emotions that are out of control. Mania has been described as uncontrollable and even dangerous joy for some, or as paranoia, excessive anger, or "hell" for others. Depression is bottomless sadness. Anxiety is overwhelming fear. Obsessive and compulsive states arise as attempts to control that fear. Psychosis occurs when our emotions exceed the bounds of our stories to contain them.

If our stories about emotions determine how we will perceive those emotions, then a narrative psychiatry must hear those stories. Under what conditions will a person fly into a murderous rage? Or attempt to "fly" off a rooftop? Under what conditions and in what circumstances is sadness profound enough to warrant suicide? When does fear become severe enough to be paralyzing? All of the "disorders" of emotion are connected to stories about the world in which we live. These stories help us understand how to feel in response to specific situations. These stories guide our sorting of people into hierarchical power relationships—the well versus the sick, the sane versus the insane, the appropriately emotional versus the overly emotional. Our stories about emotion and its origins also tell us what to do about people who appear to feel different than we expect.

Psychiatry represents a current major means of controlling "disordered" emotions. The predominant story of conventional psychiatry about emotions is that they naturalistically arise from genetic chemistry within and under biological control. I believe the opposite perspective—which is also that of most indigenous cultures, including my own—that emotions arise from social relationships and are controlled by our social networks that are continually shaping and reshaping our brains to function as desired within constraints imposed by the brain itself. Metaphorically, we could see the brain as the hardware (relatively plastic, capable of much, but useless without software). Story represents the software. Emotion arises as we live our stories as biological beings on this physical earth.

When I met Ekman, he told me that many years ago his last psychotherapy supervisor had said, "If you can increase the gap between [a person's] impulse and action, you can really help your patients. It's very difficult to achieve." In narrative psychiatry, we attempt to help the person become aware of the underlying stories that guide his or her emotional response and then to develop competing stories that generate a different and more desirable emotional response. When we are in fight-or-flight mode, we must quickly pick a story with the most survival value to guide our reactions and perceptions, thereby generating our emotional responses. Many traumatized people never step out of fight-or-flight mode. They never feel safe or secure or don't have the skills to reflect on where and how they learned to see the world as they do. This is the luxury of healing through the power of story—that we can become aware of the stories that are living through us and change them. I believe this is done by every form of psychotherapy, including CBT and psychoanalysis, when they are working well.

I have a story about that, too.

> The Choctaw people of Mississippi say that when the people first came up out of the ground, they were encased in cocoons, their eyes closed, their limbs folded tightly to their bodies. This was true of all people, including the Bird People, the Animal People, the Insect People, and the Human People. The Great Spirit took pity on them and sent down someone to unfold their limbs, dry them off, and open their eyes. But the opened eyes saw nothing, because the world was dark—no sun, no moon, no stars. No moonlit beaches shimmering at night. All the people moved around by touch, and if they found something that didn't eat them first, they ate it—raw, for they had no fire to cook it.

This opening strikes me as a parallel to the way we come into the world. Our eyes are metaphorically closed. As infants, we grope about as blindly as the first people did. Our relationships are basic. No subtleties have been introduced yet—no cooking, no fire. It's also fascinating how many cultures begin their creation stories with blindness, coldness, and darkness. Perhaps this is a wonderful description of the human journey: our species is charged with transforming darkness and coldness and blindness into seeing and light and warmth on all possible levels. I see this as a metaphor for discovering emotions and their richness and complexity. Without emotion, the world is cold and dark. Emotionality brings us into encounter with color and warmth.

All the people met in a great pow-wow, with the Animal and Bird People taking the lead and the Human People hanging back. The Animal and Bird People decided that dark was cold and miserable. A solution must be found! Someone spoke: "I have heard that the people in the East have something that makes them warm and happy. It allows them to see where they're going. They call it fire." This caused a stir of wonder; "What could fire be!?" It was decided that if, as rumor had it, fire was warm and gave light, they should have it too.

How similar this is to the indigenous California story of Coyote stumbling around in the darkness and cold, bumping his head against trees and rocks, and hearing from Squirrel about people in the East who had a big yellow ball that made things visible and warm and cooked food. These people from the East, these keepers of the Sun, are the ones from whom we must wrestle our desired traits. Are these the spirits? Are these the obstacles put in our way to cause us to grow? Wouldn't it be so boring if everything were just given to us? Perhaps it was sheer boredom that led Eve to taste the apple in the Garden of Eden.

Another voice said, "But the people of the East are too greedy to share with us." So it was decided that the Bird and Animal People should steal the fire. But who should have the honor? Grandmother Spider volunteered, "I can do it! Let me try!" But Opossum said, "I, Opossum, am a great chief of the animals. I will go to the East and will take the fire and hide it in the bushy hair of my tail." It was well known that Opossum had the furriest tail of all the animals, so he was selected.

A whole series of stories contain this element of a difficult task, including the related Cherokee story in which Grandmother Spider gained fire for the people by walking across a lake and spinning a web to carry back a burning ember left on an island by the Creator. The Creator never makes it easy for us—making sure that we generate epic stories and heroic drama, perhaps providing great entertainment for the spirits and angels. Sometimes I imagine us all on spirit television and how the spirits love to tune in for the next episode of our dramas.

When Opossum came to the East, he soon found the beautiful red fire jealously guarded by the people. He got closer and closer until he picked up a small piece of burning wood and stuck it in the hair of his tail, which promptly began to smoke and then flame. The people of the East said, "Look, that Opossum has stolen our fire!" They took it and put it back and drove Opossum away. Poor Opossum! Every bit of hair had burned from his tail, and to this day, opossums have no hair on their tails, except in Australia where they didn't steal fire and still have beautiful bushy tails.

Isn't this a lot like how we learn about emotions? We enter into social relationships to make discoveries (Opossum volunteered to go get fire), we try things out (Opossum stole the fire), and sometimes we get burned. Nevertheless, that teaches us a lot. Perhaps we had to steal emotions such as fear since they weren't always with us in their present-day form.

Once again, the People gathered to find another volunteer. Grandmother Spider again said, "Let me do it!" But this time a bird was elected, Buzzard. Buzzard was very proud. "I can succeed where Opossum has failed. I will fly to the East on my great wings, then hide the stolen fire in the beautiful long feathers on my head." So Buzzard flew to the East on his powerful wings, swooped past those defending the fire, picked up a small burning ember, and hid it in his head feathers. His head began to smoke and flame even faster! The people of the East said, "Look! Buzzard has stolen the fire!" And they took it and put it back where it came from. Poor Buzzard! His head was now bare of feathers, red and blistered looking. And to this day, buzzards have naked heads that are bright red and blistered looking.

For me this story illustrates the trial and error that constitutes emotional learning. The People are struggling to understand fire (emotion), but are still getting burned. Nevertheless, you can see a social consensus in their efforts to find it and in the efforts of the People of the East to thwart them. Of course, these stories also explain how things came to be.

We now know why Opossum has a naked tail and Buzzard has a naked head. And their nakedness can forever remind us of the risks of trial-and-error learning. "Don't be like that buzzard and get your beautiful head feathers burned off," I can hear Choctaw mothers telling their children. "Don't be like Opossum and end up with a naked tail." These remind me of the ways my grandmother and great-grandmother told stories to influence my social learning, my discoveries of emotional learning and danger.

> *Next the people sent Crow to look over the situation, for Crow was very clever. At that time Crow was pure white and had the sweetest singing voice of all birds. But he stood so long over the fire, trying to find the perfect piece to steal from it, that his white feathers turned black from all the smoke. And Crow breathed so much smoke that he could no longer sing, but could only make a harsh "Caw! Caw!"*

Again the animals are struggling to understand fire (emotion) through their trial-and-error process, still getting burned. Nevertheless, someone is learning: "And don't be like Crow and get your clothes turned all black," was a familiar Sunday morning discourse for me growing up.

> *The council of Animals sat in circle again and said, "Opossum has failed. Buzzard and Crow have failed. Who shall we send!?"*

Of course you have to reach a certain level of desperation before you can open up to the person (spirit, ancestor, helper) who can really get the job done. This person might not be the one you expected.

> *Tiny Grandmother Spider jumped up from her seat and shouted with all her might, "LET ME TRY IT, PLEASE!" Though the council members thought Grandmother Spider had little chance of success, it was agreed that she should have her turn. Grandmother Spider had a small torso suspended by four sets of legs, with two pairs turned forward and two pairs turned back. She walked on all of her wonderful legs toward a stream, where she had found clay. With*

those legs, she made a tiny clay container and a lid that fit perfectly with a tiny notch for air. She put the container on her back, spun a web all the way to the East, and tip-toed to the fire. She was so small that the people from the East didn't see her. She took a tiny piece of fire, put it in the container, and covered it with the lid. Then she tip-toed along the web, back to her people. Since they couldn't see her hidden fire, they said, "Grandmother Spider has failed."

Since Grandmother Spider lacked power and strength, the other animals overlooked her cleverness and stealth and just assumed that she had failed. But, as is usual in these tales, brute strength fails. This story is meant, I believe, to champion the power of the small: we learn about emotions and how to manage them slowly, carefully, and in small increments!

"Oh, no," she said, "I have the fire!" She lifted the pot from her back, opened the lid, and the fire flamed up into its friend, the air. All the Bird and Animal People began to decide who would get this wonderful warmth. Bear said, "I'll take it!" But he burned his paws and decided fire was not for animals . . . for look what had happened to Opossum!

Past trauma can certainly color our choices. And overenthusiasm ("Fools rush in where angels fear to tread") can lead to pain. Who will step up to the plate? Who will volunteer to be in charge of fire?

The Bird People wanted no part of it, as Buzzard and Crow were still nursing their wounds. The insects thought fire was pretty, but they too stayed far away from it. Then a small voice said, "We will take it, if Grandmother Spider will help." The timid Human People, whom none of the animals or birds thought much of, were volunteering!

We humans are in charge of emotions and their vicissitudes and complexities. We volunteered somewhere at the beginning of creation to get these big hearts and big brains to invent the wonderful stories that thrill and sadden and entertain us. Welcome to our world.

So Grandmother Spider taught the Human People how to feed the fire with sticks to keep it from dying, and how to keep the fire safe in a circle of stone so it couldn't escape and hurt them or their homes. She also taught the humans about pottery made of clay and fire, and about weaving and spinning, at which Grandmother Spider was an expert.

Always, we learn much from our study of Nature. Grandmother Spider is an amazing teacher who taught the Cherokee and the Dene people about weaving. When we are dealing with emotion (fire), we need to know how to contain it, as Grandmother Spider did. We need to know how to keep it from raging out of control and hurting people. That's what Grandmother Spider can teach us—how to bind, contain, control, and stay safe.

From this time on, the People made a beautiful design to decorate their homes—a picture of Grandmother Spider, two sets of legs up, two down, with a fire-symbol on her back. This is so their children never forget to honor her.

5

The Meaning of Pain and Depression

In any field, find the strangest thing and then explore it.

JOHN ARCHIBALD WHEELER

Both physical and psychic pain, such as in depression or other forms of mental illness, partake of a certain element of mystery. As their subjective nature makes them difficult to quantify, to verify, and to treat, we need to hear a story to understand what people mean when they say they are depressed or suffering or in pain. Through hearing their story, we can do what theologian John Donne called "passing over," meaning that we can try on, identify with, and ultimately enter for a brief period of time the perspective of their experience and consciousness. In so doing, we can experience in a fully embodied way what they mean when they use the words *pain* or *depression* or *sadness*.

Such words are merely symbols that point toward experiences, which can only be told in the form of stories. Hearing these stories of people in pain or depression change us. When we "pass over" and "return," we bring back an enriched perspective on the human condition. Our brains are primed to achieve this understanding of both the commonality and uniqueness of human experience through listening to stories.

How Do We Learn What to Call Pain?

In order to realize how our understanding of pain develops, we turn to Wittgenstein's discussion of "logically private language" and his demonstration that the very idea makes no sense. Whatever silent conversations we have within our heads, these are based on language we have learned and use in social interactions. Our thoughts are like our speech without motor movement (though the corresponding areas in the motor cortex that produce speech are activated as we think). The difference between our private inner world and the outer world is only the discovery that we can speak without sound.

Vygotsky believed that the distinction between public and private action and discourse was the result of a human practice, reflecting the art of keeping things that one thinks, feels, and plans to oneself, a skill acquired in the second or third year of life. In this terminology, *private* refers to the internal conversations we have with the panoply of characters that exist within our brains, while *public* refers to the external conversations we have with physical others with whom we have relationships. In Vygotsky's view, an infant wouldn't recognize the distinctions among personal, private, and public. I would suggest that the infant remains in an unbroken stream of sensation and perceptive awareness in which such boundaries have not yet formed. This view seems to reflect the past twenty years of research on infant psychology.

Vygotsky wrote that we should understand sadness, pain, or fear by reference to an interpersonal conversation about it. People have exchanges about sadness, fear, and pain that are more complex than their mere expression. Most conversations are meant to go somewhere—toward obtaining relief from sadness, worry, or pain; toward diagnosis of the cause for that symptom; or toward sympathy and behavioral change on the part of significant others.

Anxiety, depression, and chronic pain are performances rather than "things." I do not mean this in the sense of secondary gain. I mean that every aspect of life is performed in a world of social others. Dr. Peter Brown noted that horrific injuries sustained in battle where immediate help is not available (where there is no "other") may be entirely painless, whereas a relatively minor injury during a football game can have a player writhing in agony.[1] Toddlers who fall check the reaction of the observing parent. If the parent laughs, the toddler will often laugh. If the parent looks alarmed, the toddler will cry. Whatever we feel is being presented to the world. We are changed by the reactions of our audience (which is everyone with whom we come in contact). Our inner world is no different. As outside, so inside. We imagine ourselves performing for significant others whose opinions and evaluations and responses to us matter very much.

As an example, I participate in the traditional ceremony of my Lakota heritage—the sun dance. The sun dance includes a certain expectation about the communication of pain. As part of the sun dance people do what others could consider painful acts. In my sun dancing, I have had wooden or buffalo bone pegs inserted into the skin of my chest and back. In modern times, this is done with a scalpel that is disposed of each time. The expectation is that the dancers will accept this without any visible signs of discomfort. Paradoxically, the expectation appears to remove most of the discomfort and, as in hypnosis, it becomes "an interesting sensation" (Milton Erickson's term) instead of pain. After the insertion of the pegs, they are either tied to the tree in the center of the ceremonial grounds (the arbor) and we eventually dance backward past the point of strain of the rope until the peg breaks free, or our pegs are tied to seven buffalo skulls that we pull around the arbor while people cheer behind us, or a buffalo skull is attached to our backs for a day or two.

When I do these things, I imagine how the people who are watching will see me, particularly the ones I care about: the elders who invited me to the dance, who take pride in how well the dance proceeds, or those who have given me favors such as letting me use their eagle fan. I think about their response, and I plan or visualize how I will conduct myself based on how I wish them to react. I want them to be proud of me, so I resolve to perform the ritual in a way that will make them proud. I adjust my performance of pain to match how I want to be perceived, and para-doxically, it becomes minimally painful. Other considerations are much more important. Perhaps this is also how hypnosis works.

What pain means cannot be learned by attention to an example of the word's referent. It is best learned by watching another person's performance of pain. We understand best when people act as if they are in pain and poorly when they simply say they are in pain. If pain were only verbal, words for private sensations such as pain could never be learned. But they are learned. So there must be something wrong with a theory of meaning that exclusively interprets meaningful words as names for things.

Rom Harré, a philosopher and psychologist at Georgetown University's Center for the Brain Basis of Cognition in Washington, D.C., wrote, "In the case of private sensations, there are two things wrong with the traditional puzzle of how someone can know about another person's private and personal experiences. There must be some other way that words get a meaning than by being something to which a teacher can point and a student can notice."[2] The discovery of mirror neurons now offers us a fresh explanation: we compare the inner state of our brain as it mirrors another person's to memories of what that state has felt like to us, then conclude how they are feeling based on how we would be feeling if we were performing the same behaviors. We can be wrong, however: when people's social learning is radically different from ours (as with Lindy Chamberlain) we can draw strikingly wrong conclusions, which we will never know without further dialogue and interaction with that person.

Wittgenstein developed an ancillary argument to show that whatever private sensations are, they should not be taken to be mental things. Pain is not a mental thing. It is not an object. There are no mental objects to play the role of exemplars even if we could overcome the impossibility of using someone's private experience as an exemplar for learning a word. Pain is a conclusion drawn from a complex mixture of language, movement, and social interaction.

Wittgenstein's solution is powerful. We learn such words as *pain* by being taught to substitute a verbal expression for behavior that others around us interpret as what they would feel if they were having what they call pain. We could think of this as conditioned learning. Whenever a child produces certain grimaces and groans and reactions and behaviors, its parents say that he or she is in "pain." Here is where culture interacts with biology. Harré writes, "Part of what it is to be in pain is to be disposed to groan and express one's feeling in other ways. Substituting a verbal expression for a behavioral one leaves the basic distinction between expression and description intact."[3] Harré calls this internal tie between expression and feeling the "holistic principle."

The internal stories that people tell about pain and their "private experiences" are only part of a larger plot that we call "being in pain." If this were not so, hypnosis would not be so effective in modifying pain. I have used hypnosis extensively with people who report to me that they are in pain, and it almost always helps. When we eventually get to the stories that are related to the pain, it sometimes disappears. Even the terrible pain of terminal cancer can be modified when meaning can be attributed to the person's life and the pain can be interpreted differently. Impossible as that may sound, as recently as the month in which I write this, I worked with a dying woman to minimize her pain medication and maximize her comfort using storytelling, hypnosis, and ceremony. She wanted to be lucid to treasure each moment with her family and friends until the last. This became her story: the quest for lucidity and death with dignity, conscious to the end. She was able to do this, and everyone benefited.

We can all agree that there are noxious stimuli. Excessive heat is one. Sharp objects coming in contact with our skin is another. Excessive pressure is unpleasant. We even have circuits within the body that produce compounds to dampen our experience of noxious stimuli. These include endorphins and endogenous cannibinoids (our body makes compounds similar to what produces the "high" from smoking marijuana).

Once I have a grasp of some collection of experiences that correspond to this word *pain,* culture sets in. Depending on the demand characteristics of my situation (family, environment, community), I can be trained to lower or raise my threshold for claiming pain. Some cultures value stoicism. Others reward the quick expression of pain. Within a culture, families vary on their endorsement (or lack thereof) of values. Even without our having any awareness of the process, participation in the roles and relationships of family and community alter our interpretation of the threshold of discomfort at which we complain we are in pain. I suspect that the biological circuits designed to respond to noxious stimuli reset their "pain thermostats" in response to these influences that are suprapersonal.

Hungarian philosopher Ervin Laszlo writes that systems to which we belong "in-form" us as to how to better belong to that system.[4] The information about the state of the whole system shapes us to be better members. If the system rewards those in pain, we learn to have more pain. If the system discourages the expression of pain, we learn to have less pain. Experience is modulated by the social environment. This understanding is consistent with contemporary neuroscience, which describes how the environment changes our brains and their synaptic connections.

The Measurement versus the Meaning of Pain

We know about the world through our bodies, our organs of perceptions. Visible wounds to the body are easy to understand. If our bodies are torn and bleeding, we are wounded. Cultures differ in defining pain and suffering. They differ in prescribing the appropriate response to visible wounds: where a scratch validly calls forth cries of pain in one culture, in another, only deep wounds qualify. Culture also enters when we begin to talk about a wound or to describe a wound that cannot be seen on the surface of the body. Eurocentric cultures have tended to invalidate suffering that has no recognizable tissue damage. Conventional psychiatry has admirably responded to that by trying to locate altered tissue within the brain, to substantiate a structural basis for what has been called mental suffering. For this reason, perhaps, psychiatry has tried to locate the mind within structures of the brain to validate mental suffering.

Conventional medical writings stress the importance of accurate measurement of pain, depression, and anxiety,[5] a strange concept given the vagueness of depression, anxiety, and pain and how different these sensations must be for each person. How do we achieve accuracy and consensual agreement on a largely private experience? Charles Cleeland, Ph.D., a pain researcher at the University of Texas's M. D. Anderson Cancer Center in Houston, writes about pain:

Waiting for the patient to complain spontaneously of pain is poor practice. Patients may be afraid to report symptoms for a variety of reasons. They may feel that reporting symptoms is a type of complaint or a criticism of the physician's or nurse's clinical skills. Thus, complaining of pain may defeat their attempts to be a good patient. Differences in the ethnic and cultural backgrounds of patients and healthcare providers may also hinder effective communication about symptoms. In addition, both patients and healthcare professionals recognize that symptoms are themselves a negative prognostic indicator. . . . Patients may feel that reporting symptoms distracts the physician's attention from taking care of the cancer or is an admission that their disease is growing worse. Patients may also worry that discussing a symptom will lead to a new set of medications with unknown side-effects. Patients who are reluctant to complain of pain are at much higher risk of poor pain management. . . .[6]

The implicit biomedical assumption is that pain exists independent of the context or environment in which it is experienced, that pain is an objective reality, a thing within the body that we can assess objectively. This is the conventional medical view of pain and other private sensations. It is only intrapsychic feelings that prevent the person's expression of the objective internal experience of pain. This perspective results in the desire to measure pain in a manner similar to the measurement of other objective quantities like blood glucose or hemoglobin:

When a patient has a disease that is known to have a high risk of pain, routine and standardized assessment should be standard practice. Just as with other assays that contribute to treatment decisions, pain assessment should be initiated with pain scales or questionnaires that have been shown to be valid and reliable. The pain scales should cover elements such as the severity, location, temporal pattern and quality of pain. Some estimate of how the pain impacts on the patient's functioning should also be included. At the same time, these scales need to be brief, considering only the questions that will help drive decisions about treatment.[7]

Here we see that conventional medicine sees the private, internal experience of pain as exactly like a white blood count, *so long as the disease is known to have a high risk of pain!* This is exactly where medicine fails people: when we have no mechanism to explain a person's high levels of pain, we conclude that he or she is lying or drug seeking, or just not telling the truth. We can't imagine that terrible pain can arise from conditions that we don't think should be terribly painful. We invalidate the story of the person who presents with pain unless it makes sense within our story of what pain is supposed to resemble and how it should be performed.

Medicine's blind acceptance of questionnaires as something "objective" is true only in the sense that the paper on which the questions are written is an object. The meaning conveyed through the questionnaire exchange (or conversation) is not an object. The biomedical approach of defining internal states of mind by giving a questionnaire represents a kind of conversation in which the exchange is formalized, but nevertheless retains most elements of dialogue. Psychometrics as a science may have validity, but only within the context of that dialogue. If we see the questionnaire and the act of completing it as a conversational exchange, we come to a better understanding of its meaning. Problematic is the belief that it represents an absolute criterion or "thing" rather than providing us with another means of glimpsing fast-moving phenomena that change as culture changes. The passage of time changes the meaning of questionnaire responses, a factor that is underappreciated by their designers.

This "objectification" and almost worship of the written, disembodied response arises from a materialist paradigm or story about the nature of the world that says that it is composed of dead matter so that even living systems are ultimately formed from unfeeling, purposeless, meaningless atoms embedded in equally unfeeling, purposeless, and meaningless fields of energy. But that is only one of many possible ways of interpreting our experience of being alive.

Narrative psychiatry supports the idea that many more equally valid views exist and we don't have a way to decide who is right. We simply choose the view that best matches our assessment of the current situation and its demands. From the perspective of narrative psychiatry, the presence of pain is revealed through embodied dialogue, which is an ordered sequence of meaningful whole-body exchanges involving words, gestures, actions, and behavior, all under constraints and rules set by local stories and customs. Such a perspective is more likely to recognize pattern, purpose, and meaning.

In my practice, I always believe people when they tell me they are in pain. I want to hear their whole story about the pain and then work together to reduce it. For example, I recently saw a woman, "Sue," with severe migraines. She wanted narcotics to ease the pain. When we unpacked that request, we realized that what Sue really wanted was to feel like she felt before the onset of the migraines. While I did not ignore her wish for medication for immediate pain reduction, I also began to tease out the story of Sue's life around the time just before and during the onset of the migraines. She was making agonizing choices about her life—whether to leave her husband, who she felt was constraining her and holding her back, even abusing her, versus risk the long-term displeasure of her family, who were Roman Catholic and had told her they would disown her (a common situation in the Far North of Canada, where many aboriginal people are strict Catholics).

Sue used words like, "I felt like my head was going to explode. I felt like I was going to blow a gasket somewhere inside my brain." She was not aware of making these statements or their potential relevance to her migraines. These statements (and others like them) were just the spontaneous metaphorical expression of her body speaking the language of her experience. This is what Broom calls a "meaning-full illness," which pain often is. Broom writes:

> The meanings of meaning-full disease are those that actually predispose us to illness, that contribute powerfully to the onset of illness, and that play an important role in keeping illness going. A narrative psychiatric approach to pain assumes that it might be full of mean-

ing for the person, and understands that we can only grasp this by grasping their entire life in context.[8]

A Cree elder in Saskatchewan recently told me, "To understand someone, you have to hear every story that's ever been told about them and every story that they've told. Since that's not possible, we just do our best to muddle through." For Sue, I arranged a meeting of everyone she knew to talk about their stories about her, her migraines, and her life, and how it all might make sense that she's suffering so much. Quickly the people she invited converged on the idea that the stress of her family, her marriage and children, and her indecision was "killing her." They also spontaneously used such phrases as, "Her head is caught in a vise," and, "They're squeezing the life out of her," without recognizing the extent of their metaphors. When people talk, contexts emerge, and pain as a lived experience begins to make sense. That provided a foundation for Sue and I to work on her negative evaluations of herself and to explore her options, as a result of which the migraines resolved and she no longer wanted pain medication.

The "Story" of Depression

The medical idea is that there is an internal thing called depression that can be measured like a person's temperature. Depression is usually formally assessed by questionnaires such as the Montgomery Asburg Depression Rating Scale (MADRAS), the Hamilton Depression Rating Scale (HADRAS), or the Beck Depression Inventory (BDI). European definitions of depression and anxiety are now codified in the United States in the *Diagnostic and Statistical Manual of Mental Disorders* (DSM), the most recent edition of which is the *DSM-IV-TR* (Fourth Edition, Text Revised),* of the American Psychiatric Association, but are perhaps better conceptualized as types of suffering related to sadness, loneliness, loss of connectedness, hopelessness, and excesses of fear and worry.

---

*A fifth edition of the DSM, the *DSM-V*, is expected to be published in 2012.

What matters is how we as a culture create pathologies out of natural human experiences. Emotional or physical pain can reach such high levels that we no longer wish to feel. We want our wounds doctored and even cured. Some writers have compared what Western culture calls depression to a state of anesthesia in which we can no longer feel and are completely numb. Where do we draw the line and say that someone is too sad or that they worry too much and that they need assistance from outside themselves? How do we teach people to know if they are anxious or depressed? What are the criteria we give them? What is the template? How do I know that I am too fearful or too hopeless? How do I know when to seek "help?" When do I become "a clinical case?"

A common, contemporary term is *clinical depression,* which refers to the concept of a depression that invades the person much as a microorganism would. The implication is that it is endogenous, meaning derived from the brain, without environmental modulation or shaping, referring to a belief within Western biomedicine that brain conditions exist that are primarily brain generated without environmental input. The prototype is similar to that of a stroke, in which a clot stops the flow of blood to a brain region that dies. Function is lost. Clinical depression is characterized as being like a stroke that descends on someone. The person is helpless to change it because it is a physical process, independent of their words, deeds, and will, and independent of their social context. It requires the intervention of an expert who can pharmacologically manipulate the chemicals of the brain.

Harré offers us a different perspective in which the depressed person (or "anxious person" or "person in pain") *is* his private internal dialogue about his sadness, his private flow of sensory sensations, his private exercise of cognitive skills; equally important, he *is* his conversation with other people about his depression, his exercise of cognitive skills in the creation of further conversations about depression, and his performance of the story of being depressed in which audience response shapes future performances. The "audience" may be the physician who writes a medication prescription. Or it may be family members who become more or less convinced that the person is legitimately depressed and therefore less or more demanding that the person fulfill other functions or, as Harré might say, participate in other conversations and interactions about topics other than depression. Regardless of how much faster and how conveniently numerical a questionnaire is, it is not necessarily a better or more accurate way of conversing about depression than a verbal conversation.[9]

A man recently consulted me to determine if his sadness was "situational or clinical." He described a period of marital turmoil, heavy stress,* long commuting, and recent despair. He had just quit his job, reconciled with his wife, and was feeling much better. His doctor had put him on paroxetine (brand name Paxil, an antidepressant) two weeks previously, although this man already felt then that his sense of well-being was returning as a result of changes in his situation. He wondered if he should stop taking the paroxetine. His reasoning was that he should take it for life if his depression was "clinical," while he could stop if his depression was "situational." He expressed what is perceived to be the modern dilemma— "Am I defective or is it a result of my environment?" In his dilemma, we can clearly see the Eurocentric separation of individual from embedded context. A more common indigenous view would be to see people and their emotions as inseparable from their context.

I asked this man how we should solve this problem, and he decided we needed to discuss it with his wife. She thought he had been depressed for years. She proudly claimed that *her* previous "bad behavior" in their marriage was entirely due to her "bipolar," which finally had been correctly diagnosed. I agreed to a conjoint meeting if their marital therapist would permit it. That marital therapist would not, nor would the wife's individual therapist, leaving this man uncertain how to view his distress. His wife insisted that he, like she, had a defective brain and that he should stay on paroxetine for the rest of his life, just as she was going to stay on

---

*I am using his term, *stress,* although I think it is a word we should struggle to eliminate (like *depression* or *anxiety*), for it has multiple meanings to multiple people and no verifiable common meaning. I believe most people use the term to refer to feeling overwhelmed, stretched beyond their capacities, to a feeling of being inadequate to the demands of their situation. It is rarely used in its positive sense, of being challenged creatively and rising to the situation.

medication for bipolar disorder for the rest of her life. After an agonizing month, the man decided to stop taking the paroxetine and not tell his wife, determining his brain to be his private domain and not requiring disclosure within the marriage as to whether it was being medicated. He felt much better without the paroxetine and concluded that his depression was situational.

My reading and that of others of modern neuroscience does not fit the culturally derived distinction of clinical versus situational, since there are no isolated brains and the environment is continually changing brain structure and genetic expression. The logic that increasing the concentration of serotonin in the synaptic cleft should perpetually "cure" depression also seems unfounded within the feedback loops between brain and environment. Environment is capable of altering gene expression to reduce serotonin despite the presence of SSRIs (selective serotonin reuptake inhibitors, a class of antidepressants) like paroxetine, thereby restoring the brain to its pre-SSRI state of serotonin. Indeed, the psychiatric literature includes an awareness that most antidepressants work for eighteen months or less and then must be switched, the so-called poop out, or tolerance phenomenon. Perhaps this is how long it takes for the environment to counteract the effects of the medication in circumstances where nothing has changed in the relationships of the person with the outside world.

Traditional elders have told me that depression is not a tangible thing. You can't touch it; you can't pet it or eat it. It doesn't walk across your field. We construct a concept and then measure it, but that doesn't mean that it is a thing we can see or touch. Depression is not an entity of any sort, mental or otherwise. Instead, it is an agreement made by people to gather a collection of sensations, experiences, and behaviors and to assign them a particular label. The collection of sensations, performances, and stories that compose it are deeply meaningful, but their assemblage into a label is arbitrary. The elders point out that whatever we call depression cannot be stored, measured, or drained like a water tower.

Each person's experience is unique. We collect unique experiences into labels and force these labels onto these experiences to produce these things we call depression or anxiety. When we give depression a number on a rating scale—say 18 on the Beck Depression Inventory—that is just an arbitrary statement, not an actual measurement of how high the fluid level is. The statement, "I'm really sad, almost unbearably so," may be useful, but a rating scale of depression does not make it any more real than saying, "I'm in unbearable, excruciating pain," which qualifies for a higher rating.

We can come close to sharing others' experiences, but never fully and completely. This distinction is important in how people see themselves. A dentist came to see me, thinking he had depression. He figured he needed a medication. When we began to explore a variety of ways of viewing depression, it opened up the discourse to his whole life instead of whether or not he had a thing called depression. We began to explore the ways in which he found his life tedious, his marriage stultifying, his fear that he would grow old and die and this would be all that he ever experienced. Having depression wasn't so important as living a life of boredom and wanting to feel a sense of meaning and purpose. Over six weeks, his perspective rapidly changed without too many major shifts. We got him and his wife together to explore how to reconnect emotionally. His wife was aboriginal and attended ceremonies. He never had and decided to start going with her, which thrilled and excited her. He committed to doing some dentistry in rural and remote communities, regardless of the lower income. One year later he was a transformed man. This was a much better solution than saying he had depression and needed medication. (I did give him a Beck Inventory, and he did qualify for a moderately severe depression, but that was a superficial story compared with the one that emerged.)

We need to understand that labels such as "depression," "anxiety," or other recognized "disorders" function as a way of organizing stories that have a similar plot or theme, a way of introducing order into the chaotic nature of experience.[10] We are prompted to make such stories by our need for meaning. Psychological development is correlated with the ability to elaborate narratives in an increasingly complex way.[11] The efficiency of memory also depends on how well we can construct a story about what happened to us.[12]

From a very early age we impose meaning on daily experience through *our making stories that tell what happened.* At a very early age children develop the ability and need to represent their daily meaning through narrative processes.[13] And recent work has shown that abused or neglected children have impediments in their ability to make narrative.[14] Children develop a grammar[15] through which they impose a narrative structure for both real and symbolic daily events. Through their play, they reenact traumatic experiences, telling stories about what happened or what they wish would happen. These can be deeply healing. Adults often lack the means to do this, which sometimes ceremony, psychodrama, drama therapy, or community theater provides.

Depression, pain, or anxiety is not an object but a conversation. It's not a single photograph, but a movie. Depression is a plot or a theme that arises in "conversation" through a series of ordered and meaningful exchanges defined by local rules and customs. The radical departure of this idea from common practice is the assertion that symptoms and signs in health and disease are all topics that emerge in people's interaction with each other and that physiology is influenced (even driven) by the conversations of those interactions.

The notion of depression or anxiety as conversation asserts that the way individuals think about sadness, fear, or pain, experience sadness, fear, or pain, and act to change sadness, fear, or pain is explained by reference to aspects of the interpersonal conversation that they have appropriated. If the distinction between public and private life is the result of human practice, in which we learn how to keep things that we think, feel, and plan to ourselves, then the private experience of sadness, fear, or pain does not exist separately from the corresponding enactment with other people—both in general and for the person specifically.

My sadness, fear, or pain is a work in progress, a story, a novel, a play presented to an audience for feedback, appreciation, consumption, and countless other purposes. The audience response affects my private experience—which is my private conversation about what I am experiencing, my private use of symbols about sadness, fear, or pain, and my private exercise of cognitive skills. Through the mystery of biology my private experience (shaped by my public conversations) is also expressed in tissue processes (as in the imaging studies). We don't have to know how this happens in order to know that it does happen.

Conventional Medicine and the Loss of Soul

Conventional medicine plays a tricky game when it argues that a correlation or a relationship between different levels of explanation is meaningless unless the relation is describable in physical terms. Medicine has operated as if biology is unrelated to human relationships and is not influenced by the results of human interactions. In true Cartesian fashion, biology is seen as uninfluenced by what happens in our lives. The metaphor is that of a steam engine: the body is the engine and mind is the steam, seen as somewhat accidental and certainly not capable of any direct influence.

Depression is problematic because its definition is arbitrary, not the same for each person, and not the same in different cultures. The best attempts to reify depression have come from imaging studies that show differences in metabolism in particular brain areas in association with the classic symptoms of depression. The fact that they resolve with psychotherapy or drugs strikes at the heart of this reification; the imaging studies say nothing about cause, and the brain doesn't care how it changes. Similarly, in the field of chronic pain, pain without tissue damage has been relegated to categories such as somatization disorder, depression, secondary gain, malingering, and other progressively more demeaning labels. Patients in pain are perpetually suspect of being addicts, merely manipulating to gain their drugs.

Broom wrote that this materialist and physicalist worldview of biomedicine "has been paralleled by a general loss of 'soul' from clinical practice. [A] crucial element of soul is the human experience of *meaning*."[16] If we can engage people in conversation in which their stories can be told, they "somehow know that they are sick *because* of the meaningful things that have occurred in their lives."[17]

The dominant discourse of contemporary psychiatry recognizes pharmacological treatment as the mainstay for depression, contributing billions of dollars to the pharmaceutical industry and to established psychiatric services. More simply, depression is commonly treated with medications. This form of practice allows fifteen-minute office visits and maximizes both income and the number of patients who can be seen. More important is an intangible aspect that is difficult to describe—the illusion of the pristine nature of drug therapy, a clean intervention in which the messiness of emotions and of unbearable affect can be ignored. It is the route to status in psychiatry. It is the essence of the symbol of the white coat. It is the objective distance to which modern medicine aspires. Yet, it is more than income, or capitalism, or convenience, or number of patients seen, or status. It is a fundamental value of modern medicine—the removal of humanity and "messiness" from human interaction. The celebration of the objective, the distancing of relationships, the removal of human interaction from the equation, is central to this movement.

The construction of depression as a biological-genetic disorder allows psychiatry to flourish. The accompanying idea that depression can best be treated with medication allows the pharmacology industry to flourish. Lip service is paid to psychotherapy, but physicians primarily approach depression with medications instead of the harder work of changing people's perspectives and worldviews. People diagnosed with depression who subscribe to the biological story can relinquish much of their need to participate in any conversations about themselves except about how the medications are affecting them. Larger communities are excluded from dialogue except to educate the family about "how to live with a mentally ill member," as a class is described at the Arizona hospital where I once worked. If depression is entirely biological and is treated entirely biologically, then little value comes from conversations between affected parties, except to educate them about the expert paradigm.

Psychiatry has provided a service to the common mainstream narrative in which suffering without a "physical" disease is evidence of moral inferiority, of weakness, and worthy of shame. In this worldview, painful emotional feelings are to be avoided and are useless. Mainstream American and European thought has separated the body from subjectivity and language, rendering the body mechanical. In the time of René Descartes this helped free people from the oppression of the Church. It liberated the body from the Church so that physicians could operate. Psychiatry completed the task of liberating the mind from the Church and destroying the soul. This is why indigenous perspectives are so useful; there was no Church from which to be liberated, so the shame in emotional suffering and the mind-body split never occurred (at least, not until the Church arrived!).

However, within our modern world, for those who see depression as simply a weakness of those who lack self-sufficiency and refuse to discuss it, the biological perspective can at least allow them to start a discussion about their lives and experiences. Having escaped from the "weakness" model, the person can begin to move toward changing relationships.

Gergen writes, "Enormous problems inhere in distinctly psychological modes of explanation."[18] The same can be said for distinctly biological modes of explanation. We could say that privileged explanations are usually inadequate. In this model, what do those clients who do not respond to psychiatric drugs do within the biological narrative? Psychiatry usually responds by trying other medications or combinations of medications until something works, but this can be a lengthy process. A trial-and-error process is usually typical when selecting psychiatric medications. When one or more do appear to work, we still cannot say that they actually worked. We cannot separate the treatment from the context in which the treatment is delivered and the people who deliver the treatment.

In one study I did, the third treatment was most effective, regardless of what it was. The three treatments were acupuncture, massage therapy, and guided imagery. This harkens to the idea that "three's a charm," or the idea from American football that we get three tries to make a first down, and if we are not successful, we have to punt. Or people can simply get tired of the process and tell the doctor what he or she wants to hear in order to politely go away.

My observation is that the purely biological paradigm flourishes because of everyone's search for the "right" medication and people's conviction that it can be found. Unfortunately, this discovery happens more rarely than is believed. I have observed that many clients pursue a variety of alternatives, perhaps most commonly the strategy of self-medication via chronic alcoholism or drug abuse. Some use hidden talents and resources to excel in communities where their mood swings become attractive eccentricities. Some pursue other types of healing, spontaneously lose their depression, die, become soldiers, have spiritual transformations, and otherwise remain hidden from the dominant discourse, though several of their stories will be told in the remainder of this book.

Changing the Conversation: Telling New Stories

Creating more stories about depressives creates more depressives. If we want to reduce depression, we need to reduce the circulating stories about depression. That means finding a different conversation between those who are labeled as mental patients and those who are labeled as therapists or psychiatrists. These conversations re-create themselves with new players so long as they remain circulating stories in our social circles. Training more psychiatrists creates more depressives because psychiatrists need patients to treat. The threshold for being treated decreases. Once diagnosed and processed by the psychiatric system, people are now mental patients and are forced into that role. Their capacity to work is limited, and the expectations on them are diminished or nonexistent. Continued depression and disability becomes the easiest way to make a living.

Moving toward a narrative view of illness, whether or not we can find tissue damage, will liberate us from notions of shame and inferiority. It's not that we are bad, we just grew up with bad stories, meaning that these stories are no longer the most efficient way to see the world and satisfy our needs and wants. When social labeling of people as criminals, patients, victims, perpetrators, and so on is eliminated, relational partners can search for meaning outside of the usual conventions or roles offered by society. The goal is to eliminate roles and scripts that shape our conversations in habitual directions. We need conversations in which unpredictable outcomes emerge. If the solutions to depression were simple, we would have better ones by now. New stories must emerge to guide this search for solutions.

6

Story and the Shaping of Identity

A plurality of independent and unmerged voices and consciousness, a genuine polyphony of fully valid voices is in fact the chief characteristic of Dostoevsky's novels. What unfolds in each of his works is not a multitude of characters and fates in a single objective world, illuminated by a single authorial consciousness; rather a plurality of consciousnesses, with equal rights and each with its own world, combine but are not merged in the unity of the event.

MIKHAIL BAKHTIN,
PROBLEMS OF DOSTOEVSKY'S POETICS

Now that we have looked at emotion and how we learn about it, learn to express it, and learn to control it, let's look at identity, a crucial concept for psychiatry. Russian philosopher Mikhail Bakhtin lays the foundation for our discussion about how we develop a sense of identity, which he saw as a sometimes heroic act to construct a story to make sense of many voices and characters. When it cannot be done or we lose our way and can no longer maintain the story of a unitary character, we are called psychotic (or mystical or enlightened). Any adolescent can tell us what hard work it is to construct an identity. The challenge of adulthood is to keep one. We might say that the work of spirituality is to transcend one.

Bakhtin believed that good novels could inform psychology and psychiatry better than textbooks, with Dostoevsky being a prime example. Dostoevsky nicely presents what lies within consciousness—"a plurality of independent and unmerged voices . . . a genuine polyphony of fully valid" characters telling their story—all the stored voices and characters, preserved in stories modified by our recalling and restoring.

The presentation of a single, unitary self is something at which we must work. Mostly it is a performance for others in which we forge a single story to conform to the expectations of the situation and to achieve goals specific to that encounter. Today's self in one context is not tomorrow's self in another context. Each presentation is a new performance. This is why clients do not present the same from day to day. But creating an identity is also a reflexive performance involving an awareness from which we can watch and critique our efforts to forge a story. Regardless of what we do, we rarely get away without an argument from one of our internalized characters.

Psychotic people cannot readily create a believable (to others) story to explain themselves. They cannot manage the many voices within their brains that they have internalized. They imagine their internal characters and consciousnesses as existing "out there" instead of within. The voices seem to come from outside.

Our social relationships and experiences create what we call *mind* instead of mind existing within a brain. Mind, self, and identity are not internal objects to be discovered in the manner in which an archaeologist extracts a relic from the ground. Rather, the external world comes to be represented within our brains and actually forms our physical brain's synaptic (nerve) connections so that we have a model or a mirror of the external word. As outside, so inside. As above, so below. This happens through our internalization of the stories that are being told around us. "*To be* means *to communicate*. . . . *To be* means to be for another, and through the other, for oneself. A person has no internal sovereign territory, he is wholly and always on the boundary; looking inside himself, he looks *into the eyes of another* or *with the eyes of another*."[1]

The Story We Tell Ourselves

From my discussions with indigenous elders, I have come to share their understanding that identity is the story we tell ourselves in order to make sense of all the stories we have ever heard about ourselves. That makes sense to me and sounds very much like Bakhtin. No single, unified, essential self has appeared in my meditations and reflections. Nor have I seen one appear from another person. The people who come closest to having a consistent, unified, essential or "true" self seem the most rigid and least interesting to me. Their repertoire of potential performable stories appears limited, and they seem to restrict themselves to a subset of situations and characters in which their stories fit.

We develop our identities gradually from early infancy as we hear and internalize more and more stories about ourselves. Specific patterns of behavior, attitudes, and values that enter into our stories about our identity are fostered in the family and in all of our ongoing life experiences.[2] Identity can be defined as our "official" life story, the one that we prefer to tell.[3] A life story has been defined as "an internalized narrative integration of past, present, and anticipated future, which provides lives with a sense of unity and purpose."[4]

When I have asked the elders, "Who is the being who tries to make sense of all these stories?" the best answer I could get from them was that this being is the "me" that exists when all thought ceases. That "me" is like the stem of the flower; it connects with the roots of all other beings underground. It supports the leaves and the flowers that hold the conversations with all other beings in the world. The elders said we confuse what happens in each relationship in which we find ourselves with our soul, which has no thought (because it doesn't need language; it just knows).

"People have told each other stories and listened to stories in all cultures at all times."[5] In doing so, we arrive at an understanding and ordering of the world and the self. As we tell and retell our life story, our personal identity is continually revised. This is part of our ongoing meaning-making.[6] The story of "who we are" is a lifelong ongoing "*narrative project.*"[7] This process not only offers a sense of order to an individual's life but also a sense of continuity over time. It allows periods of major disruptions to be seen merely as turning points.

"We define our identity always in dialogue with, sometimes in struggle against, representations by others."[8] Adolescents' stories reveal how their identities are constantly being re-created, coming forward or retreating to the background in response to the politics and relations that characterize changing social situations.[9] In an ethnographic study of how high school students conceptualize their ethnic and racial identities across varied curricular settings, a change in sociocultural context was shown to have a profound effect on an adolescent's self-image. Moving from an inner-city middle school in St. Louis to an urban high school in California transformed the identity shown by an African American youth from one that was oppositional to one of academic engagement. He referred to his previous self as "the *old* me," making it a part of his life story and constructing a bridge for how he got to "the new me."[10]

Self is a multiplicity of distinct identities rather than one integrated self-identity. Symbolic interactionism defines the self as "a structure of identities organized in a hierarchy of salience . . . by their differentiated probabilities of coming into play within or across situations."[11] Identities are "internalized sets of role expectations, with the person having as many identities as roles played in distinct sets of social relationships."[12]

Gergen has identified a global trend toward developing multiple selves.[13] He traces the changing worldviews in the West from romanticism to modernism to postmodernism. Even though the individualistic view of the self associated with modernism still persists, Gergen proposes that we are increasingly becoming the possessors of many voices and that these multiplicities of voices do not necessarily harmonize. "Increasingly the individual has been deprived of traditional markers of identity: rationality, intentionality, self-knowledge, and sustained coherence."[14] Still, Gergen thinks this may be only a transitional period of unrest and fracture, which will work toward a different form of integration.

Along with Gergen, I sense that we are witnessing an ever-increasing flexibility for individuals to hop between cultures and worldviews. However, research evidence has continued to show a strong desire on the part of individuals to maintain a unified and coherent identity. In my view, flexibility assumes a different meaning when an individual blends together and integrates elements from varying cultures. Members of various cultures will be better able to share and understand cross-cultural stories, making the world a more compassionate and accepting place in which to live.

The Development of Cultural Identity

Culture can be defined as all of the stories being told in a geographical environment coupled with all of the results that occurred from the performance of these stories (buildings, books, bridges, farms, and so on). Group identity has been proposed to be "the outcome of the interaction between the capabilities, limitations, and identities of its individual members, the structure of the group including the network of social and power relationships it entails, and its position in relation to other groups."[15] A collective identity is not the summation of the identities of the constituent members, but its structure similarly comprises a content dimension and an evaluative dimension. Its formation is guided by four principles: self-esteem (to be evaluated positively), continuity (to give a consistent account over time), distinctiveness (to be unique), and self-efficacy (to strive to be competent).

Like individual memories, collective memories are selective and subject to internal and external influences.[16] Since collective memories are constructed in social contexts, group identities are subject to certain constraints, such as "the group's existing social representational systems, other groups' constructions of the past, and the physical/material artifacts of the past." Nevertheless, enormous distortions do occur.[17]

A group's cultural identity changes through historical time in a remarkably similar manner as that of self-identity. The story of a cultural group is maintained by a tapestry of customs, religion, geography, philosophy, and narrative (myths, legends, and historical texts) told in a common language. The shared story provides the individuals with an understanding of cultural norms and values and, most important of all, what constitutes a good person. In Chinese culture, for example, "self," or "identity," is experienced and conceptualized as part of a network of related persons, in a similar way as in North American indigenous culture. This is in distinct contrast to conventional Western European and American mainstream thought, which separates individuals by clear self-other boundaries.[18]

The cultural ideals serve to guide personal behavior, and how one's group is regarded by outsiders affects the collective self-esteem.[19] According to social identity theory,[20] people in general strive to achieve and maintain a positive self-evaluation, and members of a group tend to evaluate themselves by comparing the status of the in-group with that of a relevant comparison out-group. If one's own group holds an inferior position, one would experience a "negative social identity" and be propelled to act so as to upgrade the whole group. Because personal self-worth and group esteem are tied together, the individual and the collective act in a mutually enhancing manner. In a similar manner, political leaders in a modern nation-state are able to galvanize the citizenry to fight for the integrity and prosperity of the nation. They may select or even manufacture myths and legends to instill collective consciousness and patriotism. The national educational system becomes a powerful vehicle of transmission and manipulation.

University of Saskatchewan anthropologist James Waldram describes the ways in which European researchers created an "aboriginal personality" that was largely a cultural projection.[21] Their attempts to define the "noble savage" mostly reflected their own cultural self story; the "perceptual representations of their unexpected cultural experiences" reveal the writers "distance from, unworthiness of, contempt for, disbelief in, or transcendence over the cultural Other." These "perceptions" are offered "not as their belief or personal opinion, but as factual representations of direct experience."[22] The impressions were presented in "us-versus-them" binary constructs such as "normal/deviant, public/private, ecologically sensitive/insensitive, responsive/unresponsive, and so on."[23] "Almost always, the European cultural self was identified with positively valued (from that Western point of view) traits or behaviors, while the cultural Other, Chinese, or North American aboriginal is identified with negatively valued ones."[24]

Human suffering has been enormous in reference to these us-versus-them distinctions. People arbitrarily define themselves as similar or different in accordance with the stories they tell themselves about what constitutes significant similarities and what constitutes significant differences. Like personal identity, cultural identity is just a story that most people share about what makes people similar. Who we locate as part of our culture changes in accordance with where we are. One student pointed out that when she was living in Turkmenistan, anyone who spoke English was part of her culture. When she returned to Canada, that definition no longer applied; she then restricted her culture to being people with the same political and religious views.

The stories of a minority group may be sufficiently different from those stories common to most of the people in a region as to mark them as different. For example, Hasidic Jews and Hutterites both have stories about themselves that result in a performance of their dressing differently from most modern-day white North Americans. Because Hasidic Jews and Hutterites look different from North Americans—looks being one of the main ways people have historically defined culture—they stand out as a different group and are accorded status as a different culture.

In contrast, however, some homeless people who are dirty and smell are marked in more pejorative ways. If they talk to themselves and frequent public places, they are likely to get taken to jail or to a psychiatric hospital. They look sufficiently different so as to be perceived as threatening. Our job is to find out what stories these people have to guide their behavior or, sometimes, to determine what stories they lack about social behavior. I have made headway with some of my younger male clients by drawing their attention to their lack of dates. Then we can puzzle over why no women want to date them. Then we can ask one of my female colleagues to come to our session to explain why she wouldn't want to date them. Most of these reasons typically relate to hygiene and grooming. Then we can puzzle over how they can change so as to be more acceptable (and more likely to have their proposals for dates accepted). A storied approach allows this discovery of hygiene and grooming to be less threatening than a "something is wrong with you" approach.

New Story, New Identity

The relationships that affect our identity are not only with other people. Identity can also form around, or in relation to, an illness, such as in the case of "Antonio." In retrospect, Antonio had been bored with his life, but he only became aware of this after he got sick. Before he was ill, he didn't think about it. One month led to the next month and years passed. He was a psychodynamic psychotherapist; he asked people questions to help them see how their past determined their present. Before he got sick, Antonio was starting to question whether he helped people, or whether they just disappeared, unsatisfied and afraid to tell him. He had been married twenty-one years. He had wanted to adopt when he and his wife learned that she could not conceive, but she did not.

Things rarely changed. He saw the same clients each week in the same order. He watched the same shows on television. He often ate the same meal at the same restaurants. Without fail, he and his wife went to California to meditate once a year, and visited his and her parents, who lived on the East Coast. That used up her three weeks of annual vacation. As the French say, his life was *metro, bureau, dormir*, literally, "subway, work, sleep." Every day was the same.

His illness changed all that. Antonio became a man on a mission. He was searching for the correct diagnosis and for the right therapy that would change his illness and allow him to return to his "every day the same" boring life.

This was my entrée. "Why would you want to return to that life?" I asked. "What was so great about it?"

"Well, nothing," he answered.

"Then why do you want it back?"

"I don't want to die?"

"Why?" I asked. That stopped him. He didn't know. He had survival instinct, but when he stopped to think about his life, he found it meaningless, repetitive, and uninspiring.

Antonio had right-sided neurological symptoms. His right side felt heavier and weaker than his left. It was harder to initiate movement on that side. In walking or sitting, he drifted toward the right. His first neurologist had proudly proclaimed amyotrophic lateral sclerosis (ALS), also known as Lou Gehrig's disease, while telling Antonio about his own high cholesterol and about how he was waiting to die. Then Antonio had gone to the chief of neurology at the university medical school, who did not necessarily agree with ALS as a diagnosis. He told Antonio that an intravenous infusion of immunoglobulin would help make the differentiation between neuropathy and motor neuron disease. Then Antonio went to a "well-known healer" who used a machine to help diagnose. The "healer" diagnosed Lyme disease. This led Antonio to find a "Lyme doctor" in a nearby city, who gave him herbal antibiotics and wanted to start him on a year of intravenous therapy. Antonio bought a machine for several thousand dollars to heal himself with energy and was considering consultations with even more alternative practitioners.

"Your life now is certainly more interesting than it used to be," I said, smiling so he would know that I was joking with him in a good-natured way. "I don't know if I'd want to give up that illness so quickly. It seems to have improved the overall quality of your life!"

Antonio thought about this. It was hard to deny. He had done more things and met more interesting people during the past year than in the previous twenty.

"Maybe this illness is your friend," I suggested. "Maybe Creator sent it as a message, a kind of wakeup call. Maybe you shouldn't be so quick to send it away until you've heard the message it has to send." I say things like this in a nonconfrontational way, not threatening, not critical, but humorously. Humor is very important. Healing cannot proceed very easily without humor. This was a new perspective for Antonio, who had believed that he had a destiny and he needed the courage to face it.

"What if there are many possible futures?" I asked him. "What if you could slip seamlessly among them and end up where you wish the most? What if you can't predict the course of an illness from knowing its name? What if it depends more upon you and the context in which you find yourself?" This is based on what the elders tell me, which amounts to saying that disease is contextual, that it can't exist outside of the context in which you find it. In essence, they are saying, "If you want to change the outcome, change the context."

I asked questions to inspire Antonio to think, to feel the affective tone of his life. I asked what movies or plays he'd seen or what books he'd read in which the main character seemed like him.

"None," he said.

"Then you're not the hero of any story?" I replied. "How about a movie that made you cry?" He immediately remembered the movie *Whale Rider.* "What's your wildest escape fantasy?" I asked.

"To move to California," he said, "but I'd still have to be a psychotherapist. I'd still have to pay the mortgage, and that's all that I know how to do."

"I didn't know that escape fantasies had to be realistic," I said. "I thought they were entitled to be a bit outlandish." He laughed at his insistence on practicality even in his wildest fantasy.

He needed a good healing story to transform the boredom of his life before his illness into something more interesting. "What's the wildest thing you've ever done?" I asked him. He told me about flying to Italy to find the town where his grandfather had been born. He had not known any Italian. He'd had no idea how to get there.

"I just landed and rented a room in a house that turned out to be owned by a journalist who eventually wrote an article about my quest." By the time Antonio got to the small farming village where his grandfather had lived, everyone had read about him.

"Tell me about other outrageous accomplishments," I said. "Tell me about the times you transcended Antonio. Tell me about the Antonio you've always dreamed of being." We were teasing out some other identities, like the adventurous Antonio who went to Italy. I wanted to find more Antonios who could compete with "sick Antonio."

"I wanted to be an astronaut," he said. "I wanted to blast into space, find strange, new life forms, and befriend them. I wanted to save the world, invent a vaccine for cancer, cure AIDS, create world peace, win the Nobel Prize, write the great American novel, and more."

"That's so much more exciting," I said, "than boring psychoanalytic

Antonio. What would it mean to break out of your story and become the Antonio that you've always dreamed of being?"

"I could do it," he said. "I want to live and I was dying. The old Antonio was already a corpse. No wonder I got sick."

Our continued dialogue involved creating a new Antonio who excited himself, an Antonio who appealed to Antonio, a desirable identity. I decided to tell Antonio a story about Corn Woman who lived with an orphaned boy. What is powerful about story is the hidden information that often we don't know we are getting. I have found that when I tell stories to clients, they remember the stories and mull them over, wondering why I told that particular story to them at a particular moment and in response to what they were saying. Often I myself don't consciously know why I tell a particular story at a given time or to a given person. I just have a feeling or a sense that it would somehow be what that person needed. At other times I have a conscious design and pick a particular story to make a specific point.

Corn Woman found a baby boy on the path before her dwelling. Apparently he had been abandoned. At first, he was too young to question how they lived, but as he became older, he began to wonder why they only ate baskets of corn as their main staple. When the baskets were empty, the woman took them into the corn house and came out with them full. They lived on the hominy that she made from this corn. One time the boy looked into this corn house and saw nothing there. He wondered, "Where does she get that corn? Next time she goes in there I will creep up and watch her."

When the corn basket was empty, he crept after the woman and peeped through a crack in the door when she entered the corn house. He watched her set down the basket, stand over it, rub and shake herself, and heard a noise as if something were falling off. In this way she filled the basket with corn. After that he got scared and ran away, afraid that his adopted mother was a witch.

"I can't eat that," he said. "She defecates and then feeds it to me." When the hominy was cooked, he did not eat it, and so Corn Woman knew that he had seen her. "Since you think it is filthy, you will have to help yourself from

now on. I will no longer help you. When I go back to spirit world, drag my body across the field and then burn it. When summer comes, things will spring up on the place where it was burned and you must cultivate them, and when they are matured they will be your food."

Some knowledge ends your source of easy sustenance and comfort. I take this to be a story about separation and individuation—constructing an identity different from the one into which we are born. A common plot among the world's stories is being "tossed out of the Garden of Eden" when we begin to create our own identity. So long as the young boy was naïve and didn't question the source of his food, all was good. When he questioned Corn Woman, she withdrew.

After telling this story to Antonio, I realized that it came to mind because Antonio had been thrown out of his own garden of paradise to a world in which he had to "grow his own food." He had to toil in the fields of psychotherapy to pay his mortgage and other bills and to buy groceries. He was as miserable as any day laborer, or perhaps more so because he had nothing to show for his efforts at the end of the day. At least the laborer had baskets of potatoes or a completed building or something tangible.

The boy did as he was told when Corn Woman died. He dragged her body across the field and then burned what remained as she had instructed. When summer came, corn sprang forth from her flesh, and beans and pumpkins came up through the ashes. He cultivated these plants every day. When he stopped, he stuck his hoe into the ground and left. When he would return, more ground had been hoed, and the hoe would be sticking into the ground in a different place from where he had left it. He wondered if a fox was tricking him.

Like listening to elders, traditional stories present situations in which unquestioning obedience is required. We both lose and gain something when we ask questions.

The boy said to himself, "I'll creep up and find out who is doing this hoeing," and so he did. He saw the hoe doing the job all of its own accord, and that made him laugh. Immediately the hoe fell down and would not work for him any more.

By questioning, or doubting, the source of his help, the boy loses it. Antonio's work as a psychoanalyst was like the boy's curiosity. His interest in mechanism never got him anywhere but stuck with doing more work.

Later the same day, the boy's brown log house burned down, and he knew he was not allowed to stay. He would have to move on.

I had met Antonio when the house of his life had burned down and he was suffering from the aftereffects. I told this to him as I was telling the story. "You're being forced into the same situation as the boy in the story," I said. "You are being told that the life you are living that has been feeding you is also killing you. It's been easy having the corn provided for you and the hoeing done for you, but that's stopped because you have too much awareness of what's going on. You're getting thrown out of the Garden and onto the dusty road, whatever that means for you. Let's continue the story and maybe it will become clear to you where you need to go or which road you need to take."

As the boy was going along the path, he met Rabbit coming toward him, who made friends as soon as he saw him. "Where are you going?" Rabbit asked.

In the culture where this story originates, Rabbit is the trickster—like Coyote in the Southwest, the Great Plains, and the West Coast. Rabbit is the impetus for change and transformation.

"I am going to find my mother," the boy said. "I am an orphan but my adopted mother always told me that my real mother lived close by."

Saying you are going to find your mother is a more accurate answer than saying you are going to find your true self, since you have no true self to find. All selves arise from relationships, so probably what you are really seeking when you go on a spiritual quest is your mother in every metaphorical sense of the term. Dads are fun, but let's face it, "breast is best": mother is most nurturing, and being held by mother, being returned to her womb, if only for a few hours like what we do in the sweat lodge ceremony, is fabulous, and worth the walk.

> "Let us go together," said Rabbit. "I am going into the creek to tie up turtles. Let us go back and tie up turtles together and then we will go find your mother." The boy didn't want to go, but Rabbit, who wanted to fool him, overcame his objections and he went along.

Rabbit, like Coyote, shares the powers of persuasion. That's why I've often thought that all therapists are tricksters. We must "trick" people into changing, and they must let us, for without a surprising, novel experience, change doesn't happen. Coyote and Rabbit produce these novel events. New learning requires novelty and surprise.

> When they got to the creek, they peeled off hickory bark for ropes, took off their clothing, and went into the water. Rabbit said to the boy, "When I say, 'Now!' we will dive underwater together." So they went to a place that was rather deep and Rabbit said, "Now!" The youth dived, but Rabbit went out, seized the boy's clothes, and carried them away.

As Elmer Fudd said, "Nevuh twust a wasskalie wabbit." Rabbit (aka Coyote) will always leave you naked by the stream, stripped of your conceptual framework so that you're forced to build another.

> After the boy had tied turtles together by the legs, he came out of the water and found his clothing gone. He stood thinking with his head hanging down, and then he looked about and saw a persimmon tree standing nearby. He climbed it, shook off some persimmons, and rubbed them all over his body. Then he went on.

We make do with what we can find! Who knows, maybe being covered with persimmons is sweeter than clothing. It's certainly reflective of a change and transformation, but it's transitional. You can't stay covered with persimmons forever.

The boy came to a house where the people thought he was filthy and gave him food at the edge of their yard. He then went on until he came to a place where an old woman lived. She looked on him kindly. She cleansed him, and they lived together.

Here we have the beginning of the transformation—the boy (youth) is taken in by the wise, older woman, a motif that was sexualized in *The Graduate* and in some François Truffaut movies. But the traditional motif is not sexual; the boy has come to learn from the mother in her most ancient, teacher form.

One day the old woman said, "I want some fish." So the boy went to the creek. Afterward the boy came back and said to her, "A sick fish was lying there, which I put into the canoe, but if you want it, you can go and get it." So the two went down to the canoe and found it full of fish. "If you cannot carry them all away," he said to her, "tell your kinsfolk, if you have any, and let them have some." The old woman told them and they came and carried the fish away.

When the boy enters the home of the old woman, he has entered a world of alchemy and magic. This is where the change happens—invisible to us, as onlookers, who can never know exactly how. We must guess. We can't know how the one sick fish turned into a multitude or how Jesus turned the fish and the loaf of bread into many fish and many loaves, but it happened. When magic happens, the faithful have the duty to share the benefits, the wisdom, the knowledge, with all the kinsfolk.

Rabbit heard how the young man had divided the fish. Rabbit said to his wife, "You must say, 'I want some fish.'" Rabbit's wife heard him and answered, "I want some fish." Then Rabbit went to the creek. He found a dead fish and put it into the canoe. After a while he came back.

Rabbit said, "A sick fish was lying there, which I put into the canoe, but if you want it, you can get it." Then the two set out. In the canoe they found only a swollen, dead fish with its eyes turned white, and Rabbit's wife scolded him over this.

Rabbit is giving us another teaching now, for which we must honor him. He is showing us that mere duplication of form and behavior does not reproduce the magic. You have to find the magic for yourself. Each of us must find our own old woman. We must enter into her home and become her apprentice. Only then does the inexplicable occur. Rabbit shows us that simply going through the motions doesn't produce results. Form never replaces inspiration or magic. This is what psychiatry and Antonio need to learn.

Another time the old woman said, "I want some deer." So the boy went into the woods to hunt. After a while he came back and said to her, "I finished killing a deer that lay sick and laid it in a hollow, but if you want it, you can go and get it." So, the two went after it. When they got to the place, they found it full of fat deer. "If you cannot carry them all off, let your kinsfolk take them away," he said to her. So the old woman told her kinsfolk, and they came and carried off the deer.

Rabbit also heard of that. He said to his wife, "You must say, 'I want some deer.'" So Rabbit's wife said, "I want some deer." Then Rabbit went hunting in the woods. After a while he found a dead deer, put it into a hollow, and came home. "I finished killing a deer lying sick," he said, "but if you want it you can get it," and they set out. When they came to where the dead deer lay, something had already taken out its eyes and the woman scolded him.

Going through the motions still didn't work. I think Rabbit the Wise knows that it won't work, but he's doing all of this for our benefit—to show us what works and what doesn't work. That, at least, is what I'm telling Antonio. He knows what doesn't work in his life. He knows he's just going through the motions. He knows there's no magic in his life. He has to burn his psychic house and go walking about. He must find his old woman, his magic, or he will die. Magic usually comes in threes in North American stories. We must anticipate at least one more magical event. This really gets our attention.

> *One day the old woman said to the boy, "Take your axe and split me in half." After some time, the boy said to the old woman, "Comb your hair and part it well," and she started to comb it. Then he said, "I want to build a house," and he started grinding his axe. The old woman continued combing her hair, and when she finished, he said to her, "Stand in the doorway." She did so, and immediately he struck her on the head with the axe and split her in two. Now two young women stood there looking just alike. Now he had two young wives instead of one old woman.*

Like Abraham preparing to sacrifice his son, these stories call for complete obedience. The boy didn't question this insane request. He just did it. (But that's because he knew it was a story; he knew it was metaphor.) People who are labeled psychotic often can't do metaphor. They have lost the ability to story. They think it's concrete, so they go get the axe and actually cut off someone's head.

> *Rabbit said to his wife, "Comb your hair." She combed her hair, and when she finished, he said, "Stand in the middle of the doorway." She stood there, and he struck her and she fell down dead.*

There, it happened. Going through the motions eventually leads to the death of someone.

> *After that happened the people said the boy had encouraged Rabbit to kill his wife, and they arrested both Rabbit and the boy. They tried both of them. All of the four-leggeds with hair and all of the winged ones tried them. But they concluded, "It was not the boy telling Rabbit but the foolishness of Rabbit himself that caused him to kill his wife by trying to imitate the boy," and they let the boy go but convicted Rabbit.*

I thought Antonio could think about this story endlessly. There is more to understand about the difference between Rabbit and the boy. Rabbit's imitating, copying, and parodying are clearly not desirable traits, while explicitly following the instructions of the old woman are. There's a difference here that can only be understood within the story. The mysterious old woman is the key to this difference. She holds the magic. She tells the boy what to do, and he does it. Rabbit has a different intention, and it's not his journey. He thinks he can just do the behaviors without performing the story. The boy has been indoctrinated into the story and prepared. We can't just copy someone's identity; we have to be mentored by a community through a process of change and transformation. These are good ideas to sow as seeds for changing a very stuck situation.

Don't worry about Rabbit. He always escapes, or otherwise our lessons would end. Here's how Rabbit got away this time.

The people could not think of any way to kill Rabbit, so they secretly discussed a way to deceive him. They said to Rabbit, "Go and get Rattlesnake." They thought that if Rabbit went for Rattlesnake, Rattlesnake would bite Rabbit and kill him. "Rattlesnake can't walk fast enough and hasn't come. Go and get him," they said, and Rabbit started off. But he knew they were deceiving him. He broke off a long stick, sharpened it, and came to the place where Rattlesnake lived, using it as a walking stick. When he arrived he also told a lie. "They sent me from the assembly," Rabbit said. "Many said, 'Rattlesnake is long.' Many said, 'He is short.' 'Well then,' they said to me, 'go and measure him,' and so I came along." Upon hearing this, Rattlesnake straightened out and lay flat, and Rabbit began measuring him. As he was doing so he said, "Where is the center of your life?" Rattlesnake answered that his life was in the middle of his head, so Rabbit kept measuring and while he was doing so, stuck the stick into the middle of Rattlesnake's head and killed him. Rabbit laid him over his shoulder, impaled on the stick, and carried him back.

Rabbit can even trick the snake meant to kill him into revealing how Rabbit can kill it first. That's talent. Also, of course, no one really dies in these stories. We all know that. It's metaphor.

"We told you to bring him here alive," they said to Rabbit. "What is he fit for now? Throw him away." So Rabbit threw Rattlesnake away. Again, they came to an agreement. "Let Rabbit direct the water," they thought, "and it will catch and drown him." So they said to Rabbit, "You lead the water. Make it run straight in the channel." So he caught the water and led it by means of a string. Presently the water overtook him, and he started to run. When the water overtook him again he ran a crooked course. It overtook him again, and after running from it several times he got tired, let the water go, and ran off.

Here's a good example of Rabbit's genius. This time, in escaping, he improves on the stream. Rabbit never gets away without leaving an important lesson.

When they said to him, "We told you to make it straight," Rabbit answered, "What I have done is right. Since it is crooked it makes a good place in which things can range about, and when the second bottom is made it is a good place in which to hunt. I thought it would be good to cultivate and make a farm out of, so I made it that way." They could do nothing with him, and so they let him go.

So, even Rabbit gets away, as he always does. These simple yet confusing metaphors are good for Antonio. They have the right feeling tone, they bewilder. I could have chosen other stories, but this one resonated with the affective tone of his life. It presented itself and asked to be told. When the storyteller asks, the story will come.

Antonio and I continued to dialogue about him finding new stories. "You're in Act Three of your play," I said. "You're heading toward the crisis point where the story has to peak and resolve. How should it resolve? What will your next act be? Will you live or will you die? Will you be diagnosed? Will you escape to Tahiti, flying over California, and forget about paying the mortgage? Will you run off to Katmandu like you ran off to Italy? What is the story that you want to live?"

This question provoked Antonio, who realized that he found his story about himself (his identity) boring. He said he only told boring stories. He was boring. His wife said he was boring. He realized he even took comfort in being boring. Boring was safe. It was his story.

Suddenly, having difficulty walking was not boring; it was terrifying. It shocked Antonio out of his story. My suggestion was that he couldn't get back to where he was if he wanted to be well because being sick was the logical outcome of living the story he had been living. The way out was not to retrace his steps, because that would only lead him back to where he was and, surprise, surprise, you don't actually get to go backward in time. You can only go forward.

"So," I said to Antonio, "What I want you to consider is what Act Five should be. How do you want to end? What is your desired ending? And how do you get there?"

"I want to live," he said.

"Then let's create an Act Four that will lead you to the land of the living," I said.

"Forget everything you've learned about psychoanalysis and psychotherapy, and let's stick to making good drama. What are some believable paths to living? What would interest an audience? What would make people want to sit up and cheer for you? How could you transform from the living dead into the living living?"

That led us into an extended dialogue through guided imagery and storytelling, and a discussion about a logical transformation, about what to do. Antonio decided he wanted to reinvent himself as an adventurer of life. He decided that he and his wife should sell their home and take a trip around the world. He would write a book about taking his illness to various healers around the world. It was an excuse for a trip around the world that his colleagues and family would accept. But would his wife?

Next I met with Antonio and his wife, "Janet." He had explained his idea to her. His logic had been that if he was dying of ALS or some serious illness, then he wanted to spend his last good months traveling while he was still able. Strangely to him, his wife agreed. She was ready for a change. She also wanted to do something different if he was dying. "I want different memories of Antonio than those I have," she said. "I don't want him to die. I don't want him to have ALS or MS or any S," she said, "but if he does, we need to spend our savings and do all those things that people should do and dream of doing before he dies."

She even improved the plan, noting that they didn't need to sell the house; they could hire an agency to rent it. Antonio had thought they shouldn't spend what he considered Janet's retirement, the nest egg he would leave her if he died. "I don't want your money," she said. "I want you to live like you've always wished for as long as you can. If you outlive our money, we can always come home and kick out the tenants and go back to work." Antonio was very grateful. He hadn't imagined that his wife would have such a positive response. His story about what she would think had been very different.

The remainder of my work with Antonio involved helping him to consolidate his new story—as a world adventurer of healing. I enjoyed watching him gradually change the way he dressed to appear a bit more adventuresome and even rakish. He had a model from his past for this, from the time when he went unannounced to Italy. His plan was to make his way around the world in this manner.

Antonio fulfilled his commitment. Five years later he returned to my office to say hello. He had never been diagnosed, but his strength and balance and gait had returned, and he had wonderful stories about his encounters with healers from around the world. He had turned his journey into his new career and had never looked back. I told him that the audience was cheering. He had impressed them. He had created a really good story.

PART II

Science and Mind

7

How Culture Changes Biology and Genetics

A gene generates a broad physiological substratum upon which psychological phenomena can be constructed. . . . [T]he construction process itself is not directed by genes. It is organized by cultural and mental processes. Genes are necessary to generate the general capacity for psychological phenomena; however, this is quite different from genes determining that the phenomena, i.e., the competencies, will occur and what their specific content will be. Genes only have codes for physiological matters such as "association neurons"; genes do not have codes for psychological phenomena such as grammar, love, problem solving, or . . . reasoning.

CARL RATNER,
"GENES AND PSYCHOLOGY IN THE NEWS"

When I was in medical school, we dreamed that the mysteries of disease would be unlocked once we had sequenced the human genome. Once we knew the exact sequence of molecules for every gene, we would know everything about disease. I remember endless debates with classmates about the nature–nurture argument, which has ancient origins. We took either-or stands and argued that schizophrenia, for example, was entirely due to faulty genetics or, from the other camp, that it arose from dysfunctional family dynamics. We were passionately binary. I don't suppose we could imagine a world in which every story is true, in which genes and social environment interact together to coproduce an outcome.

After I graduated from medical school, however, the new science of epigenetics broke open our understanding of how environment affects genes. It's called epigenetics because it studies effects that "sit on top of the gene" and leave the sequence of molecules in the gene unchanged. While genes provide us with a basis for many functions, our environment and our experience modify the expression of our genes dramatically. In fact, "each nutrient, each interaction, each experience can manifest itself through bio-chemical changes that ultimately dictate gene expression, whether at birth or forty years down the road."[1] Multiple genes exist whose only functions are to turn other genes on and off. For example, a person can have a genetic tendency toward developing a particular cancer, but it is never expressed because an environmentally caused modification activates a gene that turns off the cancer-causing gene. Hence, no cancer.

The effect of genes on illness is often studied by comparing identical twins (whose genetic sequences are identical). A landmark study of identical twins growing up in the same household showed that they were 35 percent different in epigenetic markers, which increased as they got older.[2] This is because experiences diverge despite the twin's genetic code being sequentially identical and their living in the same household. Twins who live apart with less exposure to similar environments become progressively more different over time, with eventually diverging health histories correlated to their different gene expression profiles.

Still, most people don't know that just because we have a gene for something, it is not necessarily expressed. And psychiatric research has spent billions of dollars looking for a genetic basis for its variously defined diseases, from schizophrenia to bipolar disorder to anxiety and beyond. No single genetic cause of emotional suffering or hallucinations has emerged. Identical twins should be equally susceptible to illnesses such as schizophrenia, bipolar illness, autism, and attention deficit hyperactivity disorder, but they are not. Multiple genes have emerged as candidates to increase the likelihood of "mental illness," but none are particularly robust on their own.

Genes provide a general schematic for who we are, what traits we will have, such as eye color, skin color, or hair color. But genetics do not provide a full or even partial explanation except in certain very circumspect situations. For example, Huntington's disease, a disease in which the brain deteriorates around age forty, is based on one gene. Phenylketonuria, a disease that causes infants to be mentally retarded, is based on one gene. These are relatively rare, and what are called polymorphisms of these conditions are slowly being discovered. These are partial modifications of the gene in which the condition is not so severe or is somewhat different than would be expected. Considerable research supports the idea that genes contribute potential and that experience mitigates or exploits that potential.

Having an at-risk genome is not sufficient to produce disorder or disease: experience and the passage of time inevitably mold our DNA, silencing some genes and promoting the expression of others, thereby facilitating the cognitive, emotional, and behavioral changes that either improve or detract from our quality of life."[3] This is where our current understanding can expand the simplistic genetic explanation promoted by psychiatry in the past. We are so much more than our genome. Our life experience changes our genetic makeup. Our social environment has a huge impact on how our genes are expressed—so much more so than in other animals. Genes give us the potential for schizophrenia or anxiety or depression, but life experience and our social environments make it happen.

Changing the Song of the Finch

I'd like to tell some stories about how I use modern genetic and epigenetic research in my work of helping people. "Sandy" came to see me for what she called "bipolar." Her mother had been diagnosed with bipolar disorder, as had her two sisters. She was sure that I would diagnose her in the same way. She felt helpless in the face of what was most certainly about to happen. Upon further exploration, it was clear that much of Sandy's current misery and helplessness related to her sense of "what was going to happen" and not what was currently happening. She dreaded a genetic inevitability of diagnosis and descent into suffering like her sisters and mother.

"What if bipolar is not your inevitable fate?" I asked Sandy.

"What do you mean?" Sandy said. "You're the doctor. You know how these things work."

I changed my voice tonality and phrasing to be more persuasive. "You just don't know the more recent science," I said. "Genes are not as powerful as we thought. Do you remember the human genome project where we were going to save the world by making a map of the human genome?"

"I remember hearing about that," she said. "When's that going to finish?"

"Ten years ago," I said. "And nothing particularly profound happened. The world wasn't saved. Do you know why?" I asked. I had more of her attention now. She was forgetting to act miserable. Curiosity does that to people. We can't be too unhappy when something sparks us to wonder. She couldn't suppress her surprise (which is a sign of cognitive adaptation).

"No," she said. "Why?"

"Because much of what really matters to people, like feeling loved, having meaning and purpose, and the like are not under the control of our genes. It's under social control. Believe it or not, we're less complicated genetically than chimpanzees. They actually have more functional genes than we do. This is because, as we evolve, more of our functions come to be under social control and not genetic control.

"I've actually got a cool story to tell you about that, and maybe it will help convince you that it's not inevitable that you follow in the footsteps of your mother and your sisters. It's a story about domesticated and wild finches in Japan, where the nobility began breeding the finch for its color. When finches were wild, breeding was under tight genetic control. If a male finch wanted to mate, he had to have a perfect song, exactly what the females expected. No room existed for variation. Finches had to sing it the same way every time. Those who ventured into improvisation never got to mate.

"But when the Japanese breeders started to decide who reproduced, the quality of a finch's song and its exact reproducibility no longer mattered. Suddenly the finches began to have amazing variations in song, and they even started imitating each other and taking parts from other birds' songs and actually improvising like jazz musicians. Within 250 years, the finches turned a simple song that never varied into a richly complex music with actual syntax—movable parts that could be interchanged in different ways. The wild finch is genetically programmed to sing the exact same song, but the domestic birds lost that tight control and began to learn their songs socially.

"Darwin figured out that birds' songs are driven by natural selection. He also thought that natural (or what he called sexual) selection was crucial for explaining unusual traits of humans. Back in those days he was fighting with another Brit, Alfred Wallace [1823–1913], who angered our friend Darwin by saying that natural selection couldn't explain the size and complexity of the human brain. But when the brains of the wild finches are compared with those of the domestic ones, it is clear that very few brain areas are required to produce a song that is genetically programmed. It turns out that the genes of the domestic finches have degraded compared with the wild ones, and many more of their brain areas are devoted to song. So, you see, Sandy, Darwin was wrong. It was the loss of genetic control that paved the way for our large brains, because our larger brains are managed through social control.

"What this means for you is that it's not inevitable that you go the way of the other females in your family. Social control plays a more significant role than you realize, just like in the songs of the domestic finches, and we're going to exercise that social control now to prevent you from ever being diagnosed with bipolar disorder."

My use of science facts is largely to construct stories to convince people that change and transformation is possible. That's what I was doing with Sandy. I continued to tell Sandy variations of the same theme: that she wasn't a slave to her inheritance. Life intervenes and changes things. The problem with contemporary science is that at any given moment it presents current theories as the truth, even though those theories are constantly changing. Having followed medical science for more than three decades, I have learned not to take any current pronouncement too seriously since it may well be overturned in a year or two. Patients don't know this and don't follow the field. Whatever pronouncement (story) sticks with them in a time of chaos or crisis is the one they will assume is true forever.

I told Sandy again, for further emphasis, how birds whose songs have tight genetic control have few brain areas controlling their song. When having the exactly correct song was no longer crucial for reproduction, then genetic control began to relax, songs become more varied, the birds started to learn from each other. "This is where you are, Sandy," I said. "You can learn new songs from others. I'm here to teach you new songs to sing that are much more interesting than the songs your mother and sisters sing."

Learning from other people (or birds) activates many more brain structures, including the auditory system. If our behavior is under genetic control, we don't need much of our brain to regulate it. The primary innate structure does all the work. Genetic control through natural selection stabilizes the behavior. As genetic control relaxes and even disappears, much more variation in behavior is allowed, and all unused brain connections become relevant. For the birds, as tight control of the song relaxes, other structures in the brain begin to play a role in singing. As this persists for longer and longer, the genetic constraints weaken, and anything that can contribute even slightly to singing begins to play a role. For us, as for the birds, what our neighbor is singing, what our dad is singing, what anyone else is singing can play a role in what we are singing. When selection is relaxed, environmental effects become much more important.

So I told Sandy, "That means that whatever you inherited from your mother and share with your sisters is relatively unimportant compared with your life experiences and what you are learning from other people. This is probably how we developed language and the richness of emotions that we humans have. It's how we became able to have something like bipolar disorder but also how we can heal whatever we have, because none of us is under such tight genetic control. With language, for example, our primate cousins' vocalizations are under much tighter genetic control than ours. Unlike them, we don't have to be aroused to talk. We talk all the time. We have far fewer innate sounds than chimpanzees do and much more freedom to experiment. This means that learning from others is much more important for us than for chimpanzees. So, Sandy, you are human, and you can learn from other people. You can learn new ways to regulate your mood and emotions, ways that your sisters and mother could not know, because they haven't met the people you know. They're not here in this office with me, where we're going to learn other ways of living than being bipolar."

We humans are under much less genetic control than any other species. That control has shifted to include social control of behavior. I asked Sandy to imagine a chimpanzee baby raised in a laboratory who has never heard another chimpanzee. That chimpanzee would sound a lot more like any other adult chimpanzee than would a (hypothetical) human baby raised in a laboratory who never heard human speech. We humans need to hear language to learn it. We don't have an innate language without social learning.

As we hear language and music, our brains evolve to produce and manipulate the sounds that we are hearing. We learn to improvise. Even our brains are much less specific for emotion than animals' brains. This is shown by the fact that, for some primates, the limbic structures—the emotional center of the brain—have specific regions associated with specific forms of arousal. For example, laughter is associated with an area on the dorsal midline of the limbic system. Humans have much less specificity; lots of areas control vocalization.

Genetic selection is only a small part of the story, not the whole story. I told Sandy another story to help her to understand how our entire human history has been about overthrowing genetic control.

"Sandy, we are here today because our ancestors in every generation rebelled more and more against genetic control. Almost two million years ago our distant hominid ancestors exploded out of Africa and found all kinds of niches in which to live. Slowly they learned how to use and then to make tools. This explosion relaxed genetic control many times. We probably have the least functional genes of any animal. We started out with a simple vocalization system like monkeys have. Changing environmental conditions allowed some of that genetic control to relax, and then the genetic system degraded and other systems played a role. Selection could then play a role by affecting these other systems. This caused a remarkable reorganization.

"Genetics made language and emotion possible, but culture and environment created and elaborated language from the simple sounds apes can make. This makes us radically different from other species. It also makes the stories into which we are born much more important in shaping our brains than any other species. You were born into ineffective stories about regulating mood and behavior. That's all you knew. Now you can learn some new ones. We're going to do some exciting things together to make you so different from your mother and sisters that you have no chance of being diagnosed with bipolar disorder. You're going to learn how to be happy and regulate your moods.

"We are like beavers building dams. By building dams beavers put themselves in aquatic environments that force them to become more aquatic. What beavers have done changes what beavers are. Our socially constructed cultural environments along with our imagination have been our beaver dams that make us better and better at manipulating symbols, like language, art, and science. As we put ourselves into a world of culture, language, and symbols, our imaginations have expanded so greatly that we can live not just in the here and now, but in a world of virtual possibilities, of many 'what might have beens.'"

I went on to work with Sandy using guided imagery to explore how her life might have been if her mother had not behaved in the ways that earned her the bipolar diagnosis. Who would she have been if conditions had been different? We easily found three or more virtual Sandy's who might have been. None of them were feeling hopeless and helpless and afraid of having bipolar disorder. We were able to learn from those virtual Sandy's enough to help Sandy become more like them.

This kind of work is effective because of the social-cultural-sexual flexibility and aesthetic sensibility that is a result of our becoming genetically degraded. In that process, we shifted control of many of our behavioral and emotional traits, our susceptibilities to social control and conformity, out of the genome and into this more distributed world.

Choosing Which Past to Listen To

Life contains the capacity to self-organize. We can adapt to the environment and often do. The argument that our social environment functions to control behaviors and activities that are under genetic control in other primates can be used in reverse, to convince people that their current suffering is not because they are genetically inferior but because of the effects of traumatic experiences that have affected their DNA, but reversibly, and that they can change. "Paul," a Native Hawai'ian graduate student, came to see me because he felt terrified that he would fail. He was ready to quit school because his fear was paralyzing. In hearing Paul's story, I learned that he was the first person in his family to graduate from high school, much less to go to college and on to graduate school. He felt inferior and defective when he compared himself with the other students. He felt ashamed to be in their presence and at the university because he felt he did not belong, did not deserve to be there.

Paul's father had been a crystal meth user and had beaten Paul severely until he went to prison. Paul's mother drank heavily and relied on Paul, the oldest, and his younger sister to take care of themselves and the other children. As far back as Paul could remember, people in his family were alcoholics. I told Paul he was a miracle of resilience to have made it so far. "But my genes are bad," he said. "I took abnormal psychology in undergraduate. I took genetics. I know that our family just has bad genes. There's no way around it, and it's going to catch up to me soon. I've been squeaking by, living a lie until now, but it can't continue."

"Let me tell you a story, Paul," I said. "It's a story that starts with the amazing people you come from. People who could navigate across the Pacific Ocean in canoes with only their songs to guide them as living star maps, people who founded an amazing civilization on these islands, people who were strong warriors with epic stories and legends and great passion. You come from an awesome people." I continued along this line with further examples.

"Now let me tell you what might have happened to your family, and here's the good news, it's totally reversible. I'm going to tell you a story about a new science of epigenetics, one that you didn't learn in undergraduate school. It's the science of how a person's experience and external environment change the expression of their genes. It's a science that can help us understand how things are going to be totally fine for you. Here's how it goes.

"The environment, events in our lives, even our emotional reactions, don't change the genetic sequence we inherit, but they can alter the structure of the genetic molecule, which in turn allows for changes in the way the genetic information is replicated and expressed. The processes that allow this are called methylation and acetylation. You probably remember this from undergraduate chemistry. A methyl group has one carbon atom attached to three hydrogens and one available slot to be stuck onto any molecule. When it attaches, it is called methylation, which is one of the main ways drugs are metabolized. It's how toxins are removed from our bodies. And it's also how the expression of our DNA is modified by experience—through adding on methyl groups to the DNA. An acetyl group is similar to a methyl group but with the addition of an oxygen atom. In acetylation, these acetyl groups attach to a specific site on histone proteins, the molecules that are responsible for maintaining the shape of the DNA. Methylation can silence, or switch off a gene, while acetylation encourages the expression of specific genes.

"This little trick of adding a methyl group or an acetyl group happens as a result of immediate experience, something that scientists thought impossible even until recently. You probably remember your biology teacher in high school making fun of the French biologist, Jean-Baptiste Lamarck [1744–1829], who argued with Charles Darwin. Two hundred years ago he proposed that the environment shaped gene expression. In his day, he was 'proved' wrong by Darwin. Lamarck thought that giraffes get long necks because of needing to reach the best leaves to eat at the top of the trees. He argued with Darwin, claiming that environmental demands contributed to the neck length, not just natural selection from random genetic mutations that led to higher chances of mating and reproducing. He may or may not have been right about giraffes, but he was correct that environment changes gene expression.

"This is important because people like you (and many doctors!) too quickly assume that there's something wrong with their genes that makes you (and them) feel hopeless because you can't change your genes. It makes you feel that nothing can be done except taking medication and quitting graduate school. What's important is to remember that what you have inherited from your ancestors has not been changed. There's nothing defective or inferior about the underlying DNA. We may suffer like our parents not because we have inherited their genes, but because we have inherited the *effects* of their life experiences, which only change the *expression* of the gene. And gene expression can be rapidly altered by life experience and will change with time! Whatever has happened to your strong and healthy genes as a result of growing up, we can change quickly in our work together. It's awesome.

"As the necessary functions for survival are covered, genes can change and generate new functions without deficit. Genes have the freedom to walk away from their original function in a smooth, elegant way, which is why we have color vision. We gained it around the same time that we lost the capacity to make our own vitamin C. Before about thirty-five million years ago, birds had color vision and mammals didn't. Having color vision is very helpful in locating foods with vitamin C, which are generally brightly colored to attract birds so that they will eat the fruit and distribute the seeds. Suddenly mammals could compete with the birds for brightly colored berries and fruits. Monkeys started to not just eat insects. Since they were climbing in trees, they began to forage for fruit.

"As primates started consuming more fruit, their need for a gene to code how to make vitamin C disappeared. The gene that made vitamin C eventually disappeared. And we became addicted to fruit. Simulations confirm this expectation. If you allow vitamin C to enter an environment, the gene for producing it very quickly degrades. If vitamin C disappears before the gene is hopelessly gone, the capacity to generate vitamin C reappears. Over time, other genes relevant to making sure that fruit is present emerged through natural selection. This gene duplication made it possible for us to identify subtle color changes that birds can also readily detect. Suddenly the duplication and variation of a gene that was involved in a pigmentation of the eye became useful because we were competing with the birds for fruit. Where one gene made vitamin C, many function to help us find fruit.

"It gets even more complicated and interesting, Paul. Some things happen spontaneously through our interaction with the environment and have no relation to genetics at all. That could be relevant to you also. I'll tell you a story about plants. The way that leaves spiral around a stem of a plant is described by a sequence of numbers called the Fibonacci sequence, which is also found in musical harmonies. Plants seem to use this numerical sequencing to place their leaves around a stem in such a way that they 'stay out of each others' way' and allow every leaf to get the most sunlight. This produces a beautiful spiraling of leaves around the branch. There are no genes for the spirals. The spirals just happen as the plants interact with the sun in an entirely self-organizing process. The plant hormones that are involved work on the basis of relative concentrations: changes in the concentrations of plant hormones produce different twists of the spiral, but the basic structure remains.

"This is important for all of our lives. We need to remember that some of what happens to us is not the result of genetics or even epigenetics, but rather quirky interactions of parts of us with the conditions of the external world. The connections between brain areas change during development based on what input comes from the environment. For example, the blind mole rat has small eyes that never open. In its brain, the areas that would process vision are taken over by the areas that process sound and touch. The available input from the environment shapes the brain. This is called neuroplasticity. Neuroplasticity means that your brain is allowed to change its structure and its connections all through your life.

"Here are some other facts that will help you to believe me. There are people with six fingers whose brains have adapted so that they use them without impediment. In blind people, areas of their visual cortex are shifted to manage sound and touch. If we cut visual and auditory input in other animals, related changes will be generated. The available sensory systems take over. For example, frogs don't have depth perception like mammals have. But if we implant a third eye in the middle of the head of a tadpole, it produces an unprecedented visual map that is similar to those of cats and monkeys with three-dimensional vision. Frogs have never had this kind of map in their evolutionary history. This three-dimensional vision emerges due to the self-organizing effects of neuronal activity on synaptic connections and not because of any genes to make it so.

"The brain changes its gray matter in response to training. For example, reading music changes the structure of the primary auditory cortex of our brains.[4] Bilingual people have extra grey matter in the brain in an area associated with language called Wernicke's area, which is in the left anterior temporal cortex. The longer they've been bilingual, the more they have.[5] This is important, because it means you will develop the brain connections to help you get through grad school. I will help you do this. We will do it together.

"Paul, natural selection as in genetics is a passive, subtractive process. It takes away freedom. What I have been telling you about are those things that increase freedom and make people uniquely what they are. You have acquired all this freedom from the efforts of your ancestors, the freedom to transcend the immediate past and to draw on what has come before."

The "Genes" of Social Learning

Stories are the way in which social learning is transmitted and in which our genetics can be modified through experience. Shared stories allow us to form a coherent intent, to all point in the same direction, and to collaborate in ways inaccessible to primates who lack our narrative capacity. In our human world, emotions are learned and understood through story, especially those emotions that we construct and modify beyond the few that all mammals share. Emotions play a vital role in directing attention, forming durable memory, and giving power to ritual and symbols. Our memory is best designed to store emotional information communicated through story. If experimental subjects are asked to memorize emotional material, they find it easier to remember words that have emotional significance. Enhanced brain activity is associated with emotion. In neuroimaging studies, when an emotional word appears, the amygdala, part of the limbic system, or "emotional center" of the brain, lights up.

Stories are the building blocks of culture, playing an important role in generating emotional states that motivate socially important actions. A Choctaw story from present-day Mississippi tells how "Little People," supernatural beings or spirits who lived near the Choctaw, sometimes seized young children to evaluate them for worthiness to receive special teachings about healing.

The Little People were less than three feet tall and lived deep in forests in caves hidden under large rocks. They were always on watch, and when a young boy wandered into the woods well out of sight from his home, they would seize him and take him to their caves. Many times the cave was far away, and the spirit that captured the child and the little boy would have to travel far, climbing many hills and crossing many streams. When they reached the cave, the Little People would take the boy inside, where he was met by three very old spirits with long white hair.

The first would offer the boy a knife; the second, a bunch of poisonous herbs; the third, a bunch of herbs yielding good medicine. If the child accepted the knife, he was certain to become a bad man and might even kill his friends. If he accepted the poisonous herbs, he would never be able to cure or help his people. But if he accepted the good herbs, he was destined to become a great doctor, an important and influential man of his tribe, and to win the confidence of all his people. When he accepted the good herbs, these three old spirits would teach him the secrets of making medicines from herbs, roots, and barks of certain trees, and of treating and curing various fevers, pains, and other sicknesses.

The child would remain with the old spirits for three days, after which he was returned. He would not tell where he had been or what he had seen or heard. Not until he became a man would he make use of the knowledge gained from the spirits, and never would he reveal to others how it was acquired. It is said among the Choctaws that few children waited to accept the offering of the good herbs from the third spirit, and that is why great doctors and other men of influence are relatively rare.

Choctaw prophets and herb doctors, however, claim to have seen these old spirits and to communicate with them. During the darkest nights in all kinds of weather, strange lights wandering through the woods portend a healer and his or her little helper looking for that special herb to treat and cure some very sick person.

Similar stories exist in other cultures. Are these dreams, visions, or could they be actual experiences? Do genetic tendencies make one more likely to "accept the good herbs," and after that, what role does the social environment have in the process of learning how to be a healer?

My sense of this story is that it was designed to help children learn to delay gratification and to cultivate the trait of waiting for the offer of the "good herbs," the impulse to serve the people instead of the impulse to take something for one's own benefit. This story was part of the social environment that taught people how to be healers and what to expect from healers.

8

How Culture Is Context and Context Shapes Behavior

Two people can react to the same idea, opinion, or data in opposite ways, and the reasons for this are often ideological, which means that the people have very different stories about how to interpret the world. Our preferred stories about how things work always have a political aspect that comes from our social class, upbringing, and all the stories that we have absorbed from our past. The stories we tell as truth are told for an audience, to position ourselves within our social context to maximize our opportunities and resources. In that respect our only difference from the alpha-male of the wolf pack is our greater range of potential narratives from which to choose.

The most privileged stories in the present time are those of "hard science." This story tells us that there is one truth to be discovered and preferred over others, that one part of our experience is "objective" (meaning that scientists accept it as real and can measure it) and the other part is "subjective" (meaning that scientists do not value it). What we have learned to call "objective" is of course a mental model built on the basis of experiences which we call "subjective." It is a social construction.

*Experience can be organized and categorized in many
other possible ways than our distinction between
"objective" and "subjective," often translated as physical
and mental.*

CHARLES WHITEHEAD,
THE ORIGIN OF CONSCIOUSNESS IN THE SOCIAL WORLD

Thinking via Experience

In a move that returns us to the indigenous perspective, contemporary neuroscience has led us back to the idea that the distinction between mental and physical is a delusion created by the brain.[1] Christopher Frith, a professor of neuropsychology at the Wellness Trust Centre for Neuroimaging at University College London, writes, "Most of our interactions with other people are interactions between minds, not between bodies. My brain constructs models of my mind, your mind, and the physical world by making predictions and amending the model when predictions go wrong."[2]

This is the same as saying that we construct stories to explain the world and use these explanations (stories) to quickly make predictions about the world and guide our behavior. They are of great evolutionary value, for they allow a speed of movement and processing that would be impossible without stories about how things work. When our explanatory stories fail us and the predictions we make based on them don't come true, we must revise our stories (amend our models). Continuing to use a story that doesn't work in the face of repeated evidence is another way of conceptualizing psychiatric disturbances.

We think via our experience, which relies on highly involved mental processes.[3] University of Auckland Professor Brian Boyd writes, "We encounter the world multimodally, through our multiple senses, our emotions, our actions, and our reflections. Cognition . . . begins . . . with multimodal simulations of multimodal memories of multimodal experiences."[4] In short, inner experience represents the world in all the dimensions in which we experience it. In our thought, we reactivate "perceptual, motor, and introspective states acquired during experience with world, body, and mind; . . . the brain captures states across the modalities and integrates them with a multimodal representation stored in memory."[5] When we recall our first love, she is not just a name, or a face, but all the multiple sensory experiences encountered in that relationship, or at least a representative sum of them, enough that we can construct a narrative of that experience and of what happened.

Boyd wrote, "[W]e think, remember, and imagine by mentally simulating or reactivating elements of what have previously perceived, understood, enacted, and experienced."[6] As mentioned earlier, mirror neurons form the neurological basis for these simulations. In discussing the widespread recognition that recall is never an exact replication of experience, Boyd points out that this is not "a limitation of memory, but an adaptive design that helps us to retrieve and recombine memories in order to run vivid simulations of future experience. . . . Where the exact memories of savants allow remarkable recall of the past, but, at the expense of their coping with the future, our normal constructive episodic memory* system can draw on elements of the past and retain the general sense or gist of what has happened. Critically, it can flexibly extract, recombine, and reassemble these elements in a way that allows us to simulate, imagine, or 'pre-experience' events that have never occurred previously in the exact form in which we imagine them."[7] Our simulations involve most of the same brain areas as recalling the past, especially the hippocampus and prefrontal, medial temporal, and parietal regions.[8] Neuroscientist Randy Buckner calls this circuitry a "life simulator."[9]

In his book *Descartes' Error: Emotion, Reason, and the Human Brain,* neuroscientist Antonio Damasio describes how we use simulation as a survival tool:

Armed with these neural circuits and capacities, we get to play out scenarios in a "test drive" fashion before actually carrying out the

---

*According to Boyd, "Episodic memory records particular events that I remember as *experienced,* as *mine,* and can more or less locate to a specific place and time in my past, like my memory of climbing a particular rock in childhood, or breaking off a poplar branch to use as a knight's lance."

behavior. I have to admit, developing these capacities has aided my ability to interact with the more resistant members of my audiences. Now, I play out the scenario of how they will respond to me if I say what first comes to my mind, continuing my scenarios until I find one that will not get me uninvited from dinner or have my lecture canceled. All of us do this. We rehearse what we wish to say to someone—our boss, wife, girlfriend, co-worker—anticipating their response and the consequences, until we arrive at a comfortable version that is a compromise between what we wished we could say and what will actually have the most favorable consequences. This represents an amazing tool for social survival. When we run our vivid simulations, we evaluate the results by the emotional weightings our bodies assigned at the time to previous experiences upon which we are using to build our simulations.[10]

How Society Builds Our Brains

Contemporary cultural psychologists have shown that the social environment affects how people conceive of self,[11] how they attribute cause to events,[12] how they attend to and remember objects in their environment,[13] and how they perceive, experience, respond to, and predict their own and others' emotions.[14] Different social environments (cultures) produce differences in all of these tasks, showing that "the human mind is intimately linked with its social world or cultural context and that culture is continuously created through the actions and products of the individual minds that comprise it."[15] Neuroscientists Joan Chiao and Nalini Ambady[16] have written about how East-West (collectivist versus individualist) cultural differences affect the ways we process visual perception, self-knowledge, and self-awareness.[17]

From a separate direction, Dr. Robert Turner, professor at the Max Planck Institute for Human Cognitive and Brain Studies in Leipzig, Germany, and Charles Whitehead are showing through neural imaging studies that our collective representations (the often crucial components of human life that have meaningful existence because we agree that they do, such as customs, money, religion, cosmology, language, games, laws, power structures, and artistic genres) have well-defined representations within our brains. Turner and colleagues developed ultrafast echo-planar brain imaging technology to record rapid changes in cerebral blood flow,[18] which led to a number of studies showing the pervasive influence of social environment on the development of functional brain anatomy.[19] Turner's group has produced good evidence to support the view that our social environment and relationships actually form our brains and their synaptic connections and functional activities.

This developing body of research furthers the notion that mind is constructed socially and even that the brains that support mind are socially generated. The brain builds interpretive maps of the outer world and its characters, which allows us to function effectively. Whitehead writes, "Western individualism has long delayed scientific recognition of the social nature of consciousness—or at least of the human mind and brain. It took cognitive neuroscience over thirty years to come up with the notion of the social brain."[20]

Doidge points out that neuroscientists used to believe that the brain's maps were fixed early in life, and describes how Paul Merzenich discovered that these brains are shaped by the environment and are changing all the time. He writes, "Merzenich discovered that [brain] maps are neither immutable within a single brain nor universal, but vary in their borders and size from person to person." Merzenich originally studied maps of our body sensations, but the same can be said for our more sophisticated inner brain maps of our social world. "The shape of our brain maps changes depending upon what we do over the course of our lives."[21] We could say that psychiatric problems are disturbances in that map.

These maps are communicated in the form of stories.[22] Social approaches to consciousness emphasize the importance of shared experiences, which occur by means of social display ranging from facial expressions and body language to music, dance, art, and theater. Conventionalized displays that serve to unify experience within cultural groups were called "collective representations" by the sociologist Émile

Durkheim (1858–1917) and include language, ritual, wealth displays, and all of the cultural arts.[23]

Whitehead was interested in the social theory of George Herbert Meade about imitating and being imitated by others and becoming aware of other people through this imitation. Whitehead thought that a uniquely human characteristic was the ability to play a role, and conducted a study using the hypothesis that areas in the brain support the performance of roles. His subjects were drama students, whom he asked to look at speeches on a screen and to quietly put themselves into the role of each of several speakers, including Shakespeare's Lady Macbeth. Control conditions consisted of reading prose versions of news headlines and instructions from equipment manuals; Whitehead thought no role-playing was involved in those tasks. Brain activation was associated with the switch from the role-playing task to the control task, providing evidence that the default condition of the human brain is the role-playing state (given that activation was seen only during the switching of roles).[24]

Whitehead concluded that our brains are actually role-playing all the time, which is consistent with my belief that we are continually playing a multitude of characters in a variety of overlapping and intersecting plays coproduced with all the members of our social network and influenced by (even embedded within) the larger societal stories in which we all participate, perhaps without even realizing it. Role-play and negotiating story are the foundations of culture, and how we continually live stories through our enactment of roles formed through relationships. This makes it clear how important childhood is as a sheltered time of "extended irresponsibility," which allows us to develop our powers of make-believe and role-play. As we mature, the right hemisphere of our brain seeks explanation of the world around us at progressively deeper levels and with more coherence on both a local and a larger scale. This leads us further and further into narrative, into developing coherent stories about our world and our lives.[25] Whitehead believes that these narratives and the skills involved in producing them are prerequisites for human cooperation, culture, and reflective consciousness.[26]

As an example of this, the Kwiao in the Solomon Islands use the same word to refer to black and to blue. Traditionally they paint their houses black, but when given blue paint, they create an "unsightly patchwork of blue and black." When asked why, they deny any patchwork, asserting that their houses are uniformly and beautifully black.[27] Without words to distinguish blue and black, the difference does not exist. They have no social mirror to help them distinguish black from blue. They are unable to develop a shared experience of this difference.

Sharing the World

Turner and Whitehead are trying to delineate the mechanisms underlying our human ability to share our representations of the world. They believe there are two major processes involved. The first is an automatic form of priming (sometimes referred to as contagion, or empathy), whereby our representations of the world become aligned with those of the person with whom we are interacting. We align ourselves with others through the sharing of narratives that help us to look together in the same direction. The second is a form of forward modeling, analogous to that used in the control of our own actions. We use our stories about the world to predict the results of our and others' actions and revise our models through comparing results to predictions. Our predictive models (stories) help us build theories of mind about other people, so that we have ideas about other peoples' motivations and probable behavior.[28]

Research conducted by Frith and his team at the Wellcome Trust Centre for Neuroimaging has led them to conclude that consciousness is an evolved adaptation whose function is social, enabling us to share our collective representations of the world, this being the prerequisite for human culture. Frith wrote, "It is not just our experience of agency; all of the contents of consciousness are the outcome of a social endeavour."[29] Indeed, Steven Pinker pointed out that in the preindustrialized past strategic social information would have all been about people we had met before and would often meet again.[30] Pinker believes this explains our endless fascination with information (and especially gossip) about other people, since it helps us understand their motivations and predict their future actions.

Mirrors in the mind imply the existence of social mirrors, upon which self-awareness depends for its existence. Mirror neurons may play an important role in the underlying physiology of how we share stories. For more than a century, Broca's area of the brain was considered only language related, but if that were so, why would it be activated when we watch another person perform a movement? Perhaps because we talk to ourselves about what the other is doing. Perhaps because we generate a story about what is going on that we tell ourselves without moving our lips. Perhaps because we only recently learned to inhibit the motor movements of speech, previously always talking to ourselves out loud, only to achieve silence relatively recently. Certainly young children have to learn to inhibit saying whatever they are thinking.

Related to this, Colwyn Trevarthen, a longtime developmental researcher at the University of Edinburgh, showed that even preverbal infants vocalize and move their lips as if they are telling a story.[31] The musicality is correct; all that is lacking are the actual words, but these will come. Indeed, infants retain memories for several months without language and can later superimpose language on previously encoded preverbal memories.[32]

University of Milan philosopher Corrado Sinigaglia believes that mirror neurons allow us to gain insight into basic forms of action understanding that are "below" and "before" any deliberate mentalizing, enriching our overall understanding by bringing to light different types and levels of information.[33] Mirror neurons thus help us understand more about how people extract attitudes and beliefs from nonverbal behavior. Max Weisbuch and Nalini Ambady, professors at Tufts University in Medford, Massachusetts, argue that this extraction is both ubiquitous and efficient.[34] They posit gesture and elaborate forms of nonverbal behavior as being necessary antecedents to language and shared conceptual understanding. They believe that subtle and largely unintentional nonverbal behaviors play a key role in building consensual beliefs within a culture. Thus, we can come to adopt the same attitudes, beliefs, and behaviors in the absence of verbal communication, and our own nonverbal behavior reflects the extracted attitudes, beliefs, and ideals of our group, serving as a means for transmitting culture.[35]

Trevarthen showed that the desire for conversation-like communication develops in infants before exploratory behavior with objects.[36] He wrote, "A child is born with motives to find and use the motives of other persons in 'conversational' negotiation of purposes, emotions, experiences, and meaning. The efficiency of sympathetic engagement between persons signals the ability of each to 'model' or 'mirror' the motivations and purposes of companions, immediately. . . . Infants . . . have this."

Unlike other primates, humans have eyes whose elongated shape and whose color contrast between iris and sclera make eye direction easy to see: in short, humans have evolved eyes that reveal rather than conceal their direction. Monkey babies lack the stimulus tools to capture and hold their mothers' attention. Chimpanzee mothers rarely gaze into their babies' eyes or communicate with them. . . . [Human] infants eyes after birth can focus only about 15 cm away, the distance between the mother's breast and her face, and unlike infants in any other species, they maintain eye contact while suckling. Newborns prefer to attend to faces more than to any other visual stimulus and under laboratory conditions they have been shown to be capable of imitating humans, but not animated models, within an hour of birth. At only one day old, they will wiggle their limbs and orient their faces in time with taped female speech, but not with disconnected vowels or tapping sounds. For the first six months, infants have a love affair with human faces, voices, and touch, a factor that allows adults to bootstrap their children's intelligence by focusing their attention. Across the world, older humans instinctively address infants in "motherese," whose higher pitch appeals and whose simple but exaggerated emotional contours, coupled with highly contrastive visual signing, can be decoded without language and can therefore recruit and maintain attention. Minds find more attractive what they can process more easily and the highly patterned and stylized language simplifies understanding and invites attention.[37]

The presence of an infant releases special tenderness in human mothers. According to Boyd,[38] infants prefer recordings of lullabies sung by mothers while a child was present to those recorded without children present and adults also judge these versions as more loving.

The phrase "theory of mind" is shorthand for the cognitive ability to recognize that other people have similar mental and intentional states as we do and that their behavior is motivated just as ours is. They have a purpose for doing what they do, and they know, believe, imagine, or pretend just as we do. We need theories of other people's minds (their intent, wishes, desires, and so on) in order to relate. Two theories, simulation theory and theory theory, claim to explain how children acquire a theory of mind. Both can be true.

Simulation theory assumes that we are first of all self-aware and that we infer that others are self-aware by mentally simulating their behavior. This fits what we have discussed earlier about the brain containing a life simulator. It assumes some measure of "theater of mind," which is the ability to run social scenarios in imagination, with a cast of internalized actors who behave as if they have minds, knowledge, beliefs, emotions, and intentions of their own.[39]

Theory theory holds that children must develop a concept, or "theory," of mental states in order to acquire a theory of mind. This concept specifically depends on mimicry. The acquisition of a mental-states concept confers reflective insight into one's own mind and the ability to read other minds at the same time. For me, theory theory just refers to the story that results from running enough simulations to build up a narrative about another person. Theory theory has been confirmed by experiments in which, for example, a child is shown an M&M's box and asked what she thinks is in the box. She says "M&M's." Then she is shown that actually pencils are in the box, and not M&M's. Then, a doll is brought into the room. The child is asked what the doll would think is in the box. She answers "pencils." If asked why she didn't say "M&M's," she will deny having ever said there were M&M's in the box. This continues until she builds her own theory of mind. Like the islanders who cannot tell blue from black, she cannot be reflexively self-aware until this theory of mind develops.

Our social life rests to a large extent on our ability to understand the intentions of others. The theories of mind that are being discussed here are ways to explain how we accomplish this. Without the capacity to develop a perception of other people's intentions, we would be completely unable to interpret other people's behavior. Autistic individuals have this difficulty, and indeed, current thinking is that these individuals lack the capacity to form a theory of other people's minds.

The recent research on mirror neurons helps us understand that they facilitate this by directly matching the sensory representation of observed actions with our own motor representation of those same actions. In a sense, we understand others by generating a story based on what we would feel and think and intend if we were performing (the motor element) those same behaviors. Earlier, in chapter 4, I wrote about Ekman's studies of the facial recognition of emotion. Perhaps it goes further than that. Perhaps we entrain each other to produce the same displays of emotion (performances) through our repeated interactions via our mirror neurons. Mirror neurons represent the neural mechanism for brains being social organs, meant to keep us connected and correctly interpreting others' behavior.

Maya Gratier and Colwyn Trevarthen took this further in their studies of mother–infant vocal interaction.[40] They researched the forms of meaningful engagement that emerge in vocal interactions with preverbal infants, particularly regarding the narrative organization of coordinated expression in time. They related culture and meaning in preverbal exchange to an "implicit knowing" involving habits, procedures, and patterns that are outside of conscious awareness derived from direct perception of the purposeful and coordinated body movements of self and other (also called felt immediacy). These may be mediated through mirror neurons. Infants may be able to "go through the motions" in their brains via motor neurons of the motor behaviors of their caretakers without yet having the capacity to duplicate these movements. This may help them to "understand" on some level the intentions and emotions of their caretakers.

Boyd has summarized how this unfolds in the human child:

By about 8 months, parent-infant "proto-conversations"—more like a song than a sentence—set the scene for the special nature of human sociality and for art. Aptly described as multimedia performances, since they use eyes and faces, hands and feet, voice and movement, these proto-conversations consist of rhythmic, finely attuned turn-taking and mutual imitation, involving elaboration, exaggeration, repetition, and surprise, with each partner anticipating the others' response so as to coordinate their emotions in patterned sequence. Though taking different forms in different cultures, this proto-conversation in all human cultures resembles a duet in which child and adult "seek harmony and counterpoint on one beat to create a melody."[41]

Although all apes note where others look, on the basis of head direction, only humans, from a year old, make eye gaze as well as head movement. Human one-year-olds engage in joint attention—following others' hands or eyes and checking to see that the others follow theirs—and in proto-declarative pointing—indicating objects or events simply for the sake of sharing attention to them, something that apes never do.[42] They expect others to share interest, attention, and response: "This by itself is rewarding for infants—apparently in a way it is not for any other species on the planet."[43]

Gratier and Trevarthen confirmed that the shared focus and emotional involvement of mother and infant in the expressions of each other attest to a unique intersubjective awareness that leads infants to participate in the activity of culture[44] (and leads culture to shape their brains to further participate in it, in aligning with the neuroanatomical findings of Robert Turner[45]). They believe that narrative is a fundamental mode of human collective thinking—and acting—and that its basic function is the production of meaning, or "world making," to paraphrase psychologist and educator Jerome Bruner.

Gratier and Trevarthen redefined the boundaries of the term *narrative* to include "narratives without words" based on processes of temporal organization in language and music. They showed indices of a narrative organization in live mother–infant interactions based on communicative musicality. They claimed that interactions between young infants and adults are not only narrative in form but also present a narrative content of "common sense." They showed narrative organization for both spontaneous mother-infant interaction and interaction based on singing for and with infants.[46]

Trevarthen believes that classic attachment theory, and the contemporary transformation of it into a theory of maternal external regulation of the infant's physiology and emotional processes, fails to grasp the importance of motives for relationships between offspring and their parents that serve shared discovery of new ways of behaving.[47] He believes that a good human mother does more than protect her baby from fear. She is more than a known and secure base from which the child explores and gains experience. She and others in the infant's world are friends and playmates. From the moment of birth there is a mental engagement between interests and purposes and an emotional evaluation of the quality of concordant activity to discover and use experiences. Meaning is discovered in playful collaborative friendships, and its discovery is motivated by pleasure in dynamically responsive company.

The young child seeks a place in a community of common sense and not just security in its attachments. The neuroscience shows that deep-seated emotional systems have a role in both the sharing of emotions and experiences with other individuals and adaptive change in the growing brain and its cognitive capacities. Trevarthen proposes that human beings have a specially adapted capacity for sympathy of brain activity that drives cultural learning.[48]

In a similar vein, we can criticize conditioning theories of behavior for neglecting the active effort that humans expend in manipulating the environment and influencing others in it to get what we want. We are not passively conditioned by our surroundings. Like infants, we actively attempt to engage others around us to co-construct a new environment more conducive to our receiving what we seek to have.

Native elders teach about knowledge production being a circular process. We figure out how to do something, try it out, get feedback, refine it, try it again, and then say we've learned something that we can teach others. Indigenous knowledge systems differ in that spirits are sources of knowledge, though the same problems of verification exist as with any produced knowledge, and methods of consensus-building through councils and talking circles have evolved to evaluate the information provided by spirits. Nevertheless, we can begin to see an overlap developing between neuroscience with its mirror neurons and its social brain and the teachings of the elders.

Killing the Pain Monster

We live storied lives. We organize experience into stories as we share life interactively with others. The plot, action, characters, and morals of the stories we hear influence our synaptic connections; they change our brains. Stories also live through us. We are born into ongoing stories—those of our families, nations, religions, and cultures. People who cannot organize experience into stories are called psychotic. Narrative psychiatry makes sense of "mental illness" within the context of all those stories being lived by the person.

"Beatrix" provides us with a story to integrate all that I have been discussing. In reading this story, pay attention to the ways in which Beatrix and her views arise from her social environment. We can see a collaborative exchanging of stories that explain and guide her behavior. Her stories, representing her inner maps of the world, are sufficient to explain her behavior. No intrapsychic structures or personality variables are needed.

Beatrix was a forty-two-year-old woman with almost-grown children who worked as a psychotherapist with a degree in social work. She came from Toronto for an intensive retreat with me because she was in constant pain and had been for twenty-five years—steadily, progressively worsening pain. Like most people with chronic pain, Beatrix had been diagnosed with everything imaginable, from fibromyalgia to chronic Lyme disease to osteoarthritis to autoimmune arthritis. She also had high cholesterol and autonomic instability, meaning that her blood pressure, heart rate, sweating, and other involuntary functions could vary enormously and without seeming provocation.

Like many people who come to see me, Beatrix had been to an impressive array of various practitioners, from A to Z, ayurvedic to zen, with every letter in between. What puzzled Beatrix was that she lived very cleanly and "did everything correctly" and still had pain. The plot here was Beatrix's idea that wellness is a reward for doing everything correctly. Of course, "correctly" must be defined by stories; it is different for everyone. For Beatrix, "correctly" meant eating vegan, organic, and bland. It meant avoiding spices, alcohol, tobacco, scents, preservatives, dyes, and colorings. It meant doing t'ai chi every day in proper form. It meant "taking care of herself."

What emerged was a feeling of rigidity. This becomes a challenge to describe, because it is what author Malcolm Gladwell calls "chunked observations." These consist of intuitions that we have, which arise from our ability to grasp massive amounts of information quickly in perceptual "chunks" in a process that is largely outside of our conscious awareness. Perhaps we do this through the use of our mirror neurons. With their help, we can sense rigidity easier than we can describe how we recognize it.[49]

When I begin working with someone like Beatrix, I often use imagery to get a grasp of the story from the illness's point of view. Native American elders have often told me that every illness has one or more spirits behind it, fueling it, giving it life, making it move. They have also told me that anything that moves must have a spirit within it or behind it. Having grown up in the Native American world, I am completely comfortable with the concept of spirits and use it in my work. Beatrix also was comfortable with that view. But I invite readers who feel differently to see "spirit" as metaphor; it doesn't matter from the standpoint of our discussion whether or not spirits and spirit communication are real or metaphor.

After relaxation (what could also be called a hypnotic induction), Beatrix was asked to connect with the spirit behind or within her illness. Beatrix spontaneously launched into past-life memories. She had been trained to do past-life regressions and valued that method. While that was not what I had in mind, I believe, as Milton Erickson did, that I should always follow the lead of my clients, so past-life regression was what we were going to do. Beatrix went to a life in Egypt in which she and her mother were gardeners together. She reflected that in this life her mother had never been willing to get dirty.

Then, with relatively little encouragement on my part, she contacted her mother, who had died two years previously from medical mishaps. Her mother was with her father, who had committed suicide fifteen years earlier. He had been an outdoorsman, a man of action, an adventurer. He had heart failure from multiple heart attacks and chose to die by his own hand rather than be tortured by his doctors to change his ways, including abandoning the foods he loved. Rather than wait for the next heart attack or for the fluid buildup to kill him, he shot himself. Beatrix announced that her parents had abandoned her, moving on to greener pastures, but not before they dumped the pain of both of their lives on her. Though her pain began before her father died, it had worsened significantly around the time of his death, and again at the time of her mother's death.

I encouraged Beatrix to seek out those who could teach us about how to reduce pain. Beatrix went along an image path to a time in the past in which she thought she was a Native man named Red Sky. He was in terrible pain because his entire village had been massacred by Europeans. The young men under his charge had raided the Europeans prematurely, and the village had been destroyed in retaliation. She described a tragic scene of Red Sky killing himself in grief and agony, stabbing himself in just the place where she felt pain intermittently, in her upper abdomen. She believed this had happened in Saskatchewan, although that was unlikely because there had been no Indian Wars there. That was an East Coast phenomenon, taking place in the area where the French and Indian War was fought. By the time the Europeans reached Saskatchewan, they had figured out that it was much more cost-effective to kill the food (all the buffalo) and starve the Natives than to kill the Natives themselves.

What emerged for me in listening to Beatrix was a heroic story in which the pain she suffered was her mother's pain, her father's pain, and the pain of a tragic but heroic "Red Indian" named Red Sky whose family had been killed, quite possibly by Beatrix's ancestors. She was the wounded healer who suffered for others. She needed this exotic explanation for her pain because it could not have anything to do with her, as someone who did everything right, including not expressing the anger that she quite obviously felt toward doctors who didn't cure her, her father who left without giving her the opportunity to say goodbye, and her mother for abandoning her.

Beatrix's story left out any personal agency or any influences of her own community and context. In her social environment she had risen to be seen as "perfect and exemplary" by members of her network. She had the perfect diet, the perfect lifestyle, the perfect husband, the perfect children, and so on. The underlying plot (or core belief in cognitive behavior therapy) of her stories is that living perfectly prevents and is completely incompatible with any illness or suffering. Therefore, she had to be sick for other reasons.

After the imagery, we talked about Beatrix's life. I learned to my surprise that there had been one year in which she had been completely pain-free. This was the year after she was introduced to t'ai chi. She described it as a magical year of effortless movement and of being surprisingly able to heal others. This "spell" lifted when she decided to become a t'ai chi instructor. Suddenly she felt that she had to prove herself to be a good instructor. She felt others watching her doing and teaching t'ai chi. She woefully told me that she lost the chi when she started seriously studying the chi. Every so often in hearing a person's story, I am suddenly aware of a core plot line. I explored this further. Never did a moment go by that Beatrix didn't feel on stage. She was the therapist/healer for her community. She was the example of "good, healthy living." She hid her pain from everyone, for it wouldn't do for her audience to know how much she truly suffered, despite all the things that she "did right." It reminded me of the hidden pain of some people who kill themselves, perhaps related to her suicide theme.

This provides us with an example of how context and culture influence brain. Beatrix's symptoms were not separate from her life, which was shaped by a social environment that demanded perfection. This emerged from our discussions about her childhood home, in which anything less than an A+ was unacceptable and anything less than first place in sports was also unthinkable. The dominant story of mainstream culture is to

blame someone for illness—either the person, their behavior, their genetics, toxins, or bacteria. Beatrix was saturated in a culture of blame. She
had to blame someone or something. In her own life, she blamed people's
"bad behavior" for their suffering. She was judgmental about people who
didn't live "correctly." She believed that she lived correctly, so she couldn't
have any agency in her pain. Embedded within this culture, she had no
choice but to seek explanations in the suffering of her parents and of a
spirit from the past. These were acceptable explanations.

In my way of working with people, I like to do an opening ceremony
and prayer. In my story, spirits talk to me. Others would call this intuition or inspiration, though the word *inspiration* derives from *in-spirare,*
"to breathe into," and is related to the word *spiritus,* or *spirit.* For years
I have worked at learning to do a Cherokee tobacco healing divination
ceremony in which spirits come in response to an offering of tobacco and
tell what's wrong. I did this ceremony for Beatrix and saw (or imagined
seeing) the spirits of her mother and father. I saw her character Red Sky,
who had to be part of the Iroquoian group of people from the upstate
New York area. He was quite funny and didn't think of himself as her
past life at all. Nor was he suffering continually, as she imagined him to
be. He didn't need or require her healing of him as she thought. He had
one thing to say.

"Tell her to hunt and kill one deer the traditional way and she will be
well. But she'll never do it." And that's all he had to say.

Beatrix was aghast when I reported what I had heard. "Absolutely
not," she said. "There has to be another way. Knowing me, why would
any spirit say such a thing?"

"I could guess," I said.

"Then guess."

"I would guess that it's an incredibly wise opportunity to do something completely objectionable perfectly well," I said. "Imagine how long
it would take for you to learn how to make a bow and arrow, learn how to
shoot it, learn how to track and stalk a deer, learn how to clean a deer, to
kill and clean just one. It strikes me as an amazing challenge for someone
who wants so much to be part of Native spirituality."

That started a repartee between us that continued throughout our time together. I saw myself as almost falling back into my dialectical behavior therapy training—to always present a fixed and rigid idea with its opposite. That is the essence of dialectics—to hold an idea and its opposite and find a way to integrate them. I didn't care if Beatrix ever ate meat or hunted, but I was trying to help her see the rigidity of her ideas, and I did think it odd that she was so steeped in Native culture and spirituality and yet so judgmental of people who hunted and ate meat.

More history emerged in our ongoing discussions. She'd had four miscarriages and had felt that she'd never carry a pregnancy to term. Only when she finally gave up on ever having a child did she have two children. Eight to nine years previously she had started menopause and had become more anxious than she had ever been in her life. She described flicking a tick off her arm three years previously and seeing a big red circle where it had been. She described debilitating head pain for the past three years, which had responded briefly to *N*-acetylcysteine* and other supplements.

Eighteen years before, she had developed a muscular dystonia, a condition characterized by muscle spasms, cramps, and pain, leading to two MRIs of her brain, which showed an enlarged cistern (part of the cerebrospinal system) that eminent experts apparently decided to be normal for her. Paradoxically, the MRIs made her feel better. All her joints hurt, as did her lower back from spondylolisthesis (in which one vertebra slips forward on the vertebra below it). She was always trying to figure out the meaning of her symptoms. On a purely physical level, she believed that the pain in her solar plexus was from scar tissue from her two cesarean deliveries. She'd had chronic asthma for the past twenty-eight years, originating when she lived in an area of Ontario in which a terrible fire had burned out of control, clouding the air with smoke.

Beatrix also told me about all of her healing activities—daily t'ai chi, listening to harmonics, beading, writing poetry, gardening, resting, and

---

N-acetylcysteine is a natural product, a sulfur-rich amino acid that is used to aid detoxification through enhancing sulfation, one method the body uses to remove toxic materials.

walking with her dogs. She went to an osteopath monthly for manipulation and energy work. She went to a shamanic practitioner monthly and
took extra plant sterols and fiber. Again, from my "chunking" point of view
(meaning grasping the whole without necessarily knowing how I do it),
Beatrix seemed to be doing too much. Her healing had a driven quality to
it, as if for an audience, as if to prove she was doing everything she could.

Next Beatrix read me eighty pages of an unfinished book that she
had written. I learned that she felt cursed in a certain way for being
named after the famous Beatrix Potter, author of Peter Rabbit storybooks
that her parents had loved as young children. What became clear from
Beatrix's rendition was her incredible absorption in herself and the significance of everything that she was going through. There were so many
layers of meaning that I became confused. It represented overanalysis,
which is what I saw Beatrix doing. She thought too much and was not
fully present very often. I thought about the one year when she had been
"thoughtless" about t'ai chi, because no one was watching. So long as she
had an audience (and she was on a pedestal for her community), she had
to be perfect. I felt sad.

The only time I felt that I could get her attention was when I was
doing Cherokee energy healing/craniosacral work on her head. "What
would it be like to do nothing?" I wondered, trying to communicate
these thoughts to Beatrix as I worked on her. "What would it be like to
start over, empty? What would it be like to stop being so conscious about
everything?" She did stop thinking briefly.

Beatrix had never participated in a social milieu in which she could
relax and be less than perfect. But the effort to be perfect in every way
was taking quite a toll on her. "What if it were not so hard?" I thought to
myself, trying to make this suggestion to Beatrix during imagery. "What
if she just needed to relax and be present in the here and now?"

I decided to tell her a story to help her to relax. I chose a Coyote story
because of her identification with Native American culture and also because
she loved Coyote stories and expected me, as her Coyote doctor, to tell them.
I picked a long rambling narrative about Coyote's adventures in the Pacific
Northwest from the Okanagan (a tribe in central Washington and lower

British Columbia). I first told her the story about how Coyote got chosen to kill all the evil monsters left on the earth so that people could live in peace. This was one of Coyote's duties, though it helps to be a trickster and a shape-shifter when dealing with monsters. I saw Beatrix's efforts at perfection as equally heroic as Coyote killing all the evil monsters and hoped she would have the same association. I was also thinking that monsters would make a good metaphor for her pain.

This is what I said:

Coyote was walking north along a glistening snow-covered trail, quietly whispering a silly song. She was looking for monsters on the bright snow-covered hills, though she wished she were looking for a husband. Dark rows of trees lined the distant mountains. One of those mountains was shaped like a heart that had previously beaten inside a monster Coyote had already killed. When she took out its heart, it turned into stone right there on the pass. The trees were really short on top of that mountain, no taller than a human.

Soon she met an old man camped by the trail, his face shrouded in shadow. Smoke twisted upward in a spiral from his campfire. Old Man said to Coyote, "Welcome. Where are you going?"

"I am on my way to travel all over the world."

"Well, you had better go back and not stay here," Old Man said to Coyote. He was cooking a rabbit on a stick over the fire.

"Why should I turn back and not stay here for a while?" Coyote asked. "I am looking for a husband."

"'Because a giant monster lives here and kills everyone passing through this valley," replied Old Man.

"That monster is named Pain," I said to Beatrix, "and it lives in the dark and hidden places like some that you may have known when you were young. Maybe it's fed by the pain of anyone who passes by. That monster snores loud, growls with hunger, and stands outside your door most nights, waiting for a way in. Pain Monster is slimy, sticky, rough, and warty, lives in a swamp, waiting to grab your ankle as you walk by and pull you under. Pain leaves a bad taste in your mouth—thick, leathery, and nasty. Pain smells awful like volcano gas. Pain moves through your mind to create things that aren't really there. You can't hide forever from Pain, and Coyote knew that, because Pain feeds on fear and makes it grow bigger and bigger."

I started this theme because I had some sense that Beatrix was tortured by fear—fear of being imperfect, of being like her mother, of not being precocious and living up to the reputation of her namesake, and of the ten thousand other items that she hadn't told me. In the story, Coyote strikes out to kill her fear. At least that's what I have in mind. I'm probably using the "kill" metaphor because she's so rigidly against it. I could have picked a story in which the heroine befriends pain, but intuitively I knew that wouldn't fit, because always "making nice" and being friends was part of Beatrix's surface story. Under the surface, I could sense her rage, like a bubbling volcano readying itself to erupt. I knew I was connecting with something important because I saw a single tear on her cheek.

"But I am strong as a mountain," said Coyote. "I will fight him and kill him instead." Coyote was as determined as her thought and was already loping down the trail.

"Like tears in a good cry, Coyote had many stories, some old, some new, and did not wish to heed Old Man's warning," I told Beatrix. "She had stories of hatred, stories of sadness, stories of happiness, relief, gladness, joy, and beauty, just like you."

Coyote noticed a single, large tamarack tree nearby on a hillside standing next to a beautiful lake. "I'll put an end to the giant Pain Monster with a hard blow from this tree," she said. "That's the way I'll kill him. I'll smash him into a muddy puddle." Fancying herself the creator of the world, Coyote pulled that suffering tamarack tree from the new ground, swung it onto her shoulder, and continued her celebrated search for Pain Monster. Soon Coyote saw an unknown man who appeared nearly dead. She asked, "What is the matter, are you sick? Or just old?"

Since it was so hard for me to reach Beatrix on any emotional level due to her need to be perfect and have no emotional problems, I was giving suggestions through the story, hoping she could go through a simulation of killing her fear and pain so she could relax.

"No, I am not sick," the man replied.

"I'm going to kill that evil Monster with this tamarack tree," said Coyote.

"You might as well throw that little tree away. Don't you know the Pain Monster already sees you and you are already a tasty bite in its belly?" said the man. Coyote was shocked. At first she wanted to claim that this was a trick. But she realized the truth—that she had inadvertently walked into the Monster's giant belly and was already inside it. That's why everyone was dying. They were being digested. Soon, so would she. "I guess that's what fear and pain does," she said to herself. "It eats us alive. We are lost in the blink of an eye."

Coyote took that man's advice and threw that tamarack tree up on a hillside, where it is still growing. The Monster had climbed up on top of the mountains and had found a way to consume all of what is now called Jocko Valley. All of it was inside the Monster's belly, including Coyote, who could now see the many people lying here and there. Before the man had spoken to her, she hadn't been able to see them. She'd needed to hear the right words in order to be able to see them. Some were already dead, others seemed about to die, or were nearly dead.

"What is the trouble with all of you people?" Coyote asked another old man whose eyes were still open. "Why did you let yourself get eaten? Why don't you just leave?"

"We were all starving to death," he answered. "That Monster tricked us with fish. When we discovered where we'd come, it was too late to get out."

"But why are you still starving to death?" asked Coyote. "I can see plenty to eat here, lots of meat and fat." That's when Coyote realized that all of the meat and fat were the insides of the Monster. That's when Coyote resolved to kill the Monster. After a few really deep breaths, Coyote proceeded to attack the Monster, cutting away large chunks of grease and fat from its insides and feeding it to all of the people. They got stronger with each bite.

I suppose I was playing with Beatrix's antimeat beliefs, not that I wanted her to eat meat, but to help her to be less self-righteous about it.

"All of you people prepare to run for your lives," said Coyote. "Run for the blue sky. Follow the breeze out. That breeze is Pain Monster's breath. Follow the trail of flowers for they grow on the path that his food follows when it enters his body. Head for the smell of grapes and blueberries. I am going to cut out his heart. You must be outside of Pain Monster when he dies or you will get squashed inside him. When I start cutting, you must all run and hide." When the animals and people started running up the trail, Coyote began cutting out the Monster's heart with her stone knife.

Pain Monster awoke suddenly as the moon was rising over the horizon. "Hey," he called out. "Please, Coyote, let me alone. Don't you love me? I love you. Go away from here. Get out!" Coyote didn't love Pain Monster, who had made Coyote and all the rest of the people gloomy, unhappy, and miserable.

"No, I won't go away," Coyote replied. "I'm inside you. I'm going to stay right here until I kill you." Then she cut open Pain Monster's blue heart and the blood poured out. As he was dying, the unhappy Pain Monster's jaws began to close tightly. All the animals had escaped except for Woodtick, who was the last one out from the monster's belly. When Pain Monster's jaws closed shut in death, Woodtick was caught between them. I guess Woodtick just didn't listen closely enough to Coyote, who had cut her own way out through the heart. But framed against the sunset-lit clouds, like in a scene from Ben Hur *or* Gone with the Wind, *Coyote caught hold of Woodtick and with all her strength pulled Woodtick out of the Monster's jaws. "We can't help it," Coyote said to Woodtick, "you will always be flat-headed from your experience."*

Coyote left and started once again on her world trip. "Now that Pain Monster is dead maybe I can have some other adventures," she thought.

I wondered what adventures Beatrix might have if her pain died. She might wander along the great divide between illness and health and count the snowflakes that cover a mountainside. She might be able to drink from exotic, healing fountains and tell me new insights that came from those elixirs.

From there Coyote continued on to what is today called Missoula, Montana. Coyote walked along between Lolo and Fort Missoula when she thought she heard someone call her name. But she could not see anyone. She trotted forward and heard her name again, thinking that maybe the voice was coming from ancient caves underground, hidden where nobody could know.

"Maybe you have some of those ancient caves," I told Beatrix. "You might want to explore your own caves while Coyote looks for her next adventure. Maybe the entrance can only be seen in moonlight. Maybe you must stand beneath overhanging branches until the moon triggers the wind to let you in. Maybe even now as I'm telling this story you can hear the cries of the hawk and the nightingale. Maybe the tides could carry you forward to underwater caves to find the source of your pain. Maybe the waves could take you there. Hang onto that tamarack tree that Coyote threw to you. There's room to dance at the base of the trunk. Let it take you where it wants to go now that you have the freedom to go there, free of fear and pain. Then enter those caves to learn about the source of that pain. Maybe you'll learn how to destroy it just as Coyote learned how to kill Pain Monster. Maybe it will let go of your hopes and ambitions just like Pain Monster let go of all the people trapped in Jocko Valley."

Through this story and several others like it, and through our continued dialogue, body work, and ceremony, Beatrix was able to invent a new story in which she could have an inner circle of close friends who would meet weekly as a healing circle when she returned home. These friends would be allowed to see her pain. She would make sure that whatever was said in the healing circle stayed in the healing circle, since that was the essence of ceremony. We also made some progress in shifting the idea of external agency for her suffering to rigidity. Her pain diminished markedly during the ten days we spent together, and continued to diminish on her return home.

Though she had flare-ups and relapses, the overall progress was toward reduction in symptoms. As she and her social network engaged in dialogue and new stories ventured forth into her world, some of the therapies that had not previously worked also began to become more comforting. Beatrix had cost the health care system enormously. Now she was consuming many fewer resources. Without story, we doctors spin our wheels, order lots of lab tests, and try therapies that don't work. With stories and armed with the knowledge that our brains, nervous system, and connective tissue are formed by the stories and the lives that we lead, we can intervene in much more cost-effective and beneficial ways.

Making the Good Life

"Scott's" story provides another example of the way in which context and culture influence personal story and behavior. Scott came to see me for severe fatigue accompanied by flulike symptoms. He had diagnosed himself as having an "immune disorder." He had spent hundreds of thousands of dollars of his insurance company's money and many more of his personal money seeking a diagnosis and searching for a treatment. After five years without success, he read my book *Coyote Medicine* and decided to contact me.

Scott had an abusive childhood. His father had been physically violent toward him. His mother was chronically ill and often in bed. This was the context in which he grew up—saturated by stories of violence and chronic illness. Scott was also influenced by the larger culture. He was caught up in patriotic furor. As a way to leave home, he joined the Navy and became a Seal. He trained further in underwater demolition and attended sniper school. He went to places and did things that he said he couldn't tell me about or we'd both be in danger. After eight years, he left the Seals and became a mercenary soldier, having become disenchanted with United States foreign policy and more and more uncomfortable with what he was being asked to do. Scott served in a number of foreign armies and then graduated to arranging arms deals.

Over time, Scott began to feel that what he was doing was wrong. He began to think about where the bullets he sold were going. He began to question the morality of his mercenary work. He described himself as having slowly developed a conscience. He couldn't fight or sell guns anymore. He decided to go to back to college and slowly worked his way through university. Then he decided to go to psychology graduate school and learn how to help people. The problem came during his third year. He was too authentic. He had seen misery, and he had seen American foreign policy in action, and he didn't accept bullshit. Scott began to tell things his way in his papers. He began to stand up to his professors and question them. Scott was not being a good student. He had views of his own. Over time, more and more teachers objected to Scott's behavior. Scott persevered and finished all his course work. Where he got stuck was in his dissertation. He wrote what he thought was an excellent piece of work that challenged many of the standard assumptions. Time passed, committee members changed, and he could never get it approved. Eventually, the chair asked Scott to leave, degreeless, but having put in more time and work than any student who had been graduated.

Scott took this hard. He had always left situations that weren't working before being asked to leave. He hadn't cared so much about other places he had left, but getting a degree and helping people were important to him. Feeling broken, he turned to hedonism. He pursued his version of "sex, drugs, and rock-n-roll." The women, the booze—none of this mattered too much to him, but his dog was important, a Labrador who went everywhere with him. At night, he threw the Lab a steak. Together they shared beer, pretzels, onion rings, and life. All hell broke loose when Scott's beloved dog got sick. White blood cells were eating the dog's red blood cells (aplastic anemia). Over the next four months Scott did everything possible to save his dog, but to no avail. The dog died, and Scott collapsed into bed. He was so tired he couldn't get out of bed. Thus, began his illness.

Scott's struggles with health can be conceptualized within the larger context of stories about "the good life" and what constitutes it. Scott had tried on various stories about meaning and purpose, including service to country, service to humanity, and then just service to self. Country disappointed him. Humanity rejected and discarded him. Then he rejected all meaning and purpose but pleasure, which is what he saw most people around him doing. For him, hedonism was nihilism.

Once I learned the story of Scott's dog, his condition became more contextualized. Even while telling me about his dog's immune system giving out and his dog collapsing and dying, he didn't see the parallel to his own situation. He couldn't see how his own collapse and fear of dying began when his dog collapsed and died. Scott had lost hope. When he came to see me he was waiting to die. Scott's story has to be positioned within the stories of the larger culture that shaped him. He had no template for grief. It wasn't allowed in the military, nor in his family growing up. He didn't know that he needed to give himself the opportunity to grieve the loss of his last investment in meaning and purpose—his dog. Nor had he really grieved the loss of the military, his sense of belonging to country, and his loss of becoming a professional who helped people.

The counter-narrative that we produced for Scott was that he couldn't heal alone. He needed community. He needed other people to help him recognize his own blind spots, such as his emptiness and grief. This was a radical shift in his story, for he didn't trust anyone around him. We explored the idea that Scott had predominantly lived other people's stories—patriotism, war, money—but he hadn't had a chance to consciously choose his own story. It's amazingly empowering to choose our own story and to move through the world enacting our own story.

Choosing our own story is close to what has been called finding the authentic self, even though from my perspective the authentic self does not exist to be found, but must instead be invented in the here and now. Finding an authentic self is doomed to conflict since we have so many sides and roles to play; finding desirable stories to live that ignite our passion for life is more doable and less likely to engender conflict. We can't do this without the help of other people. Through dialogue with others in a context of wanting to be healing for each other, Scott could find a purpose and move toward health and well-being.

I did a ceremony for Scott. In it the spirits (or intuition, depending on your personal beliefs about these things) informed him that biomedicine couldn't help right now. He didn't have anything that it could treat. He had spirit drainage from all his unresolved relationships that were sucking his life force from his body. His instructions were to forgive the people from his past so they could leave his inner world. He needed to prepare a ceremony for his dog and feel its presence in his daily life. He was invited to pick three therapies to do every day for one year. If he wasn't better by then, he should see a doctor again.

Scott liked these instructions. He realized he needed community. He didn't want to give up steak and onion rings, but he was willing to maybe juice some green vegetables and drink them even if he didn't want to cook them. He would do yoga and start to exercise as well. He would explore his artistic side, because, as Bob Dylan said, "the purpose of art is to stop time."

Hearing the Wolf's Howl

Here's a story I told both Beatrix and Scott to assist in their invention of new and improved stories. I'll tell the version I told to Beatrix and leave it as an exercise for the reader to imagine how I modified it for Scott, or how it might be modified for another person.

Coyote stopped and when she looked into the woods, she saw two handsome young men sitting beside a river that sizzled with water running through rapids. Cold, Coyote nevertheless swam across the river and went up the bank toward the men. Her paws were getting torn on that rocky volcanic ground.

"They are very good-looking young men," thought Coyote, "maybe I could have one of them." She sat down between them, but they stood up and danced down to the river. "Wait for me," called Coyote. "I'll go swimming with you. The moon is out." Beneath the bright stars, Coyote removed her jacket beaded with shells, which denoted that she was a great personage. A lone wolf howled. The night was dazzling.

To Beatrix I said, "Sometime today, I want you to listen, because perhaps that lone wolf will tell you what you seek. What else could you need at this moment but his company? He's waiting for you. Reach out your hand and touch his silver coat. Stroke his fur. Feel the creamy texture of that luxurious winter coat and let him tell you the origins of your pain. Sometimes a shivering sensation will take over as you begin to hear him talking. Maybe your pain speaks the language of a great, faraway land. Maybe you have a 'king or a queen of pain,' like in Sting's song. Later you can tell me a story about the origins of your pain. For now, let's just find that story. Let the animals help you. Let them perhaps fly you to the clouds where you can sit and look down on the biggest picture for how this came about."

I saw Beatrix making some small jerky movements and quivering a bit. I assumed this meant she was having a deep emotional experience. "It's okay to let yourself go," I said. "Let yourself enter into the dreamtime. Find the prize. Learn about your pain. Maybe it's been passed down for generations, like your mother's despair and your father's heartbreak. Maybe no one in the family knows where it is, and it's up to you to find it. Maybe, like an old medal, it's been lying in a drawer for centuries, afflicting all equally without malice or forethought, just waiting to be claimed and cleaned and put on display for all to see. Perhaps pain gets dustier and dustier until it is put on display. Perhaps pain is something that all the world needs to see. It shouldn't just lie there hidden as if forgotten. Medals are best displayed on bosoms like the ornamentation of kings and queens. Would you wear your pain on your chest for all to see, as if you'd won it through some great sea battle that the English are so famous for? Wear it as if you'd splintered against the rocks, against odds for which you never stood a chance, and you survived and prevailed anyway?"

I was clearly making suggestions that she could reveal her pain to others without shame, which would probably go far toward reducing the pain, as it was probably taking a lot of effort to pretend that she was not in pain to everyone around her.

Coming back to Coyote, those men replied, "We don't want to wait; we are having a good time dancing." They danced into the river. Maybe they were part of a dream. When Coyote joined them, they pushed her down into the water and drowned her. Later, Coyote's partner, Fox, appeared from around a bend in the river, looking for something to eat.

When Fox looked into the river and saw something lying on the bottom, he said, "This must be Coyote!" Fox plunged down into the swirling rapids

and pulled out the object, and when he was sure it was Coyote, he made a
magical jump over her, twisted her tail to make a circle, and then made a
twisting kind of circle dance, faster and faster until all that vortex of energy
swirled and whirled and brought Coyote back to life.

"As you go down into your own waters," I told Beatrix, "wherever you end up, you need to be brought back to a painless life, or at least a less painful life. Don't go swirling any further down into that whirlpool of pain. Listen to the wolf and to Fox and to others who would help you."

Coyote said, "Oh, I must have had a long sleep."

Perhaps Beatrix was also having a long sleep. I was hoping she was in a deep enough trance to accept these suggestions for revealing, sharing, and losing her pain. In my story about pain, it always diminishes when it is shared with other people.

"You were not asleep, you were dead," replied Fox. "Why did you go near
those young men? You had no right to be near them; they are from the Shell
tribe. Do you know why you did that?"
  "Because I rule all that I survey," answered Coyote. "No one messes
with me."

"Let no more pain mess with you," I said to Beatrix. "Let no more pain mess with you."

Coyote climbed part of the way up the hill and set the grass and the autumn
leaves on fire. Later it was discovered that the two young men could not escape
and died in the fire. Afterward, the trees stood like blackened skeletons, dry
and cracked, bare but restful. Coyote had only prepared them better for the
icy winds of winter.

"Perhaps you could burn away your pain, as well," I continued with Beatrix. "But let the squirrels get away to hide with their winter stores.

Let the birds collect the overripe berries. And then, before the winter snow, ice, and rains come, burn your pain down to the ground. You can step out of those ashes like the phoenix rising."

I continued to work with Beatrix, hopefully having given her sufficient suggestions to allow others to see her pain, to share in her pain, and then to overthrow her pain. I took her through the stages of discovering the origins of her pain, taking the medal that commemorated her pain out of its hiding place and wearing it for all the world to see until she was ready to overthrow it and burn it away. We finished with a sweat lodge ceremony with a local elder.

The next morning, as Beatrix was about to return home, she said that her goals had been met. Red Sky was at peace. She didn't feel responsible for ending his suffering any more. She felt more relaxed, less anxious. Again I was reminded that it is her story that matters to her, not mine. Two years later she reported that her pain was much improved.

Imagine how Beatrix's brain was shaped by her culture and social environment of origin. Her parents taught her that perfection was the goal and anything less was not an option. She could never show her pain. If pain is a conversation, then her only pain conversations were internal ones, with her images of real people. Perhaps she saw her parents disapproving. She could never tell me about the conversation. Nevertheless, I think this was how her brain was organized, and pain presented itself as the ultimate contradiction. If Beatrix were performing perfectly, why should she have pain? This was our starting question, and perhaps the opposing story and the suggestions made for telling people about her pain and for becoming aware of its message did lessen her rigidity and therefore her pain over time. However, without her ever having to explain her pain conversation to me, our work started a process that changed her brain, and her pain reduced. When we have motivation, regardless of how we got it, change happens.

9

Stories from Science:
Change Is Always Possible

He refused to associate himself with any investigation,
which did not tend towards the unusual, and even the
fantastic.

SIR ARTHUR CONAN DOYLE,
THE ADVENTURES OF SHERLOCK HOLMES

In chapter 7 I showed how I use stories from science to weave a story that is designed to convince people that their brains do not have to forever be the victims of faulty genes and that genes can be changed. These stories use ideas from science to inspire hope by overthrowing the old science stories with which we grew up. In this chapter I wish to take this concept deeper and to provide more exciting stories from science, which show that change is always possible, that we are not fixed with the brain with which we were born, but can and do change throughout our lives.

Reducing the Volume

Consider "Carry," a forty-two-year-old Saskatoon woman whom I interviewed as part of my work in Canada. I was asked to see Carry because she would periodically take half a bottle of her antipsychotic medication.

Sometimes that would cause her to be hospitalized for observation or for dystonic reactions (tight muscle spasms caused by the medication) or for urinary retention or for several other side effects. Carry attended a local day treatment program. She had grown up in Sandy Bay, a reserve in the northeast of Saskatchewan, and had a rough childhood. She had two children, a nine-year-old girl who was living with Carry's brother and his family on the reserve and a nineteen-year-old daughter who was "couch surfing" around town with her boyfriend and the couple's two-year-old. Her diagnosis was schizophrenia. When I asked her why she periodically took too many pills, she answered, "Because I hate myself."

"Why do you hate yourself?"

"Because I'm a bad person. I'm ugly. I've got this illness and I'll never change. I'll never get better. I'll be like this the rest of my life." Carry was making it clear just why it is so important that we change our current stories of science. I don't believe that Carry can't change. I don't believe that science supports that point of view, even though within the conventional biomedical paradigm the inability to change becomes a self-fulfilling prophecy. Of course, Carry will have difficulty changing if she's stuck in a social network that keeps her the same. If that network doesn't change, day treatment for the rest of her life could make little difference. Carry needs a different story that inspires hope and the possibility of a better life.

"Why are you a bad person?" I asked.

"That's what my boyfriend says," she said. "And it's what the voices say."

"Tell me a story," I said, "that will help me understand how you came to feel like a bad person."

By asking repeated questions including, "And what happened next," I slowly extracted a story about what had happened the last time that Carry had taken too much medication. She clearly wasn't used to telling stories or presenting her world in a storied manner. In her story, her boyfriend had knocked on her door. She let him in, and he asked her to cook food for him. While she was cooking, he launched into a diatribe about what a bad person she was, a bad mother, ugly, fat, and more. He continued as he ate his food. Then he wanted sex, to which she consented. He threw a towel over her face while they had sex because she was "too ugly to view." Then he left. "What happened then?" I asked.

"I felt lonely. Then I started thinking about my children and what a bad mother I am, how I can't protect them, how I'll never get better, how I'll never be with them again because of this illness which will never get better. The courts will never give my younger daughter back. My brother doesn't want me to see her or call her. My older daughter is homeless and pregnant, and her boyfriend beats her up. I try to help her, and she just yells at me. My grandson doesn't have a place to live, and I can't take care of him. I'm ugly and fat."

"And how do you get from thinking those thoughts to taking pills?"

"The voices get really loud, telling me that I'm bad and ugly and fat. I sit alone in my apartment crying. Finally I can't take it anymore, so I take the pills. They're supposed to stop the voices, aren't they, but they don't. I don't think they do a damn thing except make me a little sleepy if I take enough."

Carry's plot or core belief is: "I'm hopeless and I'll never get better." She learned this storyline from the mental health system, though her entire life also supported the idea. The problem is that conventional biomedicine and the mental health system don't believe that such people can change. The system of "care" has not been designed on the basis of the principles of neuroplasticity, neurogenesis, epigenetics, and the tremendous influence of the social environment on brain function. Instead it has been designed on the basis of an individual, defective, hopeless brain model in which people are essentially maintained and warehoused. We have to stop making people believe that they are hopeless if we want them to change.

I started my work with Carry by challenging her black-and-white thinking. She had conceptualized a dichotomy of "good mothers" and "bad mothers." I introduced a 10-point scale and asked her to place herself on it as a mother. She saw herself as a "3" for her younger daughter and a "3" for her older daughter. This led to a dialogue in which she agreed that she wasn't a bad mother, just a poor mother, since "3" was higher than "0." She had done a good job for her younger daughter by getting her to live with Carry's more stable brother, whom the daughter liked. Her younger daughter was safe. Her older daughter at least had street smarts and was able to survive with a child and being pregnant and homeless. Carry did help her when she came around, until the boyfriend showed up and fighting ensued and she had to send them away lest the police get called or she get evicted. Then we discovered that on a scale of 10 for bad and good people, Carry saw herself as a "6." This was very important because she had crossed the midline. I told Carry I would have rated her a bit higher.

Then we learned that she only had one voice and it pretty consistently said what her boyfriend (and past boyfriends) had said. It got louder after visits from her boyfriend and her daughter. It was only after these visits that she took too many pills. She saw her other alternatives as staying up all night or taking a four-hour shower.

Carry's story is not very unusual in the mental "health" system. No one had taken the time to get a story to explain her behavior. She had been told that the medication was for her voices, so it made sense to her to take more when the voices got too loud. Also no one had really worked with her to help her learn how to manage her voice except to give her medication that wasn't working. No one knew about her social network (her boyfriend, daughter, daughter's boyfriend, and grandchild). No one had talked to them or to her family on the reserve.

Of course Carry was 80 percent certain that her boyfriend was just taking advantage of her neediness and vulnerability, but he was important for her because "at least someone comes to see me and acts like he cares for me. . . . He fills the void I have. I just feel no one else will love me."

Knowing her story, we can begin to imagine more possibilities for Carry. One possibility would be to reconcile her with her family so that she could move back to the reserve and have more social support. Certainly that would be a less expensive option for the mental health system, and probably better for her in the long run, if some of the difficulties in perception between her and her family could be addressed. Other possibilities included teaching her how to reduce the volume of her inner voice. We began that process in our first meeting when I asked her to say to the voice, "Madrona and I think I am a good person so you be quiet." She was to try this as an experiment and report back her findings.

Over time, Carry did manage her voice better, and we did reconnect with her family via web camera. She began to have more contact in that manner with her daughter. She eventually did move back to the reserve. At that time, she stopped her medication because, as she said, "it never did anything for the voices." She had learned other techniques to control their loudness and advanced her mothering score to a "6" and her good person score to an "8."

This is why we need better science stories for psychiatry, so that we can believe in the possibility of healing and generate hope for people instead of despair and misery.

Better Science Stories

The conventional biomedical story said that Carry's brain was defective: genetic anomalies resulted in biochemical abnormalities; change the biochemistry through medication and Carry would improve. Why didn't it work so well? Is it just because we haven't discovered all the relevant genes or not yet found the drugs that will make up for our genetic deficiencies? The theory makes sense in a mechanical sort of way—that you should be able to drive the person's experience and behavior by intervening at the biochemical level. It is consistent with contemporary biases toward reductionism, which reflect the idea that smaller, microscopic levels of explanation are more desirable than larger, macroscopic levels of discourse: the chemistry of the synapse is more important than social interaction in explaining emotion and behavior.

However, Louis Cozolino, in his 2006 book titled *The Neuroscience of Human Relationships: Attachment and the Developing Social Brain,* writes nicely about how each of our individual brains can be viewed as one neuron in a larger social brain.[1] Expectations and context may shape brain chemistry and alter genetic expression more often than genetics modifies the environment. I suspect that genetics become less and less important over time and that environmental influences take precedence in shaping our brains by the end of the first year of life.

Psychologist Ernest Rossi describes three recent discoveries of contemporary neuroscience that will forever change how we understand human nature and that support the ideas presented in this book, including hope for people like Carry.[2] First is the discovery that novelty, enriching life experiences, and physical activity activate neurogenesis—meaning new neuronal growth in our brains—throughout our lifetime. Second is the discovery that such experiences can alter gene expression within minutes throughout the brain and body to guide growth, development, and healing. Third is the discovery that every recall of a memory reframes that memory. Recalling a memory opens up the possibility for changing that memory on a molecular genomic level within our brain. As Rossi said, "We are constantly engaged in a process of creating and reconstructing the structure of our brain and body on all levels, from mind to gene. . . . 'Genetic determinism' is . . . a myth. Nature and nurture are cooperative partners that coordinate gene expression and neurogenesis to create our life experiences and continually update our memories in fresh ways whether we are aware of it or not."[3]

American psychiatrist Eric Kandel wrote,

Insofar as psychotherapy or counseling is effective and produces long-term change in behavior, it presumably does so through learning, by producing changes in gene expression that alter the strength of synaptic connections and structural changes that alter the anatomical pattern of interconnections between nerve cells of the brain. As the resolution of brain imaging increases, it should eventually permit quantitative evaluation of the outcome of psychotherapy. . . . Stated simply, the regulation of gene expression by social factors makes all bodily functions, including all functions of the brain, susceptible to social influences. The social influences will be biologically incorporated in the altered expression of specific genes in specific nerve cells of specific regions of the brain. These socially influenced alterations are transmitted culturally. They are not incorporated in the sperm and egg.[4]

In 1932 Frederic Bartlett first showed that our memories are not eidetically exact but partially reconstructed, reshaped by the mind at every stage: in initial perception, in encoding, during storage, and in retrieval. Neuroimaging is now showing us how psychotherapy and other life experiences change our brains. Novel, interesting, surprising, and arousing information associated with new adventures can induce the expression of genes within minutes in all species studied. For example, a team at the Heinrich Heine University in Düsseldorf, Germany, put wild adult rats into an enriched environment overnight. As their whiskers are an important source of highly relevant tactile information for rats, the researchers clipped different sets of whiskers for each rat (so that they could tell which whiskers were being used to explore the new environment). The activity of gene expression increased significantly in the brain areas corresponding with the longer whiskers that were being used. Gene expression changed overnight as a result of exposure to a novel environment. The genes affected included c-Fos, JunB, inducible cycle-AMP, early repressor gene, Krox-24, Egr1, NGF1, and ZENK, all of which are highly important among humans.[5] These and similar studies help demonstrate how quickly brains can change in response to new experience.

We are actually forming new neurons and synaptic connections continually throughout our lives. Researchers at the Max Delbrück Center for Molecular Medicine at the University of Berlin-Buch, Germany, showed that the new neurons actually do function and contribute to cognitive processes.[6] Novel and stimulating experiences in various cultural activities (art, dance, drama, education, literature, music, myth, painting, spiritual rituals, storytelling, etc.) facilitate neurogenesis (the growth of new neurons), vast enrichment in synaptic connections for existing neurons, and the growth of the brain.

These brain studies provide a foundation for understanding (and affirming) the healing work we do with people. Creatively using our brains—telling stories, making plays, doing art, singing, chanting, and dancing—all contribute to new brain growth in adults as well as children. Art, for instance, "arouses pleasure . . . because, like play, it fine tunes our systems."[7] Boyd believes that it builds confidence at the individual and group levels, that we are able to shape our own destinies. It builds empowerment because we can simply choose what moves us. "Even slum dwellers or impoverished share croppers can affirm with a picture on the wall that they can shape at least a part of their lives to please."[8] "In small-scale societies—including most of the human past—all participate in the art of the community, in song, in dance, weaving, carving, make-up, and costume."[9] Therapeutic power to change brains comes from this self-rewarding play. The creative arts, including their therapeutic use in the healing stories I have been telling, provide mental stimulation for brain growth and change through patterned cognitive play, beginning with the patterned playful invitations to interact from parents to their infants.

An Epigenetic Look at Mothering

In chapter 7 we saw how the field of epigenetics, or functional genomics, which studies how environmental experiences modify gene expression and duplication, leading to individual differences in brains and behavior, has revealed that our genes are not independent biological determinants of behavior, but rather, active players, responding quickly from one moment to the next to the cues, challenges, and contingencies of our ever-changing daily experiences. "Our thoughts, emotions, and behavior modulate gene expression in health and optimal performance as well as stress and illness."[10]

Some of the most fascinating (and relevant to humans) epigenetic research comes from the study of mothering. We know that maternal touch activates genes, such as c-myc and c-max, which have immediate effects on child development by activating a target gene that regulates the activity and production of the enzyme ornithine decarboxylase (ODC). Infants with higher levels of this enzyme grow larger on the same number of calories than infants with lower levels of this enzyme. These findings show how maternal touch stimulates infants' physical growth and development.[11] Deprivation of maternal touch for ten to fifteen minutes among rat pups resulted in a dramatic decrease in ODC gene expression, with smaller pup sizes at ten days of age. Within two hours, ODC gene activity was down 40 percent, where it remained until maternal touching resumed. A graduate student's stroking of the pups lightly with a soft, tufted paintbrush for fifteen minutes was enough to turn on the ODC gene and other genes and hormones associated with biological growth.[12]

Babies in psychosocially inadequate homes who are diagnosed with failure to thrive have abnormally low growth hormone levels, associated with low ODC gene expression activity. Once the babies receive adequate maternal touch, ODC gene expression, growth hormone, and physical growth return to normal.[13] Although researchers learned this information more than forty years ago, it has been grounded in genetic studies only within the past decade and sadly still does not influence social policy. Parent–infant interaction is crucial for later well-being in humans as well. Secure attachment is protective against later emotional difficulties. Infants raised with poor mothering are at high risk of receiving psychiatric diagnoses when they are adults. Low levels of parental care accompanied by high levels of control are associated with an increased risk for depression. Abuse and neglect are associated with cognitive impairments and high risk for physical and psychiatric disorders.

Some of the most interesting epigenetic research that is relevant to human mothers and at-risk human children comes from the laboratory of Dr. Frances Champagne, a neuroscientist and assistant professor at Columbia University in New York City. Champagne particularly focuses on the social environment and how it modifies genes during mother–infant and infant–infant interaction among rodents.[14]

Among rodents, maternal separation or complete maternal deprivation results in an increased stress response, reduced cognitive ability, impaired social behavior, and hyperactivity among the pups. Variations in care lead to variations in the mothering behavior of the offspring when they become mothers. Large differences exist within mouse strains, for example, for frequencies of mothering behaviors that are measured (nursing, licking/grooming, and nest building).

Among Long-Evans rats, mothers lick and groom their babies at high levels during the first week of life. This tactile stimulation alters body and brain temperature. Rats can be selectively bred for higher and lower levels of time spent licking and grooming their pups. The more the babies are licked and groomed, the more robust is their stress response, response to reward, and cognitive abilities. When challenged by a stressor the babies of low-licking mothers showed increased release of the stress hormone cortisol, along with decreased hippocampal response (meaning that they are less able to access previous memories of coping and find adequate strategies quickly). These babies showed lower levels of dopamine in the nucleus accumbens, a collection of neurons in the forebrain that form the reward system (they are less able to be motivated by reward) and decreased preference for sugar (healthy rats like sweets, just like children). They show decreased synaptophysin, a protein that facilitates our making new synaptic connections (which is what happens when we learn), and longer times to learn how to navigate a maze.[15]

Maternal behavior in general is highly influenced by the oxytocin receptor gene and by estrogen, which regulates the gene. Low-licking and low-grooming mothers have less of a particular molecule called estrogen receptor alpha than high-licking and high-grooming mothers. This molecule, estrogen receptor alpha, binds to estrogen receptors and influences genetic transcription. The effect of this binding and transcription is to increase the receptivity of the oxytocin receptor gene, which is high in high-grooming and high-licking mothers. Oxytocin is the hormone of social awareness. Being able to bind more oxytocin leads to greater social awareness. The offspring of high-licking and high-grooming mothers continue to show high activity of oxytocin receptor gene activity in the medial pre-optic area of the brain even into adulthood.[16]

If a rat's mother is low on licking and grooming, she will also be lower on these behaviors when she becomes a mother. The characteristics of the postpartum environment are crucial in shaping future mothering behavior among offspring. If the offspring of high-licking and high-grooming mothers are placed immediately after birth with low-licking and low-grooming mothers, they will grow up to be low-licking and low-grooming mothers, despite this being contrary to their genetics. The converse is also true. It is the adopting mother who influences the future maternal behavior of the offspring and not the biological mother. The social environment of their upbringing trumps their genetic code. The same is true for humans.

Cross-fostering studies (in which low-licking and low-grooming mothers raise babies that are genetically primed to be high-licking and high-grooming mothers and vice versa) show that it is the environment that is driving differences in gene activity rather than the genetic inheritance itself. How does this work? The DNA sequence tells the cell how to make the various proteins that are essential for life. The structure of DNA (the epigenome, as opposed to the sequence of DNA) serves as an "on/off" switch for gene expression. As we have seen, DNA structure is modified by methylation, which does not affect the sequence of the gene, but does affect its expression. It is caused by life experience and can happen immediately. When the cell divides, the methylation pattern is also copied. Methylation is thus a stable modification of DNA, which can be transmitted from generation to generation. This is how the immediate effects of environmental influences are transmitted across generations.

The question that is interesting in regard to humans relates to how we can offset the effects of genetic disadvantages in mothering. For mice, one way to alter their early life experience is to give them more mothers—a communal nursing nest. If we take a single mother who has been selectively bred for low nurturing and combine her with two other low-nurturing mothers so that the pups are cared for in a group (which rodent mothers will do), then lots of contact occurs between all mothers and pups. The females can still distinguish their pups via olfactory cues but will care for all equally. This provides an enhanced maternal experience for all the pups. These offspring have increased levels of grooming and increased social activity in general (sniffing, climbing on each other).

Champagne found that female offspring who were raised communally later showed enhanced maternal behavior even when raising their offspring in a single nest and even when genetically selected for low levels of maternal behavior. They showed increased frequency of nursing, which was passed on to the next generation, along with increased licking/grooming of pups. All areas of maternal behavior were increased and were transmitted to subsequent generations of pups despite genetic predictions to the contrary.

Thus, selective breeding of rodents to be poor mothers can be reversed by an enriched environment. This enrichment can be passed down to the offspring despite the genetic code remaining unchanged. This is done, as was mentioned previously, through methylation of the DNA as a result of experience. When we compare low-licking and low-grooming rodent mothers with high-licking and high-grooming mothers, we see differences in the levels of methylation in the promoter region for the estrogen receptor gene. If we look at the level of methylation, there are numerous sites of significantly elevated levels in the low-licking and low-grooming offspring who were raised by high-licking and high-grooming mothers. Once methylated, the DNA structure is changed and thereby gene expression is changed. The new structure is replicated and passed to the next generation. These methylation changes make them behave as if their genetics were different![17]

The downside of the possibility of changes in gene expression is that traumatized parents pass their trauma through their genes to their children. If your parents were abused, the effects of that abuse on their genome are transmitted to you. If your parents grew up with alcoholics, the effects of those experiences on their genetic code are transmitted to you. You may not realize that you live as if you were abused or grew up in a family of alcoholics, even though that didn't actually happen to you! You have inherited your parents' experiences. This is especially relevant to the tendency to be excessively anxious. It has been found that the children and grandchildren of holocaust survivors behave biochemically and psychologically as if they were actually in the holocaust.[18] Within aboriginal communities, we can explain continuing family dysfunction among the children and grandchildren of residential school survivors in a similar manner.[19]

The upside of these observations is that we can change genetic tendencies through changing the social environment in which people find themselves. For example, single mothers who are at risk for parenting difficulties could be grouped in houses of three or four mothers and babies so that they could support and help one another. Or grandparents could be reintroduced into the social/childrearing mix. Instead, social policy and habit is to place single parents in single-family dwellings whenever possible. Our current, dominant cultural story is that it's a sign of success to live alone and a sign of lower socioeconomic status for multiple families to live together.

We can also compare offspring development based on birth order. In humans, mothers spend more time in contact with first-born infants than with second-born infants. This has been explained as a function of maternal age, competing demands, and changes in the brain occurring from the previous pregnancy. This change in behavior may account for the birth-order effects observed in humans and other species. Champagne observed the behavior of female rats toward their first litter. Then she took those offspring and mated them. In subsequent generations she compared experienced mothers with inexperienced mothers and each of their associated offspring. She found that whether it was a first or subsequent litter, the mothers didn't change licking and grooming but did change the frequency of nursing contact. Interestingly, the offspring of experienced mothers behaved more like experienced mothers when they had their first litter. The effect of parity was transmitted to the third generation.[20]

While mothering is fascinating in its own right, for the purposes of narrative psychiatry, we see how powerful the social environment is in changing gene expression and therefore behavior. This is important for children, but these effects occur in adults of all ages. Can we augment the human social environment later in life to change a trajectory that would be predicted from maternal care? Can we place offspring in enriched environments (socially)? Can we encourage offspring to change their story later in life with any expectation that it will work? To answer these questions, we can look at the effects of juvenile environment on future maternal behavior in rodents. From that we learn that the future behavior of the offspring of high-licking and high-grooming mothers can be changed by their environment as juveniles, and not just as infants.

Changing the environment affects the transmission of mothering qualities. Enhanced juvenile social experience increases oxytocin levels, which enhances maternal care, and is transmitted to later offspring. Additionally, simply extending the period before pups are weaned from twenty-one days to twenty-eight days has an impact on social behavior.

Early-weaned mice have lower amounts of time spent engaged in social behavior compared with late-weaned mice. Extended weaning enhances the levels of the receptors in the various hypothalamic areas, including the medial preoptic nucleus, that are associated with improved mothering.

If the "teenagers" are raised in a standard environment, they will do what they are genetically primed to do when they become mothers. However, if "teenagers" who are genetically destined to be poor mothers are placed in a socially enriched environment, they will become good mothers. By the same token, if "teenagers" who are genetically destined to become good mothers are placed in socially impoverished environments, they will become poor mothers.[21]

All of the types of characteristics associated with maternal behavior can be transmitted from generation to generation, and it will look genetic even though it is epigenetic. Social experiences can have long-term effects on gene expression across multiple generations. Plasticity exists beyond the immediate postpartum period.

It Takes a Village

This research is of course highly relevant to humans. Perhaps the kibbutz or commune idea is not so farfetched after all. When people have more support and can support each other, their stories can change. The saying, "It takes a village to raise a child," can be generalized to, "It takes a village to heal a person diagnosed with schizophrenia, or to give a developmentally challenged person a good life, or to embrace a person diagnosed with autism." When we are together, our experience is enriched and our stories change from those we would tell were we alone. This is relevant for people of all ages inclusive of children diagnosed with conduct disorders or adults whose behavior is labeled antisocial behavior. When people support and nurture each other, the likelihood of criminal behavior is reduced.

What is called antisocial behavior appears to run in families (10 percent of families are responsible for 50 percent of the crimes committed in a community). Twin and adoption studies show heritability estimates for antisocial behavior at 40 to 50 percent.[22] Julia Kim-Cohen at

Yale University has been studying epigenetic effects related to criminal behavior. In the face of definite and severe maltreatment of children, she and her colleagues have found an inverse relationship between low levels of antisocial behavior and high levels of activity of the gene that makes monoamine oxidase A (the MAO-A gene). This enzyme (monoamine oxidase) breaks down the key psychiatric neurotransmitters of norepinephrine, serotonin, and dopamine, so as to stop transmission across the synapse.[23] Maltreatment of children alters the levels of these substances. Mouse studies associate this alteration with increased aggressive behavior, which is consistent with antisocial behavior in humans.

Apparently there is an interaction between genes and environment for antisocial behavior. Among 1,116 same-sex twins, children who were maltreated before age seven were much more likely to show antisocial behaviors as adults if the activity of their MAO-A gene was low compared with maltreated children whose activity on this gene was high. Apparently physical maltreatment increases the risk for mental health problems, and the MAO-A gene moderates this association. Maltreatment behavior is likely to be heritable. The mother's gene, which influences her likelihood to maltreat, is inherited by the child. This influences the child's risk of developing mental health problems. Maternal antisocial history is associated with the likelihood of child maltreatment. The more maternal antisocial symptoms, the higher the rates of maltreatment of children (over 20 percent).[24]

For many years, research in psychiatric genetics has assumed direct gene-to-disorder associations. However, ignoring the role of nurturing handicaps our ability to understand nature. Given the same genes with a different social environment, we see different behavior. The effects of genes may moderate environmental effects, or the environment may moderate the effects of genes on brain development.[25] Imagine the innovative programs we could design for young people at risk if we took this research seriously!

Another gene getting current attention is the 5-HTTLPR gene, or the serotonin transporter gene. There is a long version of this gene and a short version. The short gene has less-efficient RNA transcription. People having the shorter version of this gene have more depression, but only if accompanied by a history of childhood maltreatment or severe current stress.[26] In a New Zealand study from Dunedin, monkeys who were raised by peers and had the short version of the gene had lower levels of serotonin in their brains. Decreased serotonin metabolism is associated with depression and suicide. Having either version of the gene and a good mother resulted in perfectly normal serotonin metabolism. Good mothers appeared to protect babies who carried the short version of this gene from developing deficits in serotonin metabolism.[27]

Aggression shows the same pattern. A short gene and a good mother does not result in increased aggression. Exposure to alcohol, having a short gene, and being peer raised instead of being raised by a mother resulted in monkeys drinking to excess. Offspring from good mothers drank less than average. During the first month of life, monkeys who do poorly with visual-orienting tasks are likely to grow up to be impulsive, aggressive, and have low serotonin metabolism, but not if they have a good mother. Individuals with the risk gene and good mothers have no ill effects. Individuals that are peer reared and not raised by mothers have profound deficits.[28]

The same phenomenon occurs with the MAOA gene. If we have a good mother, there are no problems. Good mothering protects individuals who carry risk genes from developing psychopathology. Good mothering is transmitted from mothers to daughters. Here's a mechanism through which a gene that's associated with adverse outcomes can stay in a population for generations with no ill effects.

Perception Can Change Biology

Social experience affects the brain (through perception), dampening the genes that regulate our immune competency. In a study from Ohio State University, white blood cells were taken from medical students who were experiencing examination stress. During lower-stress baseline periods, long before their examinations, medical students showed significantly higher percentages than during examination times of receptors for cytokine molecules (interleukin-2), which signal the immune cells to go to work. This rise was associated with a rise in messenger RNA, a molecule signaling that genes are active and are replicating DNA. The gene activity for molecules related to immune competency fell during final exams, showing that stress affects the genes that control our immune system.[29]

The medical students' perception of examinations affected their gene activity and their immune system. These changes all happened within hours. Our perception of the world, which is the net result of all the stories we tell ourselves about the external world, changes the state of our internal world. Changing perception, such as in finding ways to make exams less threatening by studying earlier or meditating so that they're not so important, causes changes in immune function to disappear.

The Ohio State University researchers also measured the expression of two proto-oncogenes (c-myc and c-myb) in white blood cells of medical students. Broadly speaking, these genes maintain our defenses against cancer (among other important functions). During examinations the level of messenger RNA expression for both of these genes was lower than during non-exam time. Further evidence for weakening of the immune system was noted in messenger RNA produced by the genes controlling other markers of immune competency (the glucocorticoid receptor and receptors for cytokines, gamma interferon, and interleukin-1-beta, which are messenger molecules to excite the immune system to take action). Superficial wounds healed 3.5 days longer during exams than during summer break, a change of 40 percent.

If our immune system weakens so much during just the stress of an exam, imagine how it can be impacted in a person whose daily life is mostly misery. Would it be surprising that these people might develop conditions that we call schizophrenia or bipolar disorder or cancer? This would be related to their immune system breaking down.[30]

A short story of a woman who was referred to me for severe depression will highlight these points. Besides life-long depression, "Jan" had just been diagnosed with breast cancer. After meeting her and getting acquainted, I suggested she come to a workshop I was leading. She was inspired to fight both depression and cancer on more levels than her physicians were offering. The theme of the workshop was learning how to "perform illness," so the group rallied behind helping her to perform her cancer. Preparatory to that performance, we needed the spirit behind her cancer (or driving her cancer) to tell its story. I helped her to enter into a relaxed state so that we could interview the spirit behind her cancer (as I mentioned earlier, this use of the word *spirit* can be interpreted concretely or metaphorically without changing the meaning of this story). To do creative healing most effectively, we need techniques for emptying our minds, for setting aside our usual assumptions or stories about the world, so that we can have a novel experience, just as Rossi mentioned. We need to enter into a free-floating state of openness for whatever images and experiences appear.

Jan reached a state of relaxation in which she could talk about the cancer and her life from a different than usual perspective. She said, "Cancer is attacking me. It is very disorderly, trying to get hold of me. It's very messy. Now I have to clean out the whole attic and all the things I have saved, all the junk and all the things that are not finished. I come home and am busy and never get to my writing. I've been stuck for five years and have felt very angry at myself for the past year or two. My life is out of control."

I asked Jan if the spirit behind her cancer could step into the foreground and use her vocal cords. She agreed, and the tenor and tone of her voice changed as she spoke in response to my question, "What do you look like?"

"I'm red. I look like small red needles rolling around. I like to be red all the time. I don't like the ocean. I can see it, and I try to roll away. It will kill me. I need Jan to feed me. I need something sweet.

"I'm not so big. I can see stones. I look a bit like a red thistle. I like dark places. I hate light. I hate water. Bite is my name. It's like I was taken out of a deep hole filled with tears and sadness."

I asked, "Where are the tears from?"

"From a deep sadness. Somebody cried almost every day during Jan's childhood and when she was young. I've been here with her for a long time. I've been biting her for a very long time."

I asked, "What would make you leave?"

"I don't much like light. That would make me leave. If the waters float around me, then I will leave. I don't like heat. If it gets too hot, I might have to go away, too."

I asked, "Do you do anything helpful for Jan?"

"I make her wake up and perhaps think about what is important in life. I could teach her to write and to speak, to say her truth and to talk for herself. I've tried for a long time to make her wake up without her noticing, but maybe she's ready to change her life. She would have to get rid of her fear, fear of writing down her thoughts, fear of speaking to other people. She would have to be confident in herself. She would have to do some of the many things that she has always wanted to do and didn't. She always thinks these things are far away. She has to do them now, where she is, with her friends and family and the people already around her. She has to have confidence in the power of her words. She has to be connected to the spiritual part of herself. I will leave if she really does these things, but it's got to be every day, all the time, or else I will be back again."

I asked, "What feeds you; what makes you stronger?"

"I love sugar, milk, coffee, worries, indecision, and her not being able to make up her mind about anything. She has a big doubt if I'm anywhere else in her body besides her breast because her sister died half a year ago of breast cancer. So, she still has all this fear that has to go away if I'm to go away. She wants to fight me and has to fight me if I'm to go away. She has to fight me in all possible ways. She has to stay strong despite the doctors. It's the system. It makes her give up. That feeds me."

Jan's story was powerful for me because it brought home the mind-body connection described earlier. Jan had spent a lifetime of sadness, never feeling that she counted enough to do what she wished. She believed that she should always take care of someone else first (this is common among indigenous women who have had to be strong to keep the family together, and Jan was no exception). Jan's despair came from never having done what she dreamed of doing.

To our amazement, after this exercise, Jan also told us that the traditional healer to whom she had gone had told her to spend time every day in the ocean and lying on the warm sand. The healer had told her to stop eating all foods that weren't Native, at least originally, including sugar, coffee, milk, dairy, and to only eat the foods of her ancestors. The healer wanted to do a hot stone ceremony with her to raise her body temperature and wanted Jan to attend as many sweat lodge ceremonies as possible.

At the beginning of the workshop, Jan did look downtrodden. She looked sad, tired, worn out. She looked as if people had stepped on her. Her gaze was usually downward. She mumbled so quietly it was difficult to hear her.

Having participated in all this work, her workshop group helped her construct a play about her cancer. At first, she got to watch. She chose various people to play her, her indecision, water, a stone, warmth, her dead sister, her husband, and the spirit of cancer.

All were given instructions for how to behave, and we launched into a semi-improvisational piece that was quite powerful in revealing Jan's situation to her. Then I suggested that Jan enter the play and that she force it to move toward a positive ending. We resumed, and this time she broke free of indecision and cancer and walked outdoors onto the porch of the room in which we had performed. We assembled around her, and she announced that she was now going to tell stories. She proceeded to tell us, in a strong, loud, confident voice, never looking down, a beautiful story of her people. Her transformation was marvelous. I was so impressed at the difference between the Jan who had entered the room and this powerful storytelling Jan.

Here is a vivid example of what the Ohio State researchers were finding. I have no doubt that Jan's immune system had been worn out by her life and that it was reawakening as she told her story. We can imagine how her entire life had modified her genes (epigenetics) to make her immune system more sluggish. We can imagine how the research described earlier all applies to Jan's life and to her cancer diagnosis and prognosis.

Jan needed further support, so she joined a healing circle that met weekly in order to keep her momentum going. She started telling stories in her community and began to write down her stories and her poetry and blossomed as a woman. Her depression went away, and she didn't need medication or electroshock therapy as her family doctor had suggested. She needed to tell stories.

What if her cancer had metastasized? My position is that she couldn't have lost by stepping into her power. Even if she had died early, she would have died happier. Whether she lived or died from the cancer, she needed to feel her creativity, to feel that energy moving through her, to overcome the deep well of sadness that had existed since her childhood. Luckily (and perhaps not so much luck, but the effect of life change on the immune system), she has been cancer free now for the past five years.

In his book, *Anti-Cancer: A New Way of Life*, Paris psychiatrist David Servan-Schreiber tells a story that can further illuminate this perspective. He met with a man whose cancer could not be treated. He asked the man what would give his life meaning. The man answered that he could repair the air conditioning system on the local church. He did this and got room and board from the church in exchange. He had rarely been happier. When he returned to the hospital, two weeks from his death, Servan-Schreiber visited him. He thanked Servan-Schreiber for giving him back his life, even though he was dying.[31]

I am suggesting that all psychiatric symptoms and, indeed, virtually all of the brain functioning that interests us, arise through social interaction, just as my Lakota elders taught me. Social interaction precedes and forms us. A *dialogical* view of mind and self focuses on the events occurring in the world between people and is consistent with indigenous views of mind and self, unlike conceptions that center on mental states and acts hidden inside individuals. Behavioral scientist John Shotter mentions four themes that are central to this emerging dialogical, or narrative, approach:

1. There is something very special about our being alive.
2. We should focus on what occurs in those living moments when we are in contact with others in our surroundings.
3. Among the many consequences of being in the world as living, embodied beings is that it is impossible not to spontaneously respond to one another.

4. The outcomes of such responsive activity emerge through the dialogue in ways that cannot be predicted beforehand.[32.]

Here's a note I received from someone, which can further illustrate these concepts. She had been diagnosed as a hypochondriac by her previous physician. She wrote to me:

I was going to call you this morning to ask you for some advice. I am having a somewhat major autoimmune attack—Bad pain in both shoulders, hips, and knees, GI stuff, bladder stuff, and tight lungs. Ugh! I was fairly upset this morning that it hit me with such ferocity. I haven't been sick for a long time and usually it just starts with some joint pains, not all the internal organ stuff at once. So I was a bit scared. I didn't (don't) want to see the rheumatologist—he'll just put me on high doses of NSAIDs [nonsteroidal anti-inflammatory drugs] or steroids. I made an appointment for some body work and thought I'd call you and ask for some suggestions about herbs that might help.

As I was thinking about calling you I realized what a good doc you are for people like me. I realized that the story I would tell you about how I came to be sick this week was an entirely different story than the one I could or would tell my rheumatologist. In thinking about the whole story I realized that I could probably handle this flare up myself. This is a terribly important thing! And you need to know that being willing to listen to stories differently than other doctors can be the difference between being on terrible drugs like steroids and being able to get well without them. In fact, just thinking about what I was able to tell you allowed me to see the flareup more fully and understand what was happening. You weren't even here to hear the story, but your openness to listening made it possible for me to put the whole thing together. I'm rambling, so I'll explain.

Last Monday, I was resting on the sofa watching TV when suddenly I smelled carnations and saw myself in a casket! Ugh! Chilling premonition. I didn't quite know what to make of it and knew that

I could only go forward, but it scared me. The next morning, I was driving down the highway about 65 or 70 miles an hour when suddenly a truck from the oncoming lane turned in front of me. I had nowhere to go, no time to break, and it seemed inevitable that I was going to hit him. The only thing I had time to do was to swerve into the oncoming lane, which I did only to find myself facing another car coming head-on. I managed (with only about a second to spare) to pull onto the berm. Phew! Close call. I was pretty shaken up by it (remembering my premonition) and felt awfully lucky. When I got home, I got a call to do Reiki for the daughter of an acquaintance who was in a serious auto accident near where I was. Hmm. So I started working for her.

Of course, this made me think about my own close call and I started thinking about my own phobia about organ transplants. I'm not a donor because it scares me for some reason and I was thinking about the fact that I needed to get over that. The next thing I knew, I got an email from a friend who wanted me to do healing work for a man who had a lung transplant and was having rejection problems. (By this time I wanted to tell the universe to lighten up!—wrong thought, as you will see.) So of course, I now then had to deal with thinking about transplants from his perspective.

The next day, we got hit with a really bad storm on the mountain. The wind was high and the rain was blowing in the windows, so I got up to close everything. I had just finished closing my dining room window, when BAM! a huge bolt of lightning hit directly next to that window, burning the grass and sending the hairs on my body straight up (don't tell the universe to lighten up!). Needless to say, I was rattled again. The next day the immune stuff started. I didn't put it all together until I thought about calling you for an herbal recommendation. But doesn't it seem obvious that my body is just reacting (overreacting?) to these near misses?

So I'm going to work at calming my system down. I couldn't have come to that conclusion if I had thought about talking to the rheumatologist, I wouldn't have been able to connect the events, even in my own mind. Anyway, I think I will be fine. I'm going to ride my horse, watch my diet, and do some breath work and meditations to assure my organs I'm not planning on giving them away any time soon. Thanks for your openness, even though I didn't call. Any herbal suggestions will still be welcome. I honestly don't know what herbs to use for autoimmune stuff. Any other suggestions are also welcome. Anyway, it's important that you are willing to listen to odd stories, even when you're only told the stories in the patient's mind. Remember that, and don't let anyone tell you different.

This woman had internalized me as a character in her inner world. She could now talk to her internalized character instead of calling me directly. She had enough stories about me and enough stories about telling me stories and seeing how I had reacted that she could construct a story about telling me her experience and watching me react. She has now internalized the contextual nature of our interaction. Perhaps it goes even further than this. Perhaps our minds/energies are in contact with each other across time and distance. I have heard others tell me about writing letters to long-ago therapists and, though not sending the letters, still getting answers, perhaps because the relationship structure was still in place, as it was between this client and myself.

Stories Can Change the Brain

Let's consider another example of how story changed a person's brain and life. "Ursula" was a seventy-six-year-old woman from Ottawa who was brought by her husband to work with me. Her previous physicians had thought her problem was a purely neurological disorder. They were puzzled, since she clearly had a Parkinson-like condition, but definitely not Parkinson's disease, as all Parkinson's drugs made her acutely worse. I had my suppositions about a correct allopathic diagnosis, but also knew that it would not be useful, since no diagnosis offered any real potential treatments because all possible treatments had been tried. We were therefore free to work without labels to hinder us or restrain our progress.

Ursula had been born in the Dominican Republic of a local mother and a Russian army officer, who had returned to Russia soon after her birth. Her mother had come from a good Catholic family and had been rebelling against the family values by having sex as she wished. Her mother's resulting pregnancy with Ursula was considered a disgrace to all but herself, as she continued to live a Roaring Twenties lifestyle in a country of contradictions.

Ursula began life repeating the stories of others—that she was shameful, that she was a disgrace to the family, that she should disappear. As a child, she didn't know these words, so she performed them. The words surrounded her in whispers and occasional shouts. Ursula learned her role. She learned to self-evaluate based on the stories told to her and about her. My elders would say that whenever we speak, all of the ancestors speak with us and through us. When Ursula spoke, she spoke for her Russian and her Dominican Republic ancestors. She spoke for the church, for the land owners, and for the peasants. She embodied the contradictions of her time.

What was fascinating about Ursula was that she had not evolved in her dialogue since childhood. She continued to be ashamed of being illegitimate. She continued to complain about her mother and how oppressive and disrespectful her mother had been. Ursula was trapped in a psychological rigidity that paralleled her neurological rigidity.

I met with Ursula over a period of months. What slowly emerged was an awareness on her part that she actually had a rich, fulfilling, wonderful adult life and that her misery essentially ended at age eighteen when she left home and never went back. What was remarkable was how much adult suffering she had experienced related to her perpetual remembrance of her childhood pain. Ursula fit Mark Twain's quote, "Now that I'm old, I've lived through many catastrophes, most of which didn't happen." Ursula had suffered from the retelling of her childhood story throughout her adult life, even though her adult life had been without tragedy or misfortune. She had enjoyed a good career as a biologist. She had earned her Ph.D. and had published some interesting studies. She had two successful children, both grown, and both with families. She had been married for forty-two years and had enjoyed the opera, the theater, and other pursuits. Nevertheless, she remembered her life as being absolutely miserable, although none of her misery occurred after age eighteen.

Slowly but surely we changed her story to being one of her childhood being miserable and her adult life being good. Then she was much better able to receive the other therapies being offered. The positive effects of osteopathy, physical therapy, and acupuncture seemed to last longer than they had before; they began to have lasting, cumulative results.

Our next major hurdle was to convince Ursula that she could play with alternate realities. This was introduced as sheer, unadulterated play, an important means of breaking fixed and habitual roles. Here's what I told Ursula in one of our sessions: "Ursula, I'd like to ask you to create three different stories—three different 'might-have-beens' about your childhood. But first I'm going to tell you three might-have-beens about the creation of the world, this home where we live. Afterward you can give me three stories that are plausible about a different childhood that you could have lived."

Although the three stories that I told Ursula are all similar to one another, there are progressive variations. I told three differing stories because I wanted her to realize that she too had the power to do this— to change and improve her stories about herself and her world with each retelling.

Before I began I told Ursula, "I know you may not believe these stories because you are an atheist and a materialist, and I respect that. Yet I find your stories as strange and outrageous as you find mine. Maybe you will find it hard to believe my stories about a great island hanging from the sky. I have just as much trouble believing the story about how you have been miserable all your life and that you can't change your story."

Story One

Long, long ago, the people lived on a great island floating in a giant ocean. This island, which we call Turtle Island, hung from four thick ropes from the sky, which was solid rock.

"I know you will have trouble believing that the sky was solid rock, but it was in those days. It's okay, because I have trouble believing that you can't remember even one pleasant memory from childhood. Now if you were to say that perhaps you made it seem a bit worse over the years, I might concede that the rock sky is a metaphor, but definitely not until then."

At the time there were no people, and it was always dark.

"That's just about exactly the way you remember your childhood, so I was thinking you could really relate to this story and the fact that I believe it, just like you believe that your childhood really happened in exactly the same way that you say it did. The animals had to function like people since there weren't any people yet, just like your family had to pretend to be a family even though they weren't much of one, because that was all you had."

The animals and plants were told by the Great Spirit to stay awake for seven days and seven nights but most could not and slept. Those plants that did stay awake, such as the pine and cedar and a few others, were rewarded by being allowed to remain green all year. All the others were made to lose their leaves each winter. Those animals that did stay awake, such as the owl and the mountain lion and a few others, were rewarded with the ability to go about in the dark. The others couldn't.

"Just like the animals having a hard time staying awake, you're having trouble being able to imagine a different mother and a different child-hood. But if you want to make your way out of the darkness of your misery, then maybe, like the story says, you'll have to work with me and be alert and actually consider some other stories that could have happened as if we were writing a silly novel together of a young girl and her romantic, wonderful, carefree life in the Dominican Republic.

"I'm asking you to play with me like we're playing with metaphor in this story and to relax your hold on what really happened so we can have some fun playing with what might have been. Your brain is supposed to work best in metaphor/role-playing mode, so humor me, and try it out."

Story Two

In the beginning, there was just water. All the animals lived on an island hanging from the sky rocks by four ropes, and it sure was overcrowded. Needing space, they were all curious about what was beneath the water. One day Water Beetle volunteered to explore it. Water Beetle explored the surface but could not find any solid ground. Then he explored below the surface to the bottom and all that he could find was mud, which he brought back. After he collected the mud, it began to grow in size and spread outward until it became the earth as we know it.

"The all-encompassing water everywhere is like the beginning of your story, when there was just your all-powerful mother who could make you constantly miserable. And your childhood memories seem pretty over-crowded, just like that island. The animals were curious about what might lie under the water, just like I'm curious to find out what other options you may have had for a better childhood. I'd like to explore the underwater of your past just as Water Beetle explored the underwater of the world. In this story one little handful of mud was powerful enough to become the earth. In a similar way, one little revised memory can be very powerful. Many possibilities can ripple out from there."

After all this had happened, one of the animals attached this new land to the sky with four strings. The land was still too wet, so they sent Grandfather Buzzard to prepare it for them. When Grandfather Buzzard flew over the earth, he found the mud had become solid; he flapped in for a closer look. The wind from his wings created valleys and mountains.

"So that's how the world was made. How do you want your world to be made, Ursula?"

Story Three

"Here's my final story, Ursula, and then you are going to have to tell me your three stories or I'll have entertained you in vain. I've given you plenty of time for three stories to percolate to the top of your brain and tip of your tongue."

> Long ago, before there were any people, the world was young and water covered everything. The earth was a great island floating above the seas, suspended by four rawhide ropes representing the four sacred directions. The four sacred directions are really a whole other story I'd like to tell you sometime. Anyway, the world hung down from the crystal sky. There were no human people, but the animals lived in a home above the rainbow.

"See how much better this version is? The rock sky has turned into crystals. Imagine how much prettier that would be. For where there are crystals, there are little people, also called elves, gnomes, and leprechauns. Wouldn't you like to live in a home above the rainbow? In *The Wizard of Oz,* Dorothy got beyond the rainbow, but to get above is quite a feat."

> As the earth brought up by Water Beetle stiffened, the animals came down from the rainbow. It was still dark and cold. They needed light and warmth, so they pulled the sun out from behind the rainbow, but it was too bright and hot. A solution was urgently needed. The healers/magicians were told to place the sun higher in the sky. A path was made for it to travel each day—from east to west—so that all inhabitants could share in the light. Once they did that, they could see and they were warm.
>
> Finally, people were created. The women were able to have babies every seven days. They reproduced so quickly that the Creator feared the world would soon become too crowded. So after that the women could have only one child per year, and it has been that way ever since.

"I'm tired. I've talked enough. I've made the world three times. Now it's your turn to make yourself three times. Work with me here, and give me three stories that are plausible about a different childhood that you could have lived. I'm really looking forward to hearing what comes forth; I expect to be entertained as much as I have entertained you.

"You can do this each time by making one subtle change as early as possible in your life story and then just logically flow with it as if your life had been that way."

After this, Ursula did tell me three stories of alternate childhoods. In one, her father never left. In another, her mother married and gave her a stable home. In the third, her godfather adopted her and gave her respectability and stability. Throughout this process I kept challenging her to ask everyone she knew if anyone cared anymore about whether someone was illegitimate. The answers were hilarious. Some had even forgotten what the word meant. Others talked about the fad among celebrities to become single parents. Others mentioned that being a single parent would have definitely appealed to them had they known about the divorce that would be coming. No one cared. Culture has changed. Not even her Roman Catholic friends cared: "That's old-fashioned," they told her.

Slowly but surely Ursula developed more psychological flexibility. Finally, at age seventy-six, she stopped suffering about her early life. She could focus on fifty-eight years of good living instead of eighteen years of misery. As her story relaxed, so did her muscles. Although still disabled, Ursula is getting around easier and is going to events more or less on her own. She is freer, psychologically and physically. Her neurologist has no explanation because people are not supposed to improve from degenerative conditions. My argument is that her new story changed her brain. Our novel and adventurous work led to some degree of neurogenesis and synaptic reshuffling that improved function.

These examples illustrate the storytelling techniques I use to reach people to do something they're not sure they can or want to do. All this leads up to the power of ceremonies, which are enactments of larger spiritual meta-narratives with others.

PART III

The Practice of Narrative Psychiatry

10

The Power of Ceremony

The world is not only queerer than we imagine; it is queerer than we can imagine.

J. B. S. HALDANE, "POSSIBLE WORLDS"

Ceremony, along with the relationships and community that are required to conduct ceremony, provides a social structure in which our genes can be modified. I have seen people heal from spiritual ceremony—Roman Catholic mass, Jewish prayer, evangelistic faith healing, and Native American ritual—but it is not a matter of people curing or fixing other people. As an indigenous person, I believe that ceremony opens the doorway for spirits (spiritual energy) to enter the ordinary world to do work. The credit for healing belongs to that other dimension, with ceremony serving as a kind of transducer to convert our prayers and desires into physical events. Ceremony's power arises both from its creation of group coherence and from what is now being called energy medicine, a field of study and practice within integrative medicine, that pertains to energies related to distance healing and prayer. In that field, what traditional Native elders call spirits are called subtle energies.[1]

Healing arises from collaborative conversations that exchange information that was not previously available, resulting in transformation. By information, I mean what story carries that is impossibly more complex than our usual declarative knowledge structures. When a new flow of information passes from one to the other through dialogue, it changes people. In my own work, I have at times worked seemingly fruitlessly for weeks to help a client change a situation or improve a physical symptom. Then we would do a ceremony, and the immovable problem would transform overnight. This was more than just serendipitous timing of the ceremony with when a symptom or problem was about to change. I recognized with an inner knowledge that prayer and ceremony held magic and power that could not be denied.

The official version of conventional medicine shies away from ceremony and spirituality, though many of my Christian colleagues pray for their patients and bring their spiritual symbols into their workplace. Often they attend mass with their patients or belong to the same church or temple. Similarly, in Native American communities, the doctor and nurse may also attend a sweatlodge or sun dance with their patients. Many of my colleagues quietly believe in angels and angelic healing. They believe in the power of Christ to create miracles.

Indigenous worldviews place "emphasis on spiritual realms of ancestral spirits and natural powers, bound by kinship bonds. . . . A spirit-centered world view sees the universe imbued with and intimately related to spirits and spiritual forces that have real power to influence outcomes."[2] Indigenous worldviews embed human beings in a natural and spiritual world. Spirits were part of my life from my earliest beginnings. I grew up with grandparents who believed in spirits and treated them as real. As a child, I spoke to spirits instead of imaginary friends. So it was natural for me to accept experiences that involved spirits and a spiritual dimension. It was only after being at medical school for some time that I realized that most people raised in conventional, mainstream Euro-American society weren't comfortable talking about or acknowledging spiritual forces or energies.

Because I am educated, I understand the materialist argument—that all that exists is here, nonmaterial beings are imagined, and spiritual forces do not exist. When I speak to clients, I can use words like intuition and I can treat spiritual entities as metaphors. I can speak about the healing power of nature, and almost all nonspiritual people will respond. For me, ceremony opens dialogue with higher powers, greater forces, and more transcendent beings than we normally encounter, while those committed to materialism can see ceremony as metaphor or dramatic enactment. It will work equally well in either case, so long as there is a strong belief that it will succeed. In keeping with my own Cherokee-Lakota cultures, I will speak of spirits and spiritual energies throughout this chapter, leaving the reader to translate as desired.

Ceremony, Community, and Dialogue

A community orientation makes family relationships and friendships more important than individual considerations. Generosity is more important than acquisition. Identity includes stories that connect us to ancestors, to land, and to tribe, as well as stories about our own activities. Within these views, the self is relational, intersecting and overlapping with others, including spirits and natural features of the world. We need ceremony to have dialogue with those parts of us. We are incomplete without the conversations available only through ceremony. The feeling of belonging that ceremonies create maintains health.

Part of the wisdom that the Lakota and other indigenous peoples have to offer the mainstream is exactly this awareness of the importance of the spiritual realm and of community. The conventional philosophy that emphasizes individualism and separation from the natural and spiritual world is viewed as inadequate and incomplete by indigenous people. Voss and his colleagues write, "It is difficult, or perhaps impossible, for the . . . practitioner who has been trained, for example, to assess self-esteem as an indicator of good mental health and personal adjustment to comprehend the importance of the Lakota *wo'onsila*, or, 'recognizing one's pitifulness or condition of neediness' . . . as a creature in the world, dependent on all the forces and powers of creation all around and an intimate part of the natural world, not separate from it."[3] Ceremony helps us to remember our humble place in the universe, that we are very small beings compared with the majesty and grandeur of the universe. Through ceremony we address the nonphysical energies that surround us, nurture us, protect us, enliven us, and instruct us. We formally request their help with our problems.

Anyone can do ceremony, and in traditional indigenous cultures, everyone does, but some become recognized as having special gifts or talents in specific areas. This is similar to the phenomenon that Malcolm Gladwell describes in *Outliers*—that expertise in any field comes from a minimum of 10,000 hours of practice.[4] The more hours a person spends communicating with spirits, the more proficient he or she becomes, eventually becoming known as a healer (the term in Lakota is *wicasa wakan,* or man of sacredness).

Voss and his colleagues describe this nicely:

> The Lakota . . . medicine people rely on their spirit helpers to "give them permission" to treat people and conduct ceremonies. . . . The spirits work through the healer. The medicine person is only as effective as the spirits "working through him" [or her]. He is responsible and accountable to the spirits for everything. Spirits are understood as the power, force, and source of help and healing for all medicine and healing practices among the Lakota. . . . For traditional Lakota healers, the helping process begins and ends with spiritual powers and influences. . . . The interconnections among family, tribe, and clan with moral, political, and ceremonial life all contribute to a sense of harmony and balance called *wicozani* (good total health). . . . For Lakota people, life is like a circle—continuous, harmonious, and cyclical, with no distinctions. . . . The circle of healing is formed by the interconnections among the sick person, his or her extended family or relatives, the spirits, the singers who helped with the ceremonial songs, and the [healer].[5]

This is how I was taught. Ceremony is always collaborative. I create ceremony collaboratively with groups or individuals, or I attend culturally specific ceremonies and follow the instructions given to me. In either case, I am asking for help and for information from these unseen dimensions. When help is provided it is also collaborative. The spirits decide to respond, and further dialogue ensues. As my skills and knowledge of ceremony have increased, I have led ceremonies after which dramatic changes have occurred for the participants. These results are not reproducible. Sometimes the spirits help us, and sometimes they don't (or perhaps they can't). I've always imagined or perceived that they have great compassion for us and would always help us if they could, but just can't sometimes, for reasons that are beyond what we are able to understand. When healing occurs after ceremony, the credit goes to the spirits.

Ceremonies Are Enacted Stories

To understand a ceremony, we must understand the stories surrounding the ceremony. I began my journey toward ceremonies through storytelling. When a situation or a person needs help, a story will often emerge to entertain, to instruct, and to transform. Transformation is unleashed by the right story for the occasion. When I see clients whom I am not able to help with conventional medicine, I schedule extra time in their next appointment for me to tell them a story. This often leads to a succession of sessions for stories.

Contemporary biological psychiatry has its own secular rituals, or ways of enacting the stories that compose and constitute it, though it would eschew the term *ceremony* as being unscientific. These enactments include the mental status examination, the medication check, electroconvulsive shock therapy, the format of the psychoanalytic interview, the court-administered ceremony of commitment, and so much more. While Western biomedicine is also a performance of stories, these stories usually lack spiritual connectedness or supernatural affiliations.

Most of the world's narratives about mental health and distress include an important role for ceremony and for the acknowledgment of forces that we can't control in our lives. From time immemorial, ceremony has played an important part in maintaining mental health and in recovering from emotional distress. Ceremony connects us with powerful resources largely unavailable to us in any other way. And ceremonies work! Within the Dene nation, medical patients who also receive a traditional ceremony have more rapid recovery, experience fewer complications, and are less likely to suffer depression after a bout with illness.[6]

We seem to be more profoundly affected by story when we enact it, when we feel the story moving through us. We see this power in action in psychodrama, family reconstruction work, dance therapy, art therapy, Roman Catholic mass, prayer rituals, and indigenous ceremony. Each of the elaborate Dene ceremonials in northern New Mexico and Arizona represent the performance of sacred stories that have been handed down from the Holy People.[7] The Nightway Ceremony, for example, tells the story of a hero who commits an error that leads to hardship. "The Holy People take pity on the unfortunate earth-surface-person and conduct a ceremony to restore the hero to wellness. The healed one is then instructed to return to his kin and teach them the ceremony so that, in the future, others may be healed."[8] The Nightway ceremony reenacts the story of this hero's journey, including the intervention of the Holy People. Through the recitation of the story, the Holy People come to intervene again for the person for whom the ceremony is being conducted.[9]

The purpose of religion should be to help us maintain a binding commitment to spiritual awareness within the lives of our communities. This is done through the power of ritual, which is the materialization of religion, the bearer of religious tradition, the insurer of continuity of the life of the present with the original Spirit of the past. The reenactment of traditional ritual in the worship provided by religion ensures that the past (our ancestors) continues to touch our bodies, our flesh, and to reach into the hearts of our souls.

Waking Up the Sleeping Beauty

To further this discussion, I want to tell a story about how a ceremony completed some narrative healing work. This story teaches us that ceremony provides something beyond talk alone. "Dora" came to me in despair following the breakup of a relationship. She had been with a man from Ecuador who was intensely passionate, sensual, and sexual, and had left her for another woman. Her pain was beyond measure. She agonized over what she had done wrong and how the other woman was better than she. Narrative approaches and ceremony helped her to throw aside her depression and despair and move on with her life.

I began by asking her what play she was enacting in her relationship with Miguel. What character was she playing? We settled on a Hispanic version of Cinderella. She had been swept off her feet by Prince Charming. They had traveled around his home country of Ecuador for weeks. She described the poetry he spoke to her, the sensuality and passion of this Hispanic man. She was charmed, mesmerized by his genius and inspiration. It helped that he was substantially older than she and had been her teacher.

"But what character was he playing?" I asked. "Who was he in his own story?" That stopped her. She hadn't considered that. In her story about him he was Prince Charming, holding the glass slipper. But who was he in the story he told about himself? She began to think through the story that he was living—a story of many women who came and left from his life. He had had two wives and untold mistresses. This was his pattern.

"So his Prince Charming was quite different from yours," I surmised. That's when we learned Dora's plot: that her love would change him into a monogamous man, that her passion and his were so great that he would transform.

"But no audience would believe that," I remarked. "It's just not plausible as a plot. How could that happen in a believable way? After your magical summer in Ecuador, you went home to the U.S. to finish college and he went back to his teaching job in Minneapolis. Sure, you talked on the phone and visited each other, but you weren't in Ecuador anymore. Things had changed." And that's when he took up with another woman. Then Dora revealed there had been another woman with whom he had been ending a relationship when they first became close.

"It's not sounding like he belongs in the Cinderella story," I said. "I think this story of his is an Ecuadorian story of many women and of seductive conquest. But he doesn't ever stay with the women, does he?" To that Dora responded that she had met a woman who had been his mistress for ten years.

"That's a rather bleak proposition, isn't it," I asked, "from the standpoint of the Cinderella story you were enacting?"

"The words," she said. "The words that Hispanic men use, they're so romantic, so sensual, so designed to make you feel as though you're the only one, that life turns on your every breath. It's so seductive and exciting."

I asked, "Did you speak Spanish or English?"

"Spanish in Ecuador," she said, "then English when we returned to the U.S."

"Well, no wonder," I said. "Saying things like 'You are the love of my life, my soul, my every breath, my heart, and my inspiration' means something different in Spanish than in English, at least in the story Miguel is enacting. Those words in English could be very serious, but said in Spanish in Ecuador by someone of Miguel's character, they imply something like, 'I'm being romantic, and I'm good at it.' If you translated what he really meant into English it would be quite different, something more like, 'You're cute, let's go to bed.'"

Over time, Dora arrived at the realization that she had been performing one story with Miguel, but he had been in a different play. His play was about multiple conquests. Her play was about the perfect man sweeping her off her feet and their living together happily ever after. I had to remark on the cultural mismatch: "Hispanic lover meets romantic Spanish major from a midwestern university."

The narrative perspective helps us to see that no one was bad or wrong. Miguel was living out one story and Dora another. Act One went fine, because the characters could interact even though they were in different plays. They merely had to travel around Ecuador. Miguel had his summer love. Dora thought she had the love of her life, but the lines worked for both plays. Act Two got shakier. It started when they returned to the United States. Then came Act Three, in which the story lines had to diverge. Miguel's lines called for a new lover to appear. That was his plot. Dora's lines called for Miguel to abandon all others for her. Heartbreak was inevitable.

Within this narrative approach, we could look at the stories that had shaped Dora. She had internalized the stories prominent in her culture—her favorite was *Sleeping Beauty*—and they had made her susceptible to Miguel's character.

We used imagery to find the pieces of Miguel that he had left behind within Dora. We found parts of him in her heart and threw them out. We chased parts of Miguel and various items of Miguel debris out of her ears, her genitals (including the genital herpes he had "given" her), her skin, her mouth, and her brain. When we traveled to her eyes, Dora remarked that Miguel was there showing her how to see the world's beauty. I joked with her.

"Actually," I said, "it's all you. You've created an inner Miguel, and you're using him to see the world as more beautiful, but it's always been your creation. You don't actually have many clues about how Miguel himself sees the world. You just know his beautiful poetry. He may live in a black-and-white world like a 1950s television set. All this beauty you saw when you were with him, you did it yourself." Dora was shocked by the power of this proposition.

Fully escaping an old story is aided by ceremony, which provides a new story toward which it can transport the person. If ceremony were not powerful, we would not need theater or the cinema. It would be sufficient to sit at home and read or to talk with others over dinner. But the pageantry of the theater brings an added something to our experience, something lacking in ordinary conversation.

I needed a ceremony to complete Dora's transition from "addicted to love and betrayed nevertheless" to a more resilient character. A "doctoring" would complete the process. Doctoring as done by traditional healers is equivalent to what is currently called energy medicine. Traditional healers move energy through acts such as blowing smoke over a person, fanning her with eagle feathers, sucking out energy that doesn't belong with a hollow eagle thighbone, using crystals above or on the body, touching the body, massage, and more. The symbolic meaning of these acts is potent. The power of belief and of mind is always impressive.

But I believe something else is also happening. The intentions behind these acts are ways to move energy and change the underlying structure. When I feel this energy moving, it feels very real. Words fail to describe it. Theater exercises used by acting students are more effective for experiencing how energy feels and moves than anything we have invented in alternative medicine. Within the mindset of ceremony, we suspend the skeptical beliefs of the ordinary world. It's like walking through a curtain into another dimension. I empty my mind and "hear" with my mind's ear, not the physical ears of my sensory body. In that mindset, the question, is this real? is irrelevant, though it would be harder for me to lead ceremony with skeptics watching. I would be less confident and more tentative.

There were only the two of us for Dora's ceremony, but two can be enough. I began by burning sage. We waved the smoke over our bodies. I sang a sacred song to call the four directions to come (Four Winds). I asked those beings to pay attention to us, as I did the sky spirits (the sun, the moon, the light, the darkness, and the stars), and spirits of the earth and of the sea, and all of our relatives—the winged beings, the finned ones, the tree people, stone people, two-leggeds, four-leggeds, many-leggeds, creepy crawlers, ancestors, spirits of the place where we sat, and as many others as I could think to mention.

I have learned many ways to move energy during ceremony, but I have to be in the ceremonial state of mind to know which one to use at a particular time. I found myself wanting to use tobacco and a feather to fan the smoke over Dora to chase the bits and pieces of Miguel from her body and into a doll that she had made to contain him. This doll was quite exotic—a coconut for a head, various tropical flowers adorning his neck, a *lei,* sticks for trunk, arms, and legs, garlands of green plants for clothing, a skirt of fine twigs, and two kukui nuts hanging in just the right place.

I was taught to offer tobacco smoke as food to the spirits. The smoking of the tobacco generates a feast for them. I also come from a lineage of Cherokee tobacco healers who grew this most sacred of plants and were deeply respectful of its power of serving as a vehicle for spirit communication. I lit a cigar (smoke stick), offered smoke to the four directions, and proceeded to fan bits and pieces of Miguel off Dora's body and herd them toward the doll, then blew smoke into the holes left behind by their departure so the spirits could travel with the smoke to fill those energy holes and generate wholeness.

I am aware that a written description about what's done in this kind of doctoring fails to capture its essence. It must be experienced to be fully appreciated. The verbal interpretation I have given above is only an approximation of something beyond words, something that is only energy. I have the experience of being guided. I sense higher powers and energies. The presence of my grandfather Archie is always close at hand. Sometimes my grandmother Hazel comes. Sometimes other spirits help.

In Dora's ceremony I felt an ancestral presence from Dora's maternal lineage—a wise, old peasant woman who knew how to heal. I felt the presence of sea creatures—especially turtles (not surprising since we were sitting in the sand at twilight on the beach of the Pacific Ocean). I began to chant. At first I sang a Lakota doctoring song, until slowly but surely the words evolved into just vocables. I could feel the tones produced by my voice moving the last of Miguel into the doll. Dora wished for all those things to go where they should—back to Miguel, to the Creator, to his family, to whoever needed them. She asked the spirits to assist as she set fire to the doll. We put the burning doll on a platform and then walked into the sea. When we were at chest height, we let him go. The waves were mild and the current strong. He was quickly carried out to sea. We watched him burn for some time until the ocean claimed him and he sank. Then we concluded our ceremony with a formal pipe ritual and prayer.

The next morning we did a sunrise ceremony in which we arrived at the ocean before first light and began to sing as the sky lightened. I heard a message that the herpes fed on despair and that Dora had internalized Miguel's despair. I mentioned that, and she agreed. I suggested that we banish the herpes virus as well, treating it as a story she no longer needed. I used song, feathers, and smoke to chase it from her body. We finished with another formal pipe ritual together in which we prayed for her healing.

Three years later, Dora is over her relationship trauma and is productive and happy, although she, like all of us, continues to find challenges. She hasn't had any herpes recurrences.

Essential Elements of Ceremony

The essential elements of ceremony can be summarized as follows:

1. In ceremony we attempt to transform. We have a purpose with sincere, appropriate intention.
2. In ceremony we experience without explanation, meaning that we *participate*. Experience takes precedence over thought and rationale. A ceremony is a break in our usual, incessant effort to make order out of chaos. (Or, it is the recognition that chaos is order not yet perceived.) It provides a locus in time and space where we transcend the ordinary.
3. We humbly acknowledge our place in nature. It is non-anthropocentric.
4. We reenact age-old traditions that draw on the energy of our ancestors.
5. We experience spiritual awareness, the richest, deepest, most meaningful experience of Being, or Spirit. Spiritual awareness is that attitude in which we hold ourselves most open and most receptive to an original experiencing of the Divine, without thought and without our usual cultural hangups.
6. We experience the power and novelty that comes from people and spirits being brought into relationship so as to create new and unexpected patterns "that exceed the complexity of their individual constituents."[10]

1. Sincere and Appropriate Intention

Two women recently came to me for help in connecting with a local traditional healer whom I knew. I didn't question their desire for wellness. I could feel the sincerity of their desires. Immediately the depth from which those desires emanated touched and moved me. However, when I took them to see the healer from Sturgeon Lake First Nation in Saskatchewan, they brought along a friend, unannounced. I carefully explained to the healer the reasons given me by each woman for being there. He responded attentively to the first two women, but not the third. "Enid," the first woman, suffered from relationship problems. Her husband had been seeing other women. Her daughter had been using drugs and alcohol. She wanted to determine if divorce was necessary. "Barbara," the second woman, suffered from a physical illness. "Joanne," the third woman, seemed to have nebulous goals. I found difficulty verbalizing them in a concrete manner to this man for whom English was a difficult language.

He began with a sweatlodge ceremony for us. The lodge sat beside an almost completely frozen lake surrounded by birch trees. A golden Lab barked in the distance from the house. Enid and Barbara were direct about their needs. Their prayers were straightforward and to the point. Enid prayed for her daughter's life, for her to walk away from drugs and alcohol, and for her to become a healthy, beautiful young woman. She prayed for her husband to find clarity about what he really wanted. She prayed for the Spirit to give her the strength and courage to refuse to accept abuse in her life. Barbara prayed directly and clearly for a healing of her physical illness. She prayed for the health and wellness of her daughter, whom she feared suffered from that same illness. Joanne dissembled; her statements were vague and unclear. She offered prayers for peace on earth and for people to get along better. She prayed for Russia and for Israel.

The healer could understand the concrete, emotionally laden requests for help with personal and family matters. I don't think he knew where Russia was. He could not understand abstract prayers. Elders have taught me that spirits are like this healer. They respond to what is said simply and directly. The purpose for ceremony needs to be stated concretely, simply, and directly. Help must be requested *for that problem,* or no help is given. Even if spirits or healers can read minds, elders teach us that they do not respond to telepathic communication. The request for help must be formally, verbally stated. By formal I mean that we begin a ceremony by asking the leader in a straightforward, direct manner for what we seek. Even when I do a ceremony that is private or personal, I begin similarly, by stating to the spirits present why I have come to that place, what I intend to do, and for what I will ask.

"Appropriate" means in respect and harmony with the environment, particularly with the spirit of the place in which the ceremony will occur. This awareness of appropriateness comes from an inner awareness of being in harmony with that place. The first step in a ceremony, then, is to sit where it is going to be done and quietly, slowly, feel the essence of that place. We learn to harmonize with what is present. We enter a place tentatively, asking its permission to be there. Learning to harmonize sounds hopelessly vague until one watches and learns from an elder who is a master at this process of coming into harmony with a place. The master moves quietly and slowly, yet deliberately. All senses are tuned to the environment. Every change is noticed. A communication occurs with the plants, rocks, and animals. A sense of the purpose of a place arises.

Within this first principle of ceremony, we find an appropriate place for expressing our deep, inner feelings. We find a site that feels sacred, that evokes a sense of the great mysteries of life. The location is not as important as the feeling that it evokes. It could be in the wilderness, in our own apartment, or in an open area in a public park if we don't feel too self-conscious there. When I worked in New York City, I did ceremonies in Central Park, Madison Square, and even on the steps of churches. What I loved about New Yorkers was how they ignored me no matter where I was or what I was doing. When we choose a power spot, such as one of those known to indigenous peoples throughout the world as sacred sites, an awareness of the power and beauty of the site leads us to automatically speak and behave correctly.

2. Experience Over Explanation

We face a ceremony with the attitude of participating in a transformative gesture, of experiencing without explanation. I recently saw a woman with an advanced cancer who was doing "all the right things." "Sheila" was undergoing nutritional therapies at a local clinic at considerable expense. She had evaluated various cancer clinics and regularly visited the most popular writers and workshop leaders in the "heal yourself from cancer" movement. Nevertheless, it was clear that Sheila was just going through the motions. An essential commitment to life transformation was missing. Without that spiritual spark, I doubted that any of these other therapies would effectively help her.

I suggested that we do a ceremony because of its capacity to rekindle the faith that prayers are answered. It creates a catalyst, a vehicle, that allows us to transcend the state in which we find ourselves. Sheila, who was doing all the right things, but without commitment, asked me incredulously, "Do people really get well from cancer after a ceremony?" Her question was strange. If she truly believed in the healing power of her other therapies, she would know within her heart that such "miracles" of healing certainly do happen. I had to tell her that some people certainly do get well, but that there were no sure bets, no way to demand that God heal her, no way to make a pact with God for healing in exchange for a certain number of prayers or sweat lodges. I felt that she needed to mix some love and prayer and sweet experiential faith with the brew of her other remedies. Healing may not require the dedication of Saint Francis, but it does involve his kind of ecstasy and sense of participation and union with God and nature.

We come to ceremony with our faith, and we renew this faith through seeing prayers answered. When people construct personal ceremonies, I advise them to *be prepared to pray very specifically for things close to personal experience for which they have faith that the ceremony can start a transformation.* Ceremonies do this. Ceremonies demarcate change in the cosmic order.

3. Acknowledging Our Place in Nature

In ceremony, we humbly acknowledge our place in nature and provide an opportunity for dialogue with spiritual realms and their inhabitants to alter our neuronal connections, to change our synapses, to modify us, which is related to the state of heightened awareness into which we step. We are more susceptible, more suggestible, and more fertile for reorganization and change. Ceremony thus helps us find balance, harmony, and good health.

Here's an example from a seventeen-year-old young man who was diagnosed with autism. "Fritz" believed in spirits. He wanted to do a ceremony to contact Anne Frank, who was his hero. I told him that I couldn't guarantee that we would bring Anne Frank, but I would try. We began by smudging everyone with sage. Then we offered cedar to fill any holes left by the cleansing with the sage. Then I sang a song to alert the guardians of the four directions, the sky spirits (*wakantankan*), and the earth spirits (*ni'kun sicun*) that we were doing something important and would appreciate their paying attention.

In the morning, the sun tumbles brightly
through the Eastern windows,
dancing on dusty shadows,
sharpening the colors.
We can only appreciate the greenness of grass
in bright cloudless sunlight,
can only appreciate water
after a day of thirst.
They come from the West,
the North,
the East,
the South,
whispers on the wind, shadows,
messages from the Great Mystery.
Beech trees in the West protect us
from the setting sun.
In the East, the land slopes down
to the sea.
Wisps of mist and dew shimmer above the grass.
Songs in the distance rise and fall with the force of the wind,
prayers to the rising sun,
the sea,
the setting moon,
the fields and meadows,
the crows and swallows.
Blue herons stretch their wings at the edge of the sea.

Then I offered tobacco while Fritz spoke about what he wanted to know, which was a long litany of questions about various animation companies, requests for things that he wanted to acquire, and expression of grudges he carried. When the tobacco was gone, I told Fritz that he probably should stop since the tobacco was gone and we couldn't keep the portal open to the spirit world forever.

According to traditional teaching, smoking tobacco opens a portal to the spirit world. White Buffalo Woman or First Mother comes to sit in the smoke. She then takes the prayers or thoughts and offers them immediately to the Creator to answer. In those moments when the portal between worlds is more open, this world achieves a freshness and a power usually not experienced. Trees seem so much more profound. Even the grass can sing. I did hear a message for Fritz. The information appeared in my mind.

"Gratitude," I heard. "Patience. He needs to learn gratitude and patience." My contacts refused to answer his individual questions, saying that he could get these answers from his parents, who loved him and could help him find these answers. They also said that some of the answers he wanted would come to him in due time, but not necessarily today.

What they wished was for him to show gratitude to everyone in his life on a daily basis. They acknowledged that his brain was different from most and that he had to work to understand other people. They wanted him to approach each person in his life each day and say, "Thank you. I'm grateful that you're in my life. What can I do today to make your life better?" Fritz was not willing to do this with his parents, as he saw them as blocking him from getting his immediate desires fulfilled. He was, however, willing to ask me what he could do to make my life better. I said, "You can act peacefully around your parents and never hit them. That will improve the quality of my day for I won't worry about you so much." Then we sang a pipe song and loaded the pipe and smoked it so that Fritz would be blessed and assisted to become more aware of his surroundings, especially the other people in his world.

4. Drawing on the Energy of the Ancestors

Ceremony provides us with opportunities to experience what Lakota calls *nagi,* which I translate as "that which contains all the stories that have ever been told by me or about me or in my vicinity or by my ancestors." These stories include the deeds of my ancestors, good and bad, and perhaps the stories from the spirit world that have come with me into this world. Ceremony gives us access to usually hidden stories, which can be powerful.

The dialogue within ceremony affects all participants. We alter, as do the larger entities with whom we communicate during ceremony. We must contribute something to ceremony's shape, just as ceremony shapes us. How this is done is mysterious. No explanation can be made, although, after the fact, we know that something has transformed, something unusual has happened. In the ancient enthronement ceremonies, it was precisely through ceremony that the king became a god, no longer a mere mortal. Without the enthronement ceremony, the king was just another man with a scepter. The ceremony was the portal through which he stepped to become king. It was the alchemical procedure that transformed him from lead to gold, not his birth or the death of his father or any other external event. We see this in Lakota thought as well. The Great Medicine Bear, Hu Nunpa, becomes godlike as the result of a ceremony performed to make him so, not because the Creator wants it or because he wants it.

From an elder I learned the ceremony that is used when strangers ask to enter a camp of the people. It begins with cleansing with sage (also called smudging). Smoldering sage is brought around the circle, and the smoke is directed over each person. Then the pipes that have been brought into the ceremony are loaded. Loading the pipe begins with singing a song of respect, often called a "pipe-loading song." Once the song has been sung, then the stem and the bowl are joined and tobacco is placed into the bowl—a pinch for each of the seven directions (North, East, South, West, Above, Below, Center). Each pinch of tobacco is placed in the smoke of the sage before being placed into the pipe. When the pipe is full, sage is placed over the tobacco to "plug" it and it is placed on the altar. A "four directions song" calls the guardians of each of the four directions, along with those of the sky and the earth, to pay attention to our ceremony.

We sit in a circle and proceed clockwise around the circle so each person can tell a story of a time when he or she demonstrated courage, the first of the four virtues, associated with the West. The idea is to prove to those listening that one is worthy of being admitted to the community. When everyone has spoken, another song is sung to honor the West or the Bear who lives there. Next, cedar is burned, and a song is sung to honor the North and the Buffalo who lives there. Then going around the circle, each person tells a story of a time in which he or she demonstrated strength, endurance, or fortitude, the virtue of the North. When all are done, another honoring song is sung. Then sweetgrass is burned, after which a song is sung to honor the East and the eagles who dwell there. Then each person tells a story to demonstrate that he or she has a vision or a purpose or has received a vision or a purpose, the virtue of the East. When all are done, another honoring song is sung. Finally lavender is burned to honor the South and, around the circle, stories are told of times that demonstrate that the teller has shown the virtue of compassion, forgiveness, or exceptional love or kindness. In times past, the Council of Elders would then deliberate on the merits of each individual as presented and would decide whether or not to welcome them into the community.

I conducted a similar ceremony with a group of people in Denmark, and all demonstrated the four virtues. All were invited to join the community we were forming. The formation of our community for working together for the week of a conference in this way was much more powerful than a more typical way of introducing ourselves with stories about where we work and what we do and how important we are. The invitation to enter the community was completed by all present offering a prayer as we went around the circle; then we smoked the pipes that had been filled.

What we did next came to me in a spirit-inspired moment and cannot be deemed traditional, though it could have been. After the pipes were smoked, I spoke to the collected group and invited them to enter into an altered state of consciousness—the one where dreams originate. I continued to speak and give suggestions for openness to experience and invited each person to let a spirit who wished to help them speak through them or dance through them. I said this could be a plant, a rock, a mountain, a lake, a river, an animal, an ancestor—whatever came. I stopped speaking when the first person began speaking as her spirit. I then stepped into the background, chanting softly and drumming. Everyone present spoke for a spirit and many moved as that spirit. These spirits had advice for our community and became supporters for our work together.

Popular American culture calls these beings "power animals," but the traditional cultural concept is less firm, less fixed, less rigid. These entities are not necessarily just animals, but any aspect of the universe. The concept is that a spirit might choose to come help you. You have to listen carefully and cultivate this relationship, which will unfold in its own unique way. The meaning of the spirit who comes is not coded in a book, as a more New Age approach might indicate, but is offered by each individual spirit. The spirit speaks for itself and says what it has come to teach or communicate. I have been amazed in my workshops by how many people want to see an animal and look up its message in a book, rather than engage in the much more powerful opportunity to connect with a vibrant nonphysical entity and learn what it has to offer.

5. Growing Spiritual Awareness

Most important, ceremony creates rich, deep, meaningful experiences of Being, or Spirit. Ceremony serves to create increased spiritual awareness, which helps to achieve the purpose of the ceremony. Doug Boyd, author of *Rolling Thunder,* a book about the traditional healer bearing that name, describes how he would never commence a healing ritual before being satisfied that the patient's purpose held dignity and meaning for that person.[11] Just wanting to get well was not enough for Rolling Thunder to do the ceremony; the person's purpose had to relate to a greater good that the patient would achieve if he or she became well. The fulfillment of this higher purpose became the point of the ceremony.

6. Creating New Patterns: How and When to Pray

Ceremony signifies a discontinuity in the fabric of space-time, as if we had been given permission to request a bending or temporary suspension of the usual rules of physical reality. After the sacred pipe has been smoked in the Lakota sweatlodge ceremony the leader reminds the participants that *their prayers have already been answered.* He or she does not say that their prayers might now be answered or to pay attention to whether or not the prayers will be answered. The leader emphatically insists that the prayers *have been* answered, because of a covenant made between the Creator and the people through *Wohpe,* or White Buffalo Calf Woman. Through her gift of the sacred pipe and the promise that she made for the Creator and at the Creator's instruction, when the pipe is loaded and smoked in the sacred, traditional manner, the prayers have already been answered. Past tense.

Some people get confused by this concept, which results in their not knowing how to pray or for what to pray. An unparalleled arrogance or anthropocentrism lies within the modern, individualistic Western story about the world. I have watched this unfold in a sweatlodge in a person praying for an immediate end to war. In contrast, an indigenous person would tend to pray for an end to the fighting between two people in her family. She might pray for the land on which she lives. She might pray for the health of the animals living on that land or for their abundance. She would not tend to pray for so large a concept as the end of a war because of a general feeling that such a prayer would be arrogant. One elder said, "Think globally, but pray locally."

The notion of "local" prayers is central to ceremony and consists of experiences with which the individual is personally familiar. The larger the experience, the less familiar we are with it and the more it is formed from other people's prayers and not just our own. If consensual experience is the result of prayer (and this is what traditional Lakota and Cherokee people believe), then a large-scale experience is the result of large-scale prayers. We recognize that our prayers must take into account the prayers of the many. This is acknowledged in the wording of prayer. A person might say something along the lines of, "Creator, if it would be okay,

Larry over there is really hurting, and it makes his family hurt, and I'd really like to ask your help for him, if that would be okay."

How to Do Your Own Ceremony

I believe everyone should have a personal ceremony, and I suggest that all my students and clients create one. In planning a ritual, we should be clear about our purpose. What do we really want? How do you do this?

Most desirable would be to recall your childhood spirituality—if it is still a spiritual path with which you resonate in a positive way. We might describe this as rediscovering the faith of innocence when Santa Claus spoke to you or when you looked at Christ on the cross and felt his suffering and saw fresh tears in his eyes. Mountains are moved by the faith of a child. Find a ceremony that was deeply meaningful to you, then find someone who knows how to do that ceremony and dialogue with him or her about teaching you to do the ceremony in a way that makes it responsive to the changing needs of our current historical situation, while still honoring the ancestors who developed the ritual. I have helped clients do this and have witnessed beautiful reenactments of the Christmas story, German winter solstice celebrations, and Jewish harvest festivals. Christians may take a sip of wine and eat bread that has become the blood and the flesh of Christ to symbolize this communion gesture. (Remember the meaning of the word *communion* came from *communication*.)

If you have no ideas of your own and cannot find a teacher to guide you and you resonate with Native American traditions, try this. Obtain some sage and something in which to burn it. Find a candle and flowers and arrange them at a place where you feel peaceful and whole. Begin by stating (out loud so the spirits can hear you) why you are doing the ceremony. Sing a song to honor the spirits, remembering that ceremony is an alchemical transformation through faith. The elders say that the spirits cannot resist a song, and your ancestors cannot resist hearing your voice in song. I sing Lakota songs that I have learned from elders. Sing any spiritual songs that you believe the spirits of your ancestors would feel honored to hear. Once you have the spirits' attention, then a statement of purpose or prayer often comes next.

I pray to the seven directions—North, East, South, West, Above, Below, Center—acknowledging each of their gifts. I pray directly, humbly, and simply, acknowledging that my will may not be the wisest course. I pray for others first, then family, and last, one or two needs that I have. Then I load my pipe and smoke the tobacco for the ancestors and the spirits, knowing that the Creator hears my prayers directly. As an alternative to a pipe, you can roll tobacco in a corn husk and smoke it in that manner (without inhaling). Or you can burn incense. Then I close my ceremony with another song and say thanks to all the spirits who have come.

This simple procedure can be very powerful if approached with the attitudes described earlier in this chapter. I recently used it to ask a spirit to start my car when its battery had died. It did, and I was able to drive into town in time to make a class and have my car worked on later. "Miracles" will happen, but only when, within the consciousness of the ceremony, these events seem normal and commonplace, that is, the participants believe miracles can and do readily occur in ceremony.

What if you have no idea how to begin your personal use of ceremony? Anything can be ritualized, as long as it provides a means with which you resonate spiritually and emotionally. I have started clients in ritual through making them a visualization tape to which to listen. I ask them to begin by burning sage or incense, to say a simple verbal prayer or statement about their purpose in listening to the tape, and then to lie down or sit and let the tape do its work on them. When done repetitively, this is a ceremonial ritual.

I have started musicians in ceremony through their music. If you want to do this, find music to play or sing that evokes a sense of the sacred in you. Begin by burning sage or incense to mark that you have entered into a different context of time and space. Olfactory cues—that is, scents—can be very powerful; the human olfactory system is connected to the limbic system, or emotional center, of the brain. Demarcation of the beginning and ending of ceremony, such as through a concrete act of lighting a candle and blowing it out, burning sage to begin and burning cedar to end, singing an opening song and then a closing song, sets it apart from ordinary reality, thereby increasing its effectiveness. After the opening, make a simple prayer or statement of purpose or a request for help. Then play the music, and the ceremony is ended.

Similarly, those who are artistically inclined can make sacred objects as their ceremony. The process begins with an opening and ends with a closing as above. A statement of purpose or prayer comes next. Then an object is made while the person is engaged in contemplation of the sacred, in a meditative state of consciousness. The object could be a simple drawing, a carving, a doll constructed from natural materials, and so on. The medium and the result are far less important than the intention to use art to communicate with the Divine. I frequently remind clients that this art is not for sale and should not be judged. Personal sacred art is perfect regardless of its appearance, because it expresses a spiritual experience for that individual.

One woman started this process by carving animal totems in bars of soap. She had received dreams of carving totems, but had never done any art in her forty-three years on this planet. She began with soap because of its forgiving quality. This reduced the performance/production anxiety often associated with art (unfortunately inculcated by our educational system).

If you wish to do a ritual with friends or with a loved one, try the same formula. Pick one of you as the leader who performs the opening gesture (lights the incense, lights the candle, and so forth). Then sing together. Use whatever instruments of celebration are available to you (drums, rattles, spoons, violins . . .). Rhythm as provided by drums and rattles can be a powerful trance inducer, but all music is helpful.

Let each person make a personal statement of purpose or request for help. Start at one place in the circle and proceed clockwise (the direction in which the sun travels). Share communion with each other through offering tobacco, through sipping sacred water, through eating a special food, or through your own unique means. The idea of communion is to ingest the spirit into your physical body. Then the leader performs the closing. As you use this form, change will spontaneously occur and you will be in attunement with how ceremony has changed over the ages. Eventually your "clan" will have its own unique ceremony specific to your personalities and needs.

Make time in your life for ceremony, pray with your heart, and believe that prayers *are* answered. These are sufficient guidelines with which to start exploring the healing power of ceremony.

11

How Communities Create Change

Man is made by his belief. As he believes, so he is.

BHAGAVAD GITA, 500 BCE

Communities can create powerful shared narratives, which allow all of their members to look in the same direction, to share intentionality, and to experience the belongingness of coherence with other people. This sense of group coherence and shared intention, cultivated by being in a group that regularly does ceremony together, holds more power than do "powerful shamans" or other healers. Spiritual power arises through relationship. It arises from common prayer, from coherent thought generated by shared intention. People who pray together or share spiritual practice together week after week become coherent with one another.

When I encounter people who have experienced miraculous (by biomedical standards) healing, these people are usually members of tight-knit communities, whether on rural or remote reservations or in the middle of ethnic neighborhoods in the largest cities. What seems important is duration of relationship, longer history of exposure to doing ceremony together, and being in a cohesive spiritual relationship with each other. Where these conditions are met, miracles can occur. Elders and ceremonial leaders certainly can be wonderful people who inspire confidence, faith, and hope, and whose cultivation of relationships with spirits is helpful in healing, but their role rides on top of a solid community of long-term relationships that build interconnected-ness and a communal mind.

I suspect that the mainstream media miss the importance of community and focus on the idea of the powerful, individual healer as a result of the pervasive individualistic paradigms and the contemporary preferences of mainstream Euro-American culture to find quick fixes and answers outside of ourselves. Hollywood movies about Native people and traditional healers frequently contain scenes of a mysterious "medicine man" or "shaman" shaking his rattle over someone and chanting, after which that person is instantaneously cured. Alternately, they focus on a magical potion, which only the healer knows how to concoct from an exotic plant that only grows in a very difficult place to reach. But the most powerful ceremonies I have attended have been those with groups who had been doing ceremony together regularly for many years, regardless of who their leader was. Communities are more powerful than individuals—a consistent lesson from indigenous cultures.

Canaries in Our Social Mine Shafts

Every community, however, has its seeds of disharmony and imbalance. I see those individuals who struggle with what we call "madness" or what could be called "unacceptable behavior" as the canaries in our social mine shafts. The suffering of these individuals should alert us to be aware that we as a whole are not well. Rather than trap them and segregate them away from others, we need to celebrate their sacrifice and undertake the healing of the communities in which we live so that these individuals can suffer less. As any Dene (the tribe of Northern Arizona and New Mexico) person would recognize, we are all responsible as a group for the suffering of any one of us. Traditional people do not ostracize and separate people who are suffering, unlike our contemporary societies. Michel Foucault (1926–1984), a French historian and philosopher who studied and influenced social science disciplines, wrote about the birth of the contemporary concept of madness as arising from the birth of the merchant class and the accompanying need to remove annoying and irritating people from streets and shops and put them into asylums.*

Today our asylums (state hospitals in North America) have largely been emptied, although many of the ill simply went from state hospitals to jails or the streets. The "mad" are among us. We go out of our way to avoid them, crossing the street when we see homeless people muttering to themselves on sidewalk corners. They frighten us. They challenge our sense of order. We worry that their illness is contagious, that we might catch it. We label them as "insane" and make them different from us. We expect professional experts to take them under care, fix them, and keep them until they look "normal" when standing on street corners or entering grocery stores.

If we are to transform our society, we must change the way suffering people are treated. In *Narrative Medicine* I wrote about the World Health Organization's studies of schizophrenia in third world countries and how people who receive these labels are not taken out of their communities, but are cared for by family and friends, at home, with dignity and respect.

We have reason to fear some people who appear mad, for some are violent, though much less often than we fear. Some people do have to be sequestered away from the bulk of humanity until their stories change. Recently in Hawai'i, a man was released from the state hospital and promptly went to a store, bought a knife, and lethally stabbed a woman in the ice cream store next door, who had no relation to him. When I lived in Saskatchewan, a man who had been declared insane decapitated an innocent passenger on a bus traveling from Winnipeg to Regina. Rare as these events are (like shark attacks in Hawai'i, which happen on average once per year with one fatality on average every ten years), they fuel our fear of people who are different.

I wonder what would have happened to these people if they had been approached with love and compassion when they first showed signs of

---

*Foucault studied psychology in the late 1940s and 1950s in Europe. His first major work, *The History of Madness in the Classical Age,* was published in 1961.

disturbance. My Quechua psychiatry colleague from Ecuador tells me that the custom in his culture upon seeing apparently disturbed people is to bring them home and feed them. If we adopted this practice in the mainstream world, what would happen to violence from disturbed people? I suspect incorporating them in this way into community would make most violence go away.

We All Need Healing Circles

I think we have a universal need to belong to a healing circle. This proposal is echoed on www.mehl-madrona.com as the Hocokah Project. *Hocokah* is a Lakota word for "healing circle," also sometimes used to refer to the altar used in a circle. In indigenous North America, *circularity* was a more useful explanatory concept than *linearity*. People in ceremony sat in a circle. The four directions were conceived circularly. The horizon is a circle. We must turn ourselves around 360 degrees to see all directions. The compass is a circle. I suspect the medicine wheel began as a representation of the horizon.

Nature is full of circles—the sun, the moon, the earth and other planets, the base of a mountain, bird nests, beaver homes, and more. Even from its rising to its setting, the sun traces an arc across the sky. A wonderful Dene story from northern Arizona tells how the people learned to build their homes as circles (hexagons) by studying how all the animals built their homes. I am even told by hunters that animals' territories are circles, marked as such by the animals as they roam. Circularity conveys repetition more than linearity. The repeating of the seasons exemplifies this.

Circles are useful for understanding life's mysteries. We know that circles better explain open systems than straight lines. Feedback loops are circular. Traced out over time, the circle becomes the sine wave, with its waxing and waning, its peaks and troughs. Circles help us to better understand how our behavior affects others, whose behavior in turn feeds back to affect us. One classic example in ecology is the waxing and waning of coyote and rabbit populations on the Kaibib Plateau of Arizona's Grand Canyon. Rabbit populations rise when coyote populations dwindle. The rise of rabbits gives coyotes more food. Then coyote populations rise. Too many coyotes mean not enough rabbits. Rabbit populations fall and cannot sustain the coyotes. Coyote populations fall and rabbits rise again. This is life, as any biology student can tell us.

In the Lakota world, everyone belonged to a healing circle, usually organized around an elder. The healing circle took care of its members. It was an opportunity to be healing for each other. In larger gatherings (such as for a sun dance) people traveled with their hocokah and camped together and ate together and did sweatlodge together even as they prepared to enter the larger group. The healing circle was a constant supportive presence and also provided each person a group with whom to do ceremony.

I read a beautiful account of a clinical psychologist, Joyce Vesper, in Scottsdale, Arizona, doing a ceremony with her patient to complete her healing from dissociative identity disorder (what used to be called multiple personality disorder).[1] The ceremony was done by the client and the psychologist in a park in Scottsdale. It would have been so much more powerful if it had been done as a part of a healing circle, with other people. It was still healing for this patient and therapist, but if it had been part of a healing circle, it could have been healing for many others in different ways at the same time. When we share ceremony as a community, we create larger narratives in which we all participate that draw us closer together forever.

Talking Circles

Healing circles often used "talking circles." Within Lakota culture, the talking circle was a tool for communication, better decision making, and strengthening of a hocokah or the entire community. The talking circle occurs both within the context of a healing circle and independent of a healing circle. A common format is for one person to call the circle to order. Sage that is smoldering is passed around the circle. Each member blesses himself with the smoke by symbolically using his hands to direct the smoke over his body.

When the sage returns to its beginning, the initiating member states her intent for the talking circle. The intent starts the circle, though the circle can go anywhere. Examples of intents could be: "I need help with reducing the severity of my colitis." "I need help getting a voice under control that is tormenting me every day." "I need help figuring out how to financially survive the month now that I am out of work." Or, "I need help figuring out what sense to make of my recent doctor visit and all that she had to say and recommend."

Then the initiator says a prayer to make the circle sacred. Sometimes a song is offered to the beat of a drum or rattle. Then the convener starts the movement of a sacred object around the circle, giving each person the chance to speak. The talking circle is done when all have spoken and no more words are left to say. Usually a consensus or a consensual understanding has been reached by then. Sometimes a talking stick is used as a way to indicate who is speaking. When one is used, it is usually a staff that has been made sacred by prayers and decoration. Whoever is holding the stick is entitled to speak as long as he or she wishes without interruption, which is an amazing, almost never occurring experience in modern culture.

Imagine eight to twelve people sitting in a circle. The sage has been passed. The smell lingers. The initiator of the circle has stated her intention and has said a prayer. You can still feel the beat of the drum from the song that hasn't yet left your ears. The stick has been passed to the person on the initiator's left, who is free to talk as long as he wishes. When he is finished talking, he passes the stick to the person on his left, and the process continues.

Rather than a talking stick, some circles use an eagle feather, a stone, or a crystal. Other circles use no object. The speaker simply states that she is finished. Objects symbolize and embody the wisdom of the group. They spiritually empower the holder of the object to speak her or his truth as an offering to the circle. They help us speak from the depths of our soul, but in the end, we can always pray and heal without any objects whatsoever. Objects are extras, sometimes powerful through their absorption of all the good prayers and intents in all the ceremonies in which they have been used.

What is said in a talking circle is unpredictable. People's potential responses change as they listen to each speaker. No one ever says what she thought she was going to say. When people have to listen, they are changed by each speaker. Something new emerges from this dialogue that could not have occurred without it. Talking circles provide opportunities for "listening without judgment" in the words of French psychiatrist Jacques Lacan, or "deep listening" in the words of Australian Aboriginal people.

A talking circle provides a means for the diversity of views and talents present in the group to emerge in a nonthreatening way. Communication in which people talk over each other and interrupt cannot accomplish this. In a direct, cross-talk format, people are too busy thinking about what they want to say, instead of listening to the person speaking. The talking circle prevents this.

The talking circle is part of a healing circle, which is so much more. The healing circle can use the talking circle format to break the ice, introduce new people, and explore each other's stories. It can use the talking circle to establish the guidelines for what will happen and how its members will behave. Action is initiated from the dialogue that ensues from the talking circle.

I have seen healing circles use the talking circle format to plan ceremonies and have done this in workshops. As the stick goes around the circle, each person contributes something from his or her traditions of origin. A joint ceremony that is part of everyone slowly emerges. What is amazing is that everyone knows how to create a ceremony if given permission to do so.

Restoring a Lost Art

I believe people have always been part of healing circles and in recent times there has been a trend to return to various types of healing circles. We could probably trace the loss of healing circles to the development of the Industrial Age and the birth of nuclear families, isolated from one another. This has gone too far. We are unnecessarily isolated in contemporary North

America. We are so lacking in people with whom to do ceremony, to cry, to laugh, to act out skits, to drum, to dance. We are alone amid an ever-growing population, trapped in our little boxes (apartments, homes, farm-houses), isolated.

My cousin picked me up from the airport when I went to visit my mother for the weekend before Thanksgiving. We were reminiscing about the big family get-togethers we used to experience. "Nobody does that anymore," she said. "We haven't done that for years."

"What do you do to get together?" I asked.

"Maybe we have hors d'oeuvres," she said. "We stop in for a few minutes on Christmas Eve."

"What about Thanksgiving?" I said. I hadn't attended Thanksgiving with my mother for years since I have my own children and they are scattered about and are unlikely to congregate at my mother's house. I was out of touch with how things had changed.

"We don't get together anymore," she said. "We don't do that." My large family had disintegrated into small nuclear groups that rarely encountered one another. The idea of being spiritual with one another was even stranger. Following my grandmother's death, spirituality for my family had become going to church on Sunday morning: the usual Christian affair of all sitting facing the front (so different from sitting in a circle) and rising at the proper time to sing songs from a songbook, listening to a sermon, and mumbling a prayer from a book. When I joined them, I felt no depth. No connectedness happened between us, although I could believe that many people were able to connect with Creator through this ceremony, however vapid I found it. I was grateful that my mother had stopped going to church regularly, because I found it so boring. Like most people, I crave connectedness, not superficially going through the motions.

I suggested to my cousin that she start a healing circle. Maybe even people in my family would want to come. She doubted it. Describing the way I start healing groups, I made the following suggestions to her.

First, you call everyone you know and invite them to come to a meeting at a specific time and place for the purpose of being healing for each other. I suggest that the person who convenes the meeting start by stating his or her intent and inviting others to join in making that intent manifest. The talking circle is a good way to begin, since it provides a structure from which healing can emerge. Through the format of the talking circle, people present their unique talents to offer to healing. Some may know Reiki or massage. Some may know how to sing healing songs, while others may know how to drum. Others may be familiar with ceremony. Through the passage of the stick around the talking circle, people become familiar with each other's talents and abilities. When the circle ends, perhaps it is time for a healing to take place.

One person can enter the center of the circle for healing, if that is what the group decides. Imagine how it would be to lie in the center of a circle of ten people. Some are sending Reiki, others are massaging you, others are singing for you, others are drumming, and others are saying soothing words (storytelling, guided imagery, or just helpful talk). This is really what we need—to feel connected in this way.

Besides a talking circle, healing circles can include meditation, guided imagery, yoga, Reiki, massage, drumming, singing, reflexology—in short, just about anything that's healing. Groups naturally tend to share in ways that relate to the needs of the members. It's wonderful to build into the evening a simple tradition of treats and fellowship afterward.

What I have learned from participating in healing circles from Croatia to Australia is how wise and healing people can be for each other. The hocokah movement that we are creating recognizes this. Healing circles need to be nonhierarchical. They need to overthrow the "medical expert" paradigm that has been so carefully constructed in the North American health care system. (Medical experts are important for their "know-how," but they are not necessary for most of the healing that we need in our lives, especially preventive transformation to avoid or avert disease.) If everyone belonged to a healing circle, we would take our aches and pains there first. We would explore how to help each other in that context. We would reserve the aches and pains we take to biomedical physicians to those that our healing circle can't help us reduce and for which our healing circle members feel a biomedical perspective would be useful. We would use our healing circle to figure out what we would do with the recommendations that biomedical physicians make for us.

A Healing Circle Story

"Mary" was part of my healing circle in Saskatoon, Saskatchewan. She suffered from debilitating pain during her menses, so much so that she was occasionally hospitalized for pain management. She had suffered for seven years. She was unable to work during her cycle and had been reduced to home-based businesses and part-time work, since employers would not tolerate long monthly absences. Her doctors had diagnosed endometriosis (in which the lining of the uterus extends into the abdominal cavity) and insisted on surgery. (This is so typical of how doctors think—structurally. I have often questioned such a diagnosis, which leads to uterine removal, since I suspect many people have equally severe signs of endometriosis, but no symptoms. While I have sometimes seen surgery be curative or helpful, I have also seen it fail.)

Mary joined our healing circle. During her first visit, she talked about her symptoms incessantly every time she had the talking stick. By her second visit, she talked about her sadness and misery and unhappiness. By the third visit, she talked about her boyfriend and how he didn't want to have children and how much she wanted to have children, how terrified she was to lose her uterus, and how angry she was that the doctors didn't seem to care. By the fourth visit, she talked about being raped seven years earlier. Light bulbs lit above everyone in the room except for Mary.

"Don't you think that might have some relationship to your pain?" asked the next speaker as the talking stick passed. Others echoed similar sentiments. When the stick returned to Mary, she was confused. How could that experience cause her to have this disease? She had mentioned this idea to one of her doctors (a woman gynecologist), who had belittled her for even suggesting it. The speaker to her left suggested that doctors don't always know everything about the mysteries of sickness and health. The next speaker suggested that we work as a group to help Mary heal her past and her pelvis. Someone suggested that we make a collage to express

Mary's pain. Mary agreed and brought magazines and images to the next meeting (her fifth). Everyone participated. We didn't need the talking circle that week, because we had a task to do. Mary created a collage about her rape, about her pain and her uterus, and about the life she wished to have.

At the next circle (Mary's sixth), we began again with a talking circle to discuss the collages and the experience of making them. During that circle, family reconstruction was suggested. Mary revealed that her father had sexually molested her and beaten her as a child (a far-too-common occurrence). The group encouraged her to act out some scenes from her childhood that would help her understand how her past was still active in her present. We talked about some particular dramatic moments from her childhood (not the molestation itself) coming from times when both of her parents had been drinking. We planned two scenes to enact the next week. Mary asked to observe and chose another circle member to play her.

Mary's seventh circle was powerful and intense. Group members played Mary, her father, her mother, and her brother, first in a powerful scene in which her father had stabbed her mother while they were fighting drunk and the police had come. Her mother went to the hospital. Her father went to jail. She and her brother went to equally drunken relatives nearby. Everyone recovered physically. Her mother's wounds were not severe. Her father eventually was released from jail. But the family never recovered emotionally. Her parents separated, which perhaps was a good thing.

The second scene we played was a time when Mary's mother was passed out drunk in the living room after falling down and hitting her head on the edge of the sofa. Mary was seven years old and was terrified, with no clue about what to do. She was afraid her mother was dead, but she was more afraid to call for help because her mother had told her never to do that because social services would take Mary away from home if they came to the house and found her mother passed out drunk. Mary's brother was gone. What was she to do?

Enacting these two scenes with the group was powerfully revealing and healing for Mary. We spent Mary's eighth circle discussing these enactments, with group members proposing a healing ceremony. Mary agreed. We finished the eighth circle discussing what to do in the healing ceremony. A plan emerged, with each person contributing an element from his or her own past and culture.

On Mary's ninth circle, we did the ceremony. An entrance was constructed so that it looked as if Mary was crossing a bridge to enter the room. She was ceremonially smudged with sage smoke. Participants sang to her. A member sang a song to call in spirits. He then talked to the spirits and said we had come together to cleanse Mary's soul and to request that her pain be removed and that she be allowed to get well. We had come to ask that her past be healed so that it no longer tormented her. Then Mary spoke. She tearfully described what had happened and asked for healing and for forgiveness. We then offered tobacco to the spirits and sang and drummed. The assembled group worked collectively on Mary for more than an hour, doing energy healing, Reiki, and any other techniques that anyone knew. Everyone stopped at once. Mary sat up. "I'm a different person," she said. "I'm clean."

She looked different. Everyone hugged her. Tears were shed. Mary then burned her collages of her past, keeping the one of the future she wished to create. We finished with a Lakota pipe ceremony that I was asked to lead for the group.

Everyone was willing and happy to devote several meetings to healing Mary's pain, probably because it helped to heal pain in each person on some level. Mary's pain stopped soon after her ceremony. She continued to come to the healing circle, but she no longer needed to be the center of the group's attention except for the occasional week when she felt part of a crisis or had some difficulty and asked for the time. Over the course of the next year, she left her boyfriend and met a new guy who wanted to have children and seemed like a much better marriage prospect. She was able to get a full-time job as a beautician (which she had trained to do) and began to study art at the community college. She was a much happier and healthier person.

This healing circle was cost effective. It didn't cost Mary anything. Imagine how much she had cost the healthcare system up to the time of her ceremony and what her surgery would have cost. And it might not have even worked! This is another reason why everyone needs to be in a healing circle—so that we can save the healthcare system, since it's sinking like the Titanic even as I write these words. It costs too much due to its emphasis on structure and disease and not on healing and relationship. Paradoxically, it will sink regardless of whether it is a single-payer system like Canada or a multiple-payer system like the United States. It simply is too heavy to float.

Healing Circle Dynamics

One person described her healing circle to me in this way: "[We] feel so thankful to be there. We share the experience of it being somewhere we really look forward to going. One of us called it an 'anchor'—that no matter what else was happening we each knew 'that's where I go on Wednesday nights!' We all feel that we are there to be equally healer and to be healed, and that by following the 'flow,' so to speak, we come away with what we need that night. We all feel comfortable in any role—perhaps being vulnerable and 'unavailable' one week and strong and 'available' the next. We experience no judgment from each other around this, and no one person seems to shoulder more than another."

Peter Blum, my friend from Woodstock, New York, notes that in a healing circle, "There is no way to know what will present itself. Sometimes there seems to be no particular focus. We might practice receiving energy as healers, for instance. Sometimes we drum and sing and dance or tell stories of miraculous moments in our lives. Other times a person or two will communicate that they wish to be the focus of ceremony for a personal healing. It's a fine line between form and formless."

What is hardest about our contemporary healing circles is the question of leadership. Once upon a time, in the indigenous world, elders presided over healing circles. If you are lucky enough to find an elder to join you, great. But it is often hard to find a good elder. And leaderless healing circles work fine. This is good to keep in mind in the situation that sometimes arises when the available elders are stifling and restrictive of progress. I have seen elders prevent creative movement and change.

I remember two particular Cree elders who insisted on their definition of tradition over any other. They scolded any women who wore dresses that did not sweep the ground. They insisted that no one could come to their ceremonies if they ever drank alcohol or even if anyone in their extended family drank. They had too many rules and prohibitions to keep track of them all. Needless to say, the youth, who really needed to spend time with elders, never came. Those who came were obsequious and didn't question the authority of the elders. This was not my idea of elder leadership. In my view, anyone should be able to come to a healing and be accepted. I don't want to tell women how long their skirts should be. I don't mind if homeless people come, and I welcome people who live at the margins of society, practicing alcoholics and drug addicts, people who are psychotic, and anyone else who shows up.

A "postmodern" perspective on healing circles is necessarily different from a traditional cultural approach, even if it looks the same most of the time. What makes us postmodern is our awareness that no one can claim to have the truth. We can only argue on the basis of what works, what is practical, and what is aesthetic. A traditional cultural approach can remain in a premodern perspective that whatever they think is right and true. This is what I saw these Cree elders doing, although I wondered how traditional long skirts were, since the idea of covering every bit of potentially exposed female flesh seems more Christian than aboriginal North American.

So, in our move to start healing circles in every living room, we are decidedly postmodern. A Quaker healing circle might involve people sitting in silence together until someone feels moved to speak and might not involve a talking circle or stick at all. A Christian healing circle might start with Bible reading and prayer. Each group will have its own way of proceeding based on local customs and practices.

The question of leadership remains. My feeling is that someone must convene the healing circle. Someone must explain the rules for a particular circle, however simple they are—and the simpler, the better. Someone needs to set the initial intent for the circle and say the starting prayer (or prayer equivalent). Someone needs to say the closing prayer. Ideas that seem to work include the servant leader model and the idea of rotating facilitators.

Regarding circle facilitation, my friend Magili Chapman-Quinn, a family doctor from Maine, wrote, "Whether with humor, the weaving of words or silence, strong leaders stay present and committed to what is actually taking place, rather than invested in the circle being 'successful.' . . . Good facilitation is usually 'transparent,' in the sense that members leave the circle less impressed with the wisdom and power of the facilitator(s) than with a strong feeling of the movement and connectedness of the whole circle."

I can't emphasize enough the power that individual people find when they meet together for healing. People are amazing. Imagine what would happen if everyone belonged to a healing circle. If you are reading this and want to start a healing circle, be the initiator. Call everyone you know and invite them to join you at a specific time and place to explore how to be healing for one another. Once everyone convenes, as the convener, you need to create the initial structure. You can say that the goal is to create an environment where people can be helpful and healing.

Then you can explain the idea of the talking circle and propose starting in this way until you have settled on your own structure for what you will do and how you will do it. You can begin by setting the initial intent as figuring out how to proceed to be healing for each other, and then pass the stick around so that each person can contribute his or her thoughts. You can continue going around the circle until everyone has said what he or she feels the need to say. Then you can summarize what you have heard and send the stick around again for people to add to or subtract from your remarks.

Then together you can develop a structure and resolve the question of leadership: will you rotate being the person who starts the meeting, have the same person do it each time, or have the person at whose house you are meeting do it? Once a structure is created, you can periodically revisit it through the talking circle format to make sure that everyone still likes it and that it is working for everyone.

I'd like to finish by describing a ceremony that one healing circle in which I participated created to say goodbye to one of its members who was moving to another country. The ceremony began with a procession from inside the room where we did our work to a beautiful pond in the forest that surrounded the facility where we met. We walked the five minutes to the pond accompanied by drumming and chanting. Coffee was very important to this woman, so the group began its ceremony by sharing coffee, passing a cup around the circle for each person to take a sip.

Then we were cleansed by having drops of fresh water sprinkled over us. Then each person tossed a flower into a pot of water in the center of the circle, symbolizing that we were each offering our energy to the whole. The idea was to take a thing from nature to generate a blessing for the entire group. Then we did a folk dance, which is called a braiding dance, since arms are intertwined as people move around a circle. Next each member of the group spoke about the person who was leaving.

Then we danced as the helper animals that we had discovered during previous meetings, and each animal offered a piece of wisdom or advice to the woman who was moving. I remember some of the blessings given by the animals:

"May the light of the sun reflecting in the deep ocean make you think about God's reflection in you."

"May the rose petals remind you of your own lightness and fragrance."

Then I sang a song of thanksgiving and we all shook hands and hugged the woman who was leaving. As part of the handshaking, each person looked deeply into every other person's eyes, which was also deeply moving.

12
To Story or Not to Story

"One can't believe impossible things."
"I daresay you haven't had much practice," said the
Queen. "When I was your age, I always did it for half an
hour a day. Why, sometimes, I believed as many as six
impossible things before breakfast."

LEWIS CARROLL, *THROUGH THE LOOKING GLASS*

Standard Treatment for Psychotic Disorders

Historians argue that the introduction of neuroleptics (also called anti-psychotic drugs, beginning with chlorpromazine) in the 1950s made it possible to empty the mental hospitals.[1] In *Mad in America*, Robert Whitaker writes that the belief that the introduction of chlorpromazine (marketed in the United States as Thorazine) made it possible to empty state hospitals stems from research by Brill and Patton. In the early 1960s, they reported that the patient census at state mental hospitals in the United States declined from 558,600 in 1955 to 528,800 in 1961. Although they did not compare discharge rates for drug-treated versus placebo-treated patients, they nevertheless concluded that neuroleptics must have played a role in the decline since it coincided with their introduction. The fact that the two occurred at the same time was seen as the proof.[2]

Whitaker points out the obvious confounding factors. In the early 1950s, the Council of State Governments in the United States urged the federal government to share the fiscal burden of caring for the mentally ill and proposed that "outpatient clinics should be extended and other community resources developed to care for persons in need of help, but not of hospitalization."[3] As part of this agenda, states began developing community care initiatives, funneling the mentally ill into nursing homes and halfway houses. This change in social policy could easily have been responsible for the drop in patient numbers observed by Brill and Patton.

One state did compare discharge rates for schizophrenia patients treated with and without drugs during the time period of 1956 and 1957. The results do not support the historical claim that it was medications that allowed the emptying of the state hospitals. In a study of 1,413 first-episode male schizophrenics admitted to California hospitals, researchers found that "drug-treated patients tend to have longer periods of hospitalization. . . . Furthermore, the hospitals wherein a higher percentage of first admission schizophrenia patients are treated with these drugs tend to have somewhat higher retention rates for this group as a whole."[4] In short, the California investigators determined that neuroleptics, rather than speed patients' return to their communities, actually hindered their discharge. A significant aspect to note about these studies is that they could never be done again, because we will never fill up the state hospitals again (though we are filling the prisons with people diagnosed as schizophrenic).

The true period of deinstitutionalization in the United States was from 1963 to the late 1970s, and the exodus of patients was clearly driven by social and fiscal policies, providing the impetus for Ann Braden Johnson's book, *Out of Bedlam.*[5] In 1963, the federal government began picking up some of the costs of care for the mentally ill who were not in state institutions, and two years later, Medicare and Medicaid legislation increased federal funding for care of mental patients, provided they were not housed in state hospitals. Naturally, states responded by discharging their hospital patients to private nursing homes and shelters so as to transfer the costs to the federal government. In 1972, an amendment to the Social Security Act authorized disability payments to the mentally ill, which further accelerated the transfer of hospitalized patients into private facilities. As a result of these changes in fiscal policies, the number of patients in state mental hospitals dropped from 504,600 to 153,544 over a fifteen-year period (1963 to 1978).[6] Another large exodus occurred in the early 1990s, when state hospitals delivered patients to homeless shelters.

Since deinstitutionalization, the standard of care for schizophrenia and other psychotic disorders has consisted of indefinite maintenance on drugs based on research demonstrating their effectiveness in treating acute psychotic symptoms and in preventing relapse.[7] However, the effectiveness of long-term drug treatment has been questioned.[8] The long-term outcomes with schizophrenia remain poor and may be no better than they were a hundred years ago, when water therapies and fresh air were the treatment of the day.[9]

In 2002 that paradox stirred an unusual editorial in the journal *European Psychiatry*, in which the author, Emmanuel Stip, posed this question: "After fifty years of neuroleptic drugs, are we able to answer the following simple question: Are neuroleptics effective in treating schizophrenia?" He wrote, "Actually, the answers yielded by these simple questions by meta-analysis should elicit in us a good deal of humility. If we wish to base psychiatry on evidence-based medicine, we run a genuine risk in taking a closer look at what has long been considered fact."[10] Whitaker's review of the research literature goes even further, concluding that the preponderance of evidence shows that the current standard of care—continual medication therapy for all patients so diagnosed—may do more harm than good.[11]

Further critique of sole reliance on medication for schizophrenia is beyond the scope of this book, which aims to present the more positive alternative, the discovery of narrative and of healing in conjunction with replacing medication, whenever possible, by social relations. The message of this book is that social relations are more powerful in changing brains than medications, though medications can provide a bridge for those suffering people who have no social relations as they develop and nurture them.

New Stories for Old

A narrative approach to psychiatry involves finding better stories to replace deficient stories that do not perform well in making sense of the world and telling us how to behave. Our perspective is that much of what the biomedical world calls "mental illness" results from having and performing deficient stories or from not having a story at all with which to make sense of the world and operate in it effectively. While this idea may sound simple, it signals a profound shift in psychiatric thinking from the currently prevailing story of abnormal brain chemistry to a story of social brain and neuroplasticity.

York University neuroscientist Raymond Mar has reviewed the available literature and concluded that nothing activates more areas of the brain than a good story. Even with multiple areas of brain damage, we usually retain our ability to appreciate and tell story.[12] In narrative psychiatry, stories, rather than individuals, are our fundamental unit of discourse. Many people share the same story; other stories are unique for each person. Some stories work very well. Others barely work at all.

For example, if I have lots of stories to prove that I don't belong, then I will tend to behave in groups as if I don't belong and people will treat me as if I don't belong. This was one of the stories of my earlier life. I didn't realize that the stories that proved I didn't belong were being performed by me whenever I entered a new group, with the result that I eventually didn't belong and was excluded from the group. Friends and talking circles and ceremonies helped me change the stories that I performed when I entered new groups. I still have to work at this because of the tendency to fall back into the habit of acting like I don't belong.

From infancy, we are seeking to command the attention of others and to shape it more finely to get what we want, including a sense of belonging to a community who cares about us. If we don't have the skills (stories to tell us how to do this), we suffer and may come to be diagnosed as mentally ill.

Sometimes deficient stories result from brain-environment mismatch. Dyslexia and child development specialist Maryanne Wolf at

Northwestern University in Chicago has written an entire book about the mismatch between the brains of children who have difficulty reading and the environment of the printed word. She wrote, "I look at dyslexia as a daily reminder that very different organizations of the brain are possible. Some organizations may not work well for reading yet are critical for the creation of buildings and art and the recognition of patterns—whether on ancient battlefields or in biopsy slides."[13]

Wolf provides an entire chapter (3) about Michael Merzenich, who developed a computer program (FastForward) that matched the brain organization of dyslexic children and progressively shaped their brains toward the organization required for optimal reading. Those who are labeled mentally retarded may similarly need specially structured environments in order to meet their full potential and to lead rich, productive lives (from their point of view). Similarly, people labeled autistic often need ways of translating the contemporary social environment into their own stories or maps about the world as well as ways of telling a story that make sense in the social environment in which they find themselves.

Biomedical models have not settled on one single cause of schizophrenia and have attributed it to everything from genetic predisposition to abnormal brain chemistry, home environments, and even cat-borne viruses. Schizophrenia and other psychotic disorders are often associated with a lack of story or lack of capacity to structure a narrative from life experience. In this perspective schizophrenia is associated with a difficulty in forming a rich narrative about experience.

The Negative Power of Labels

No two brains are the same because, as I have shown in earlier chapters, brains are created, shaped, and maintained by a perpetually changing social and biological environment. The brains that produce the cluster of symptoms and signs that are labeled as schizophrenia or psychosis share in this uniqueness. Schizophrenia is not a unique biological identity; it is a social construction about brain and relationship and behavior. When we group a wide range of problems together under a single label, we are making a story. The idea of comorbidity, in which people are given multiple diagnoses, is a poor way to address the problem of individual uniqueness. We do better to envision one brain participating in multiple stories. Depending on how we view those stories, we can generate many perspectives on how that person does not fit well into the world or on how he or she suffers. Nevertheless, this is one person performing multiple intersecting stories for multiple audiences.

"Psychiatric diagnoses are based on a set of false assumptions stemming from the nineteenth century," says Professor Richard P. Bentall, author of *Madness Explained*.[14] These assumptions include "the idea that there is a clear division between 'mad' and 'sane' people, and that distinct psychiatric categories like 'schizophrenic' actually exist." Bentall also notes, "Because psychiatric patients are seen as having a biological brain illness which affects their rationality, they are not usually allowed a say in the matter [about their diagnosis or treatment]."[15] We used to joke that psychiatry is the only field in which the customer is always wrong.

Giving a person a label like schizophrenia allows us to dismiss him as a human being. It allows us to assume (incorrectly) that we know him and the stories that preceded his current state of misery. The German philosopher Friedrich Nietzsche criticized Plato and Socrates (in *Beyond Good and Evil*) for believing that their views were true accounts rather than merely one of a number of ways of seeing the world. French philosopher Michel Foucault carried this idea further in writing that people "construct the objects of which they speak" through their conversations. In this context, we must wonder whether contemporary biological psychiatry constructs schizophrenia from a multiplicity of biological anomalies associated with people who are different or "annoying." It presents its ideas as if they are truths that stand outside of history, as having a unique, all-encompassing authority that is free from history or context.

"Rather than diagnosing and treating people on the basis of psychiatric categories, which actually contain many people with no symptoms in common, we need to look at each sufferer's symptoms individually from a psychological perspective," writes Bentall. "It then becomes relatively easy to understand why they [the symptoms] might be happening and how the sufferer can address and cope with them."[16] This more individualistic practice is more compatible with the evolving narrative movement and with indigenous knowledge systems.

I don't like our contemporary psychiatric diagnoses because of what they do to people. I challenge anyone reading this to talk to people who have been diagnosed. I am sure that you will discover how the weight of such a label becomes a self-fulfilling prophecy. We can say that those who are labeled schizophrenic have been offered a specific story to explain their painful "being in the world." When the description of their suffering conforms to that provided by the DSM, they are labeled schizophrenic, which is akin to offering them an explanatory story of their unexplainable experiences. But this story is one that just creates a cage in which the sufferer is imprisoned. The label is injunctive; it tells people how to act and what they can expect from their lives. It limits their potential. It takes away their real stories. When your stories are gone, you have nothing.

Boyd says, "Stories help train us to explore possibility as well as actuality effortlessly and even playfully, and that capacity makes all the difference."[17] This is why our job in working with desperately suffering people is to restore their capacity to make stories and tell stories, progressively shaping those stories toward ones that allow them to live and work and love in a world of other human beings and to be happy. Healers have been offering sufferers other narratives to explain their suffering for centuries. Here is an example from the eleventh century of an early narrative psychiatrist, Avicenna (also spelled Ibn-Senna) (ca. 980–1037), a famous Persian physician:

Avicenna treated a prince of Persia who had melancholia and suffered from the delusion that he was a cow. He would low like a cow, crying, "Kill me so that a good stew may be made of my flesh," and would not eat anything. Avicenna was persuaded to undertake the case, and sent a message to the patient, asking him to be happy, as the butcher was coming to slaughter him, and the sick man rejoiced. When Avicenna approached the prince with a knife in his hand, he asked, "Where is the cow so I may kill it?" The patient then lowed like a cow to indicate where he was. By order of Avicenna in his role as the butcher, the patient was also laid on the ground for slaughter. When Avicenna approached the patient, pretending to slaughter him, he said, "The cow is too lean and not ready to be killed. He must be fed properly and I will kill it when it becomes healthy and fat." The patient was then offered food and medicine, which he ate eagerly and gradually gained strength, got rid of his delusion, and was completely cured.[18]

Avicenna knew how to do what psychiatrist and hypnotherapist Milton Erickson recommended a thousand years later: always work within the patient's story. Erickson said that therapy is substituting a good idea for a bad idea.[19] Avicenna might have said that healing is substituting a good story for a bad story. Jungian analyst James Hillman wrote that psychotherapists are workers in story and that "successful therapy is a collaboration of fictions,"[20] just as Avicenna demonstrated.

Working in Story

Working within the patient's story to relieve pain is what we do in narrative psychiatry. "Rowen" was one of the most pained people I ever met. He invented ritual after ritual to make his voices go away. Those voices told him the most hideous things—that he had murdered his little sister in his sleep, that he should cut off his penis in atonement for his lustful thoughts, that he would burn eternally in hell.

Initially I used medication with Rowen, but, most importantly, I offered him deep listening to all of his stories. He deserved my attention and the attention of others, not our dismissal through labeling. Eventually neural imaging will be so sophisticated that we will be able to identity the imbalances in brain circuit activation that are associated with the kind of misery he suffered, but even that will not change the necessity to hear his story. I suspect that neural imaging will confirm that every brain is unique and that deep listening changes brains. When enough of us can sit with people like Rowen, surrounding and engulfing them, their stories will change, and with them their places in their social networks, which will change their brain organization and reduce their suffering. Eventually they will no longer suffer so acutely. In Rowen's case, community, through talking circles, healing circles, ceremonies, and just listening, did heal him and made his medication unnecessary.

Rowen slowly let us bring family members into our work together (I say "we" and "us" because I work mostly with students and colleagues, rather than alone). His sister shed some light on Rowen's preoccupation with sex and with cutting off his penis. His father had molested her for a prolonged period. She was quite angry but also was shocked that Rowen seemed to know. "How did he know?" she asked. "Not even my mother knew."

"Everyone knew in their own way," I answered. "This way was Rowen's."

Bentall asserts, "Identifying and addressing the problems the sufferer, rather than the psychiatrist, perceives creates an understanding of each person's condition which is far more scientific, humane, and effective than a blanket diagnosis. . . . It also allows us to identify people at risk of psychological breakdown earlier, and keep them out of the traditional cycle of diagnosis and treatment."[21]

Rowen's biggest problem, as he identified it, was the fear that someone else, or he himself, would cut off his penis. His worst voice commanded him to do so and sometimes left him shaking under his bed. He asked us to tie his hands to the bedposts to prevent him from hurting himself or someone else. It turned out to be just as effective to pretend to do so. Our solemnly pretending to tie up his hands was wonderfully comforting for him.

We also created a drama in which Rowen watched one of us play the commanding voice and one of us played him and we demonstrated ways to resist the voice. He got very involved in helping us to create the costume of the voice and its mask. We began to construct a story about where the voice originated and how it had found him. The more details we added, the less powerful it became, until it was a voice just like any other voice. Slowly but surely this voice merged with a memory of his father's voice telling him to run because his father was going to cut off his "pee-pee." Whether it was true or not didn't matter. Rowen now had a story about that voice and a means to resist and ignore it that dramatically reduced his suffering.

Rowen, and others like him, refute the idea that one best approach exists for dealing with schizophrenia or any psychiatric condition, suggesting that there are as many "treatments" as there are stories, causing me to reminisce about the introduction to an old television show the *Naked City*, which began by saying, "There are 5 million stories in the Naked City." And counting! More stories than people, for sure.

Listening—the Radical Alternative

If (as traditional elders tell us) identity is a story that people tell and retell that is then reinforced, modified, reformed, revised, and revisited by the audience's reactions, then we must learn to listen very carefully if we are to understand a human life. When we give a person an identity story in the form of a diagnosis or a label, if they believe us, they will proceed to live out that story, and it will confirm to us that we were right in giving them that label. When I met Rowen, all of his family had dismissed him except for his aunt, who insisted on dragging him to new doctors and healers. Rowen had adjusted to a life of misery in a board-and-care home. This was the best for which he could hope. Today he is an accomplished artist, supporting himself through the sales of his paintings and sculptures. We were able to help him overthrow the story provided by his diagnostic label.

Jacques Lacan (1901–1981) wrote that the listener should be free of all interpretative elements, theories, presuppositions, so as to really *hear* the other person.[22] When we listen in this way, he said, we offer the patient a priceless gift. This kind of listening is rare in our modern experience. Today, the narrative approach has picked up this torch to carry— that healing does involve deep and very active listening and that this deep listening forms a context in which the teller of her story expects to be healed. Listening forms the context in which healing unfolds. This listening is what we gave Rowen.

Here is another story to guide our understanding. "Carter" was a twenty-four-year-old man who had been hospitalized for confusion. When I met Carter in the hospital, he was completely befuddled. He had been away from his family for four years of college and was in his senior year. His parents had begun to worry because of his strange phone calls (a common presentation of madness). They went to get him at college in Winnipeg and found him naked in his apartment surrounded by stacks and stacks of newspapers, take-out food cartons, and an empty refrigerator. He had decided clothes were unnecessary and tried not to wear them. This didn't work so well when he needed to go to the grocery store, so he started having all his food delivered. He had stopped going to classes and had finally given up food. He apparently hadn't eaten (or hadn't eaten much) for almost one month, inspired by stories of yogis who lived only on air. Carter was hospitalized and then driven home to Saskatoon to recuperate.

Carter was discharged from the hospital on 20 mg of olanzepine (Zyprexa) daily, 100 mg of trazodone (Desyrel) at bedtime, and 2 mg of lorazepam (Ativan) three times daily for restlessness. When I first saw Carter in my office, he could hardly talk. "Zombie," he mouthed. "Too much meds. Too strong." Carter didn't have much more to say in our first appointment, but I got the message and cut his olanzepine to 10 mg and began a plan with the family to wean him off the lorazepam.

When I started working with his family I discovered the shared theme of all the family members had to do with consumption. Carter was embodying the opposite statement from his parents, who were very concerned with status, wealth, having the best cars, getting Carter's brother into Harvard. We could have called the family dialectic between Carter and the others as, "To have or not to have—that is the question."

Of course, from the standpoint of everyone else in Carter's family, he was crazy. From the standpoint of the doctors and nurses in the hospital, Carter was crazy. However, he was performing a story. He couldn't reflect on his story, which is what has been called pre-narrative awareness. He could not tell us the meaning of the story or explain the metaphors he was using. He was, however, from my point of view, completely engrossed in an enactment. Unfortunately, it had taken over his life. He had no other stories from which to draw. His choices were severely limited. He reminded me of a client I had once who walked all day around the block where his parents lived lugging a big wooden cross on his shoulder in imitation of Jesus marching toward the crucifixion. That poor man's choices were also severely limited.

I continued meeting with Carter both alone and with his family (and with as many of his friends as would also come). While the theme of the first two months was conspicuous consumption, the theme of the next four months was intrusive control. Carter's family seemed to have tried to plan every moment of Carter's life even though he perpetually disappointed them. Carter's brother went to Harvard. Carter only went to the University of Manitoba. Carter's brother, "Henry," was pre-law and getting straight As. Carter was doing only average in a commerce program. Carter's brother's girlfriend was one of the prettiest coeds in Massachusetts. In fact, she had been first runner-up for Miss Rhode Island. Everyone was impressed with Henry and everything he did. Carter had no area in which he could be superior to Henry.

In this context, Carter's long-meandering soliloquies on Hindu spirituality and yoga made more sense. Of course, R. D. Laing (1927–1989) was saying this in the 1970s—that if you could put the "crazy" person's words and deeds into context, they didn't appear so crazy, and were often social commentary on a world gone mad.* Laing even explained why madness was often found in the more intelligent patients. They were able to comprehend the impossibility of their lives, generating all the more suffering and desire to communicate their condition.

We were six months into our work together when Carter began to be able to oppose his parents without the need for indirect theater (my term for his behavior). He was actually beginning to tell them what he didn't

---

*Ronald D. Laing was a Scottish psychiatrist who studied psychosis extensively. Contrary to prevailing thought in his day, he accepted that a client's expressed psychotic experiences were valid, lived experiences, rather than medical symptoms. He and his colleagues were responsible for implementing alternative healing environments for people who were psychotic in the United Kingdom. Laing was not antipsychiatry; he saw psychiatry differently than just drugging people.

like about their lifestyle and about the differences between how they treated Henry and him. He was able to talk to me about a girlfriend who had been dominating him almost as much as his parents did. Just before he had deteriorated he had finally rebelled and quietly, passively had done infuriating counters to her demands, and she had left him. Unfortunately, when she left, he had felt all alone. He hadn't intended for her to leave, just for her to get the message that she was being overly intrusive, though he only realized that almost ten months after the fact. After six months of work, Carter's olanzepine was at 5 mg daily and he was off all other medications.

The next four months of contact were all about Carter's developing a sense of agency and independence—that his story wasn't bad or wrong just because it wasn't his brother Henry's story. I used my "Act Three" story, which Carter liked. In this story, I tell people we can only compare ourselves to others after the play is entirely over. Comparisons made prior to or during Act Three aren't valid because we don't know what's coming. I remembered a colleague of whom I was once jealous. He had written more books, given more prestigious talks, and made more income. Then suddenly I heard he was dying of cancer. I told Carter and his family what a teaching that had been for me. I had been making Act Three comparisons, when so quickly and suddenly my friend's Act Five had come and gone. Looking at his overall life, I realized that I wouldn't have wanted to be him. Carter understood my point. "You don't know Henry's story, nor its ending," I said. "If you did, you might not want to be Henry." We began to construct an identity for Carter that was unique and different from Henry's. In fact, Henry ceased to have any relevance to Carter's identity. We began to explore what values Carter wanted to live regardless of the values of his other family members. His olanzapine was then 2.5 mg per day.

One month later Carter stopped taking olanzepine, and three months later he returned to Winnipeg to finish his degree at the University of Manitoba. I hear from him occasionally, and he continues to do well living his own life. Upon graduation, he began to date and is now living with a woman he loves. She is not as gorgeous as Henry's trophy wife, but

Carter told me that he prefers her by far. Carter's parents are grateful for his recovery, but remain disappointed that he will never be the son that Henry is. Much of my work with Carter was helping him to construct a story in which that was just fine.

Homes for Healing

I want to finish this chapter by acknowledging some of the trailblazers who have struggled to put story to psychosis in the context of community. They have written about their work in listening and finding meaning in even the most distorted communications of psychotic and disturbed people. One of my heroes, whom I will quote extensively, is American psychiatrist Loren Mosher (1933–2004), a pioneer in helping people with diagnoses of schizophrenia to recover. Mosher and his generation of avant-garde psychiatrists excelled in providing us with a continuing legacy that we aim to carry forward under the banner of narrative psychiatry. Mosher's writings are instructive in demonstrating how he learned to bring a "what you see is what you get" bias to his interactions with patients and a sensitivity to the issues of degradation and power, especially as embodied in conventional institutional practices.

Mosher wrote that the institution itself gave him master classes in the art of the "total institution": authoritarianism, the degradation ceremony, the induction and perpetuation of powerlessness, unnecessary dependency, labeling, and the primacy of institutional needs over those of the people it was ostensibly there to serve.[23] His efforts to be helpful to people were interrupted by these institutional needs. When brought up, they were denied, rationalized, or simply invalidated: "You're just a resident and aren't yet able to understand why these processes are not as you see them." From a series of such experiences, he began to believe that psychiatric hospitals were not usually very good places in which to be insane.

Psychiatric hospitals generate more psychiatric illness because this is what they expect; this is their context. Psychiatric patients learn to perform the role expected by the institution. Mosher asked, "If places called hospitals were not good for disturbed and disturbing behavior, what kinds of social environments were?" In 1966 and 1967, this interest was nourished by R. D. Laing and his colleagues in the Philadelphia Association's Kingsley Hall in London. The deconstruction of madness and the madhouse that took place there generated ideas about how a community-based, supportive, protective, normalizing environment might facilitate reintegration of psychologically disintegrated persons without artificial institutional disruptions of the process. This resulted, from 1969 to 1971, in the design and implementation of the Soteria Project near San Francisco for the benefit of psychotic individuals. *Soteria* is a Greek word meaning "salvation" or "deliverance." There, Mosher showed that psychotic people responded to positive social relationships embedded in an expectation that they would respond and stop being psychotic and that the psychotic experience would be transformed through the dialogic interaction into something meaningful and valuable to the affected individual.[24]

In Mosher, R. D. Laing, and Joseph Burke's alternative social settings, very psychotic people gradually learned how to play different roles and eventually could not be identified as "mental patients." Regardless of the biology of their brains, the social environment changed that biology to permit better functioning. They became what they were expected to become. They were able to change the story that society had previously given them.

Soteria House was designed as a medication-free treatment environment and was as successful as antipsychotic medication treatment in reducing psychotic symptoms in six weeks.[25] Mosher was able to demonstrate the importance of context for people suffering from a psychotic episode.[26] He showed that 85 to 90 percent of acute and long-term clients deemed in need of hospitalization could recover in the community without conventional hospital treatment. In a modified form, in facilities that Mosher influenced called Crossing Place and McAuliffe House, where so-called long-term "frequent flyers" were treated, people treated by a supportive social environment improved as much as hospital-treated patients and at considerably lower cost.

These and other studies and projects showed that social alternatives to acute psychiatric hospitalization were as effective or more effective than medication in psychiatric hospitals for the short-term reduction of psychotic symptoms and also for longer-term social adjustment. The outcomes from the original medication-free, home-like, nonprofessionally staffed Soteria Project demonstrated that people without extensive hospitalizations (less than thirty days) were especially responsive to the effects of a positive social environment, so much so that these well-defined healing environments were replicated in other places. Reviews of other studies of diversion of people deemed in need of hospitalization to "alternative" social programs consistently showed equivalent or better clinical results, at lower cost, than from medication and hospitals.

In the years since the Soteria Project's successful implementation, a variety of alternatives to psychiatric hospitalization have been developed in the United States. Their results have been extensively reviewed, with each review finding consistently more positive results from a variety of alternative interventions as compared with control groups.[27] R. B. Straw, for example, found that in nineteen of twenty studies he reviewed, alternative treatments were as, or more, effective than hospital care and were on average 43 percent less expensive. The Soteria study was noted to be the most rigorous available in describing a comprehensive treatment approach to a subgroup of people labeled as having schizophrenia. It was also noted that, for the most part, the effects of various models of hospitalization had not been subjected to equally serious scientific scrutiny.

I take this to mean that social engineering is more effective than biochemical engineering in controlling biology. Our brains respond better to beneficial environmental changes and warm, loving human relationships than they do to external biochemical manipulation. Despite these clinical and cost data, alternatives to psychiatric hospitalization and extensive use of medication have not been widely implemented, perhaps due to the pharmaceutical industry's excessive control of the medical profession, the capitalistic preference for product over human service and relationship, and the American-European story about magic potions that quickly cure all of our woes.

Soteria House

Soteria took place from 1971 to 1983, during the time when I was in medical school in the San Francisco Bay Area and afterward when I worked in the area. Many of us in the region followed this project with great interest. A two-year follow-up study compared randomly assigned people who had undergone the "Soteria method of treatment" with those who underwent "usual" general hospital psychiatric ward interventions.[28] All potential participants were public-sector clients screened at the psychiatric emergency room of a suburban San Francisco Bay Area county hospital. All subjects met the DSM Axis 1 criteria for schizophrenia, as rated by three independent raters. The earlier onset (eighteen to thirty years) and marital status criteria were designed to identify a subgroup of persons diagnosed with schizophrenia at statistically high risk for long-term disability. Both Soteria-treated and control subjects were young (average age of twenty-one), mostly white (10 percent minority), at least high school graduates, raised in typical lower-middle-class, blue-collar suburban families.

Mosher characterized the Soteria method as the twenty-four-hours-a-day application of interpersonal phenomenologic interventions by a nonprofessional staff, usually without drug treatment, in the context of a small, homelike, quiet, supportive, protective, and tolerant social environment. He described the core practice of interpersonal phenomenology as focusing on the development of a nonintrusive, noncontrolling but actively empathetic relationship with the psychotic person without having to do anything explicitly therapeutic or controlling. In short, it was characterized as "being with," "standing by attentively," or "trying to put your feet into the other person's shoes." The aim was to develop, over time, a shared experience of the meaningfulness of the person's individual social context—current and historical. There were no therapeutic "sessions." However, a great deal of useful social interaction took place as staff worked gently to build bridges between individuals' emotionally disorganized states to the life events that seemed to have precipitated their psychological disintegration. The context within the house was one of positive expectations that reorganization and reintegration would occur as a result of these seemingly minimalist interventions.

In 1974 Mosher and colleagues opened a "replication" facility called Emanon in another suburban San Francisco Bay Area city, because they saw that the Soteria method worked. They wanted to immediately replicate their good results with another group of staff and clients in another house in another community to address the potential criticism that their results were a one-time product of a unique group of people and of expectation effects. Despite their consistently positive results, funding for the Soteria Project ended in 1983.

Because Mosher conceived the Soteria program as a recovery-facilitating social environment, he used the Moos' Ward Atmosphere Scale to compare Soteria, Emanon, and the usual treatment hospital ward milieu.[29] He found that Emanon was remarkably similar to its older sibling, Soteria House, on all measures and that both Soteria and Emanon were very different from usual psychiatric treatment.[30] At two years after admission, people who had lived at Soteria House were working at significantly higher occupational levels, were significantly more often living independently or with peers, and had fewer readmissions. The vast majority never received a single dose of antipsychotic medication during the entire two-year period.

Mosher's results highlight the ways that social relationships shape the brain and its responses. Even more significant are the ways that profit motivations shape the health care system, for, clearly, drug treatment is more profitable for those who control health care, even if it doesn't work as well (or at all for many) and even if it ultimately costs society more. But the preponderance of drug treatment and not social relationship treatment for schizophrenia and psychosis is not just driven by profit motives; it is also driven by a story that isolates these phenomena into defective, individual brains whose biology must be altered by biological means. It is a linear, cause-and-effect story, a simple mechanics approach that assumes biological causation that then requires biological treatment. Psychiatry will not change until its master narratives change.

Crossing Place

In 1972, Mosher became the psychiatric consultant to Woodley House, a halfway house founded in Washington, D.C., in 1958. In consultation, staff were often distressed when describing house residents who went into crisis and there was no option but to hospitalize them. They saw recovery from such institutionalizations as taking nearly eighteen months. So, in 1977, a Soteria-like facility, called Crossing Place, was opened by Woodley House Programs. It differed from its conceptual parent in that it:

1. Admitted any nonmedically ill client deemed in need of psychiatric hospitalization regardless of diagnosis, length of illness, severity of psychopathology, or level of functional impairment
2. Was an integral part of the local public community mental health system, which meant that most patients who came to Crossing Place were receiving psychotropic medications
3. Had an informal length-of-stay restriction of about thirty days to make it economically appealing.

So, beginning in 1977, a modified Soteria method was applied to a much broader patient base, the so-called "seriously and persistently mentally ill."[31] Although a random assignment study of a Crossing Place model has been published, it was clear to Mosher from early on that the Soteria method "worked" with a mixed client group. Because of its location and "open" admissions, Crossing Place clients, as compared with Soteria subjects, were older (average age of thirty-seven), more nonwhite (70 percent), had multiple previous admissions, were long-term users of the mental health system (averaging 14 years), and had been raised in poor urban ghetto families. There were no suicides among clients in residence and no serious staff injuries. Although the clients were different, the two settings (Soteria and Crossing Place) shared staff selection processes,[32] philosophy, institutional and social structure characteristics, and the culture of positive expectations. By 1997, more than 1,000 people had been admitted and discharged directly to the community, completely avoiding hospitalization.[33]

In 1986 the social environments at Soteria and Crossing Place were compared and contrasted as follows:

In their presentations to the world, Crossing Place is conventional and Soteria unconventional. Despite this major difference, the actual in-house interpersonal interactions are similar in their informality, earthiness, honesty, and lack of professional jargon. These similarities arise partially from the fact that neither program ascribes the usual patient role to the clientele. Crossing Place admits "chronic" patients, and its public funding contains broad length-of-stay standards (1 to 2 months). Soteria's research focus views length of stay as a dependent variable, allowing it to vary according to the clinical needs of the newly diagnosed patients. Hence, the initial focus of the Crossing Place staff is: What do the clients need to accomplish relatively quickly so they can resume living in the community?

This empowering focus on the client's responsibility to accomplish a goal(s) is a technique that Woodley House [the parent of Crossing Place] had used successfully for many years. At Soteria, such questions were not ordinarily raised until the acutely psychotic state had subsided—usually 4 to 6 weeks after entry. This span exceeded the average length of stay at Crossing Place. The shorter average length of stay at Crossing Place was made possible by the almost routine use of neuroleptics to control the most flagrant symptoms of its clientele. At Soteria, neuroleptics were almost never used during the first 6 weeks of a patient's stay. Time constraints also dictated that Crossing Place had a more formalized social structure than Soteria. Each day there was a morning meeting on "what are you doing to fix your life today" and there were also one or two evening community meetings.

The two Crossing Place consulting psychiatrists each spent an hour a week with the staff members reviewing each client's progress, addressing particularly difficult issues, and helping develop a consensus on initial and revised treatment plans. Soteria had a variety of ad-hoc crisis meetings, but only one regularly scheduled house meeting per week. The role of the consulting psychiatrist was more peripheral at Soteria than at Crossing Place: He was not ordinarily involved in treatment planning and no regular treatment meetings.

In summary, compared to Soteria, Crossing Place was more organized, had a tighter structure, and was more oriented toward practical goals. Expectations of Crossing Place staff members were positive but more limited than those of Soteria staff. At Crossing Place, psychosis was frequently not addressed directly by staff members, while at Soteria the client's experience of acute psychosis was often a central subject of interpersonal communication. At Crossing Place, the use of neuroleptic drugs restricted psychotic episodes. The immediate social problems of Crossing Place clients (secondary to being system "veterans" and also because of having come mostly from urban lower social class minority families) had to be addressed quickly: no money, no place to live, no one with whom to talk. Basic survival was often the issue. Among the new to the system, young, lower class, suburban, mostly white Soteria clients, these problems were present but much less pressing because basic survival was usually not yet an issue.

Crossing Place staff members spent a lot of time keeping other parts of the mental health community involved in the process of addressing client needs. The clients were known to many other players in the mental health system. Just contacting everyone with a role in the life of any given client could be an all-day process for a staff member. In contrast, Soteria clients, being new to the system, had no such cadre of involved mental health workers. While in residence, Crossing Place clients continued their involvement with their other programs if clinically possible. At Soteria, only the project director and house director worked with both the house and the community mental health system. At Crossing Place, all staff members negotiated with the system. Because of the shorter lengths of stay, the focus on immediate practical problem solving, and the absence of clients from the house during the daytime, Crossing Place tended to be less consistently intimate in feeling than Soteria, although individual relationships between staff members and clients could be very intimate at Crossing Place, especially with returning clients . . . it was easier to get in and out of Crossing Place without having a significant relationship.[34]

Neither program ascribed the usual patient role to the client. Crossing Place admitted "chronic" patients, and its public funding contained broad length-of-stay standards (one to two months). Soteria's research focus viewed length of stay as a dependent variable, allowing it to vary according to the clinical needs of the newly diagnosed patients. Hence, the initial focus of the Crossing Place staff was, what do clients need to accomplish relatively quickly so they can resume living in the community?[35]

McAuliffe House

In 1990 Mosher helped to establish McAuliffe House, a Crossing Place replication in Montgomery County, Maryland. Crossing Place staff helped train the McAuliffe House staff; for didactic instruction there were numerous articles describing the philosophy, institutional characteristics, social structure, and staff attitudes of Crossing Place and Soteria and a treatment manual from Soteria. At McAuliffe House Mosher and colleagues implemented the first random assignment study of a residential alternative to hospitalization that was focused on the seriously mentally ill "frequent flyers" in a never-before-researched "public" system of care. Because of this well-funded system's early crisis-intervention focus, it hospitalized only about 10 percent of its more than 1,500 long-term clients each year. Again, because of a well-developed crisis system, less than 10 percent of hospitalizations were involuntary. Their voluntary research sample was representative of even the most difficult multiproblem clients.

The study excluded *no one* deemed in need of acute hospitalization except those with complicating medical conditions or those who were acutely intoxicated. The subjects were as representative of suburban Montgomery County's public clients as Crossing Place's were of urban Washington, D.C.: midthirties, poor, 25 percent minority, long durations of illness, and multiple previous hospitalizations. However, many of the Montgomery County nonminority clients came from well-educated, affluent families. The alternative and acute general hospital psychiatric wards were clinically equal in effectiveness, but the alternative cost about 40 percent less.[36] This meant a savings of roughly $19,000 per year (of 1993 dollars) for each seriously and persistently mentally ill person who used acute alternative care exclusively (instead of a hospital).

Fountain House

Another example is Fountain House in New York City. Fountain House is a professional self-help program, operated by men and women recovering from mental illness, in collaboration with staff. "The emphasis at Fountain House is on relationships—member to member, and member to staff. Members engage with each other to regain their productivity and self-confidence, resume their lives, and re-enter society. They take part, as well, in promoting their rights, and in erasing the stigma that often separates them from their neighbors. Since its founding in 1948, Fountain House has served a total of more than 16,000 men and women. Its innovative 'clubhouse' model is today the basis for more than 400 similar programs in 32 countries around the world, assisting some 50,000 men and women. The Fountain House concept has been adopted in part by another 1,000 programs in the U.S. and abroad."[37]

The Finnish Psychosis Project

The Finnish Psychosis Project presents another way to provide story to those who have none or for those whose stories are inadequate to negotiate their lives. Paul Ricoeur believed that new lives emerge from telling stories that have not yet been told.[38] According to Ricoeur, we are justified in speaking of a life as a story waiting to be told and of a life as activity and passion in search for a narrative. This is what we do when we create narratives through the course of dialogue. To have meaning and value, lives must be interpreted through narrative. Problems arise when people are blocked and the search for a quality narrative is diminished, thus reducing the sense of agency.

People who are labeled psychotic have difficulty finding a narrative to tell. They are stuck in pre-narrative experience. The audience and other characters then conspire (in some network sense, as in a neural network) to block their access to alternate stories and to create stories to dominate the person. Any alternative story that would better encapsulate the person's pre-narrative experience is unavailable, unimaginable, unattainable, thus reducing the person's sense of agency. The person can no longer see or make choices. The person is no longer a performer, but more like a member of an audience *to* his or her own performance of a story. (I believe this is the source of the voices that make running commentary on all that the person is doing.)

When the stories in which we are enmeshed are unbearable, psychosis offers escape. The person labeled psychotic can create an alternative story (and world) that replaces the unbearable situation in which the individual is immersed. Finnish psychiatrists Juha Holma and Jukka Aaltonen believe that these stories emerge from the person's inner conversations and with the exclusion of narratives coming from conversations with external people.[39] This gives the story a sense that it is lacking in "reality testing," when those of us who share consensually narrated stories listen. They believe that elements of the psychotic person's story keep his or her identity from collapsing altogether. Even the most psychotic-sounding stories typically maintain a modicum of sense of agency, since they tell a story about a person who does interact within some world.

Holma and Aaltonen created the Finnish Psychosis Project at the University of Jyväskylä in Jyväskylä, building on the idea that health is associated with a sense of agency[40] and the idea that we have the capacity to make sense of our lives and to act in the world to improve our lives and decrease our suffering and pain.[41] They recommend integrating different treatment models in a need-adapted way: family-centered interventions with team work, including the patient; family and network in conjoint therapy meetings; and a guarantee of the psychological continuity of the treatment process through the different treatment modalities. The patient takes part in all treatment situations in which decisions about him or her are made.[42] They see this approach as an attempt to strengthen the psychotic patient's sense of agency at every stage in the treatment process.[43]

In 2000, Aaltonen's group published a two-year outcome study of two groups of consecutive patients with first episode nonaffective psychosis, both treated in accordance with their "need-specific Finnish model."[44] The two groups differed only in the use of neuroleptic medication. Three sites used a minimal neuroleptic regime, while the other three used conventional management strategies. In the experimental group 42.9 percent of the patients did not receive neuroleptics at all during the whole two-year period, while the corresponding proportion of those not receiving medication in the control group was 5.9 percent. The overall outcome of the whole group was favorable. The main result was that the outcome of the experimental group was equal or even somewhat better than that of the control group, also after controlling for age, gender, and diagnosis.

Making New Devices

Here is an example of how this philosophical approach plays out in practice:

"Cathy" was a twenty-year-old woman brought to me by her mother because she had stopped going to school and rarely left her bedroom. She had previously enjoyed a fairly active social life and a moderately heavy class load at college. She described herself as feeling depressed and sluggishly heavy and had decided that some of her former friends had obtained alien technology and were using it to suck the energy right out of her body while she slept. She thought they were doing this just to be cruel. Cathy's mother, "Felicity," had a different story. She thought Cathy was suffering from an overgrowth of *Candida albicans* (yeast) in her gut and probably had a leaky gut syndrome. Large molecules were leaking into Cathy's bloodstream and into her brain through the big holes in her gut. Felicity had celiac disease and guessed that Cathy also had it.

The original psychiatrist whom they had consulted had referred them to me because he believed that they were as crazy as I was and perhaps we deserved each other, especially since Cathy would not take medication (she feared that the medication would react with the alien technology being used on her). Nor did Felicity want Cathy to have medication. Felicity believed she should be on treatment for *Candida* overgrowth, leaky gut, and celiac disease. Felicity wanted Cathy to stick with herbs, vitamins, and prayer. One item of agreement emerged; psychiatrists were evil (I was an exception). Cathy believed that they were aiding and abetting the aliens. Felicity believed that they were in bed with the drug companies.

The structural similarities in their narratives were remarkable. Both attributed no agency to Cathy. As in the biomedical narrative, Cathy was limited to the prescribed act of ingesting substance. In Cathy's narrative that meant being eventually sucked dry by the alien device until she was dead. For both, "others" were causing the problems, either by alien technology or by bad molecules leaking through from *Candida* organisms. Both mother and daughter ignored my efforts to move the conversation toward even modest discussions about stress and lifestyle.

Following Avicenna's lead, I wondered aloud about starting Cathy on an anti-*Candida*, gluten-free, and casein-free diet. Cathy exploded. "I will not follow some stupid diet concocted by my mother. I will not take cheeksfull of her obnoxious pills. She's as bad as those damn doctors."

"Well, now," I thought. "That didn't work. What would Avicenna do next?" So I posed the question to Cathy, what could help?

"I need a jamming device," she said.

"I've been in this place before," I thought. "When in doubt, go with the flow!"

"Could we make one?" I asked.

"Sure," Cathy said, "If you know how."

"I know how, but I need your help," I said.

"Absolutely," she said. I was in luck. My son and I had just built a transistor radio from scratch. I had the schematics.

"I have some plans for just such a device," I said, walking toward my credenza. I shuffled through some papers and pulled out the diagram, bringing it back to Cathy.

"You'll have to help me make this."

"I don't know anything about electronics," she said.

"But you're clearly a smart girl and could learn." I circled one of the transistors. "I'll supply this one. I've got a special alien-resistant transistor that will jam most alien devices."

"How did you get that?" Cathy asked, suddenly suspicious, probably fearing I was an alien in disguise.

"My clients give me stuff like this," I said.

"And you believe them?" Cathy asked, incredulously.

"Always," I said.

"What do I need to do?" Cathy asked.

"Go down to Radio Shack," I said, "and have them help you find all these parts and a circuit board on which to put them. You'll also need a soldering gun and some solder. Get a basic electronics book, too. You'll have to learn more than you know now to outsmart these alien devices. We'll build this together when we meet, that is, if your mother wishes us to continue."

Felicity was confused, as she had imagined them leaving with a shopping bag full of herbs and vitamins and potions. To her credit, she appeared to be intrigued. Perhaps she recognized the power of relationship.

"I suppose I could bring her back," she said, noncommittal. "If she wishes to come."

"Do you want to come back?" Felicity asked Cathy.

"I guess," she said.

"All right," I said, "and one more thing. I'm going to need you to draw one dream every morning so I can learn more about these aliens and their devices, since most of the energy stealing is done at night. Usually these devices affect your dreams and leave clues hidden within the dreams for us to decipher. Drawing is the best way to find these clues." (I knew Cathy had been an art minor and was good at pen and ink, watercolor, and oil.)

"I guess," she said.

"And it wouldn't hurt to take some of your mother's potions," I said. "Drinking her potions will make her worry less and keep her off your back." Saying this got me back into Felicity's good graces.

"I guess I could take a couple things," Cathy said.

"You figure out what is most important and give her that," I said to

Felicity, "and only as much as she's willing to take without an argument." Felicity agreed.

Thus I began helping them to rewrite their stories, shared and separate, about Cathy's behavior. I was maneuvering to create some small space of agency for Cathy and to open space for a narrative to begin that was different from the concrete one of things from the outside making people crazy.

Cathy and I spent the next two months of meetings making a transistor radio together while we talked about the drawings of her dreams. I learned much about her life. Her parents had undergone a bitter divorce starting four years earlier and completed one year earlier. The rancor was ongoing. Whatever dad wanted, mom opposed, and vice versa. One of Cathy's dreams had her being torn apart by her two parents. Her brother had gone with her father, though the gender war had been exploding for over a decade. While Cathy found her mother annoying and silly, in an endearing sort of way, she was genuinely scared of her father and brother. She described her mother as someone's spinster aunt who happened to be a medium who drank wheat grass smoothies. She described her father as cruel and sadistic. He was a high-ranking police official destined to become a commissioner. She wanted to be no part of his life. She said he was worse than the psychiatrists. He would lock her up in a heartbeat. That's why she hadn't seen him in over a year.

On the day our device was finished, I produced the magic crystal transistor for Cathy to solder into place. We turned the switch on and music mixed with static blared forth.

"That sound," Cathy said, "that's them."

"That's good," I said. "It means we're starting to jam them and you're going to get your energy back. It sounds like a radio sometimes," I added, "but it's doing more important work. It's a jammer in disguise so the aliens won't recognize it."

"What's next?" Cathy asked. I'd already explored this question with a friend who had given me plans for a small device that could be used to triangulate a cell phone and locate it exactly. I proposed to Cathy that we build a device to locate the alien machine so we could go see where it was. For this we needed to learn more electronics. Cathy had already been reading about how transistors and capacitors worked, so she was open to that. She believed that the aliens had given us these devices in the first place.

Our next project took four months. During this time Cathy continued to draw her dreams and began talking about her largely disappointing love life. She picked incredibly attractive guys (Cathy was a very pretty blonde) who were cruel and humiliated her. When she could take no more, she hid from them and avoided them until they eventually went away.

A particularly revealing dream occurred in which her insides were being vacuumed out until she was completely hollow. "That's how I feel," she said. "That's so totally me—hollow girl."

"Maybe you need something to fill you up again," I said. "What would that be?"

Cathy began to be able to talk about situations that drained her energy and made her feel empty inside. We were making progress toward a more sophisticated narrative. Next I wanted to learn more about her friends and why she thought they would want to suck out her energy with an alien device. What emerged was a pattern of jealous friends competing over the boys that Cathy dated. Cathy felt hurt and betrayed by her friendships.

We finished the devices and began to determine if they did anything. Eventually we figured out how to locate Cathy's cell phone. More importantly, she was talking about the lack of anything fulfilling and meaningful in her life. We had come far toward a narrative understanding of her profound emptiness. We had started to include her mother again, who needed to be taught how to listen to Cathy. Felicity was much better at talking nonstop about her theories of leaking guts, *Candida,* celiac disease, and the importance of common prayer. I could see Cathy's point that much was said, but little heard. I began to teach the two how to listen to each other.

By nine months, Cathy was laughing about the gadgets we had made and her theories of alien devices. She had come to a new understanding that she had been a character in a play that she called *Much Ado about Nothing*. She was building more solid relationships and exploring spirituality in a different way than her mother and counter to the materialism of her father. She had joined a healing circle in the area and had begun to paint more seriously. She was also considering going back to college. Our electronics play had convinced her that she could actually manage science and math more than she thought.

By one year after our first meeting, Cathy had returned to school and had no longer talked about alien devices for at least three months. She was remarkably better and allowed her mother to believe that she had been healed by the leaky gut/*Candida* elixirs (which certainly could have helped). She had never taken any medication.

In my work with Cathy, just as in the Finnish Psychosis Project, the main themes of therapy are independence and a sense of agency. People struggle with these questions: To what extent is there a need to share feelings and experiences and remain independent at the same time? How can close relationships be maintained without losing the sense of agency? How far can one be similar to others and at the same time maintain one's own identity? Sharing feelings and experiences and being in close relationships is indispensable in the search for a narrative for our pre-narrative experiences. During this process it is important that the identity and sense of agency of everybody who takes part in it is retained. Thus, the Finnish Project, Mosher's work, Laing's work, and narrative psychiatry converge to point toward the effectiveness of changing stories in a social context as a means of changing brains and lives.

13

Indigenous Models for the Practice of Psychiatry and Mental Health

*What we call rational grounds for our beliefs are often
extremely irrational attempts to justify our instincts.*

THOMAS HENRY HUXLEY

I have spent much of my life learning from indigenous elders and translating that experience into more digestible forms for wider consumption. When I refer to indigenous people, I mean those people who have been present in a place as long as oral history remembers. Archaeologists can usually find someone who was there earlier, but their presence has been lost in the oral tradition of that place or it has become so stylized as to present the previous inhabitants as mythological characters, deities, or demigods.

All of the elders with whom I have spent time have been comfortable with the goal of making their wisdom and stories accessible to all and transforming industrialized culture through their teachings to something more human friendly and sustainable. Indeed, the Lakota visionary His Crazy Horse prophesized in the late nineteenth century that, in seven generations, the children of the invaders and colonizers would come to embrace Lakota spirituality and would come to the Lakota to learn how to be spiritual. Despite the objections of some racial purists, this is happening. The Lakota sweatlodge ceremony is probably the most common style practiced in North America. Many Lakota sun dances now include people of all ethnic backgrounds. Lakota is one of the fastest growing aboriginal languages. Websites, books, CDs, and courses are proliferating. The message of Lakota spirituality is changing the great-great-great-great-great grandchildren of the conquerors.

When asked about the interest of so many non-Lakota in Lakota spirituality, one elder told me, "These days, so many Indians want to come back from the spirit world, and there's not enough Indian bodies to go around. So they have to take whatever they can find. So nowadays, being Indian is more than skin deep. You have to look into the person's eyes to know from where they came."

I am one of these people, a mix of Lakota, Cherokee, Scot, and French. I believe His Crazy Horse was correct that mainstream North American and European worlds need the wisdom of indigenous cultures. I have journeyed far and wide to watch healing elders tell stories to people who are suffering—stories to uplift them, stories to transform them, stories to inspire them—in the process, giving them better stories for life. The elders want their stories told, believing that the most important experiences of life can only be expressed by stories. From stories we learn about the subtle nuances of relationship (with all beings) and about the emotions that arise within those relationships. They also know that we gain wisdom by exploring the way in which all stories are true.

One elder told me that every story has a spirit, just as does every person and every illness. For every symptom, every ache or pain, a spirit behind it drives it, fueling its fire. Therefore, when we hurt or suffer, we need to look to what is behind this suffering. Buddhists say that every illness has consciousness. The Australian Buddhist Sonam Rigzin uses the word *intelligence* to refer to the consciousness of illness. He says that "Every particle or subparticle of any material contains within it a form of intelligence which enables it to survive in a workable relationship each to the other."[1] In North America, I think we would say that every process is driven by consciousness. Symptoms and suffering can be seen as process.

Suffering and pain are part of stories that are told and retold, interpreted and reinterpreted.

Elders taught me that these stories are coauthored with spiritual and natural beings. They expand psychiatry beyond humans, opening up a psychology of nature and of spirits and the interactions of humans with all of these beings. Within the oral tradition, magic and spirits abound and power is cultivated through ceremonies. Knowledge comes directly through the experience of being in ceremony, of listening to spirits, and from nature.

Indigenous Psychiatrists

I'd like to share some stories about indigenous healers as narrative psychiatrists. First, I'd like to point out some of the essential aspects of their perspective on narrative psychiatry:

1. There are no bad people, only bad stories.
2. Bad stories can readily be replaced by good stories.
3. The more people tell and hear good stories, the more likely they are to stick and to have an impact.
4. Miracles are always possible through the Creator, so we mustn't ever succumb to the story that tells us that our situation or we are hopeless. Hope is perpetual.
5. These new stories that we are learning must be lived within community, which is what makes them real, makes them manifest, makes them able to replace the old stories of suffering, isolation, and woe.
6. Every story has a spirit, and every time a story is told, it has an effect on the listener (so tell lots of good stories). This spirit of the story stays with the person and continues to work on him or her long after the storyteller has departed.
7. Don't tell bad stories or gossip, because those stories will undo the good stories you are telling.

Being Badger

I brought a suicidal man to one of my favorite elders in Saskatchewan. "Henry" had just been fired from his job of the past six years. Henry's job as a research scientist had been his life. He had grown up on one of the Cree reservations and had lived a childhood of deprivation. School and learning had rescued him. He had devoted his life to science, and this was all that had meaning to him. When economic downturns happened and his employer decided that he was expendable, Henry's life ended as far as he was concerned. I met Henry in the emergency room. His sister brought him to the hospital because she was sure he was going to kill himself. Henry agreed. He was ready to die. We negotiated a contract for him to stay alive for at least one more week. I offered to take him to see a Cree elder (John). He agreed. I saw him each day until Sunday, when we drove from Saskatoon to Prince Albert to participate in John's healing session and sweatlodge.

John sat with Henry and asked him to tell what had happened. Henry told his story. His whole life had been about succeeding in science, which was his ticket off the reserve. His parents had been alcoholics. His brothers were in prison, and his sisters had taken up the sex trade. His family life was as bad as it could be. Throughout his life he had told himself that he would make something of his life.

John listened to him. I felt the profound depth of this listening. When Henry was done talking, John took him from the living room into his special treatment room. I was invited to come. I sat near Henry as John smudged him. Then John took both of Henry's hands in his and began to pray. He asked Creator to bless Henry and talked about how Henry had survived his childhood intact, as no other member of his family had. John praised Henry and gave him a new story—that he was a survivor, that he was a success just in being alive. John sang over Henry and fanned him with an eagle wing. In time, he finished and told Henry he looked forward to sharing the sweatlodge ceremony with him. John's first story for Henry was a nonverbal narrative of love and acceptance. His more verbal story followed.

Back in the days when the world was re-created, Badger was looking for a hill large enough to burrow into and build himself a house. The world had been destroyed by a flood. So we have that same teaching as in the Bible.

"It was kind of like your world getting destroyed by your being fired, when everything that mattered to you was taken away."

Anyway, the earth was as flat as Manitoba. It was so flat you could kick your dog and still see him running three days later. That was when Wisakedjak realized that they would have to build their own mountain to have warm and safe homes. "You will find nothing but ant hills here," he said.

"I guess I'm kind of your Wisakedjak," John said. "I'm telling you to build your own mountain. You can't trust others to give you a home."

Badger had never thought of building a mountain, but Wisakedjak had watched when the first mountains were made, so he thought he knew how to make one. Badger would have never thought of building a mountain in which to place his home without Wisakedjak's suggestion. Wisakedjak knew he needed a rock from the lower world, and wanted Badger to go get it."

I have used this story, too, particularly with people who know more than they think they know. Henry was a Badger-like character who needed to come into his own. He reminded me of one of my clients, "April," who deferred to everyone else. She rarely did what she wanted to do. She dreamed of an entirely different life than what she had. She studied acting but didn't act. She studied singing but never sang. She knew people who were successful (in her eyes), and she never felt she could measure up. I used a variation of the same story for her as part of a larger effort to foster her independence, which slowly did happen. April emerged from the shadows and began to assert herself in her world. She began to sing in public and eventually in coffeehouses. That fostered her continued transformation.

I suppose in medicine and psychology, we are always trying to get others to do their work. The problem arises when these others think that our work is to "fix them." Then we must find a way to get them to go out and do their work, like Badger, who is asked in this story to get a rock from the underworld. We need to set our clients on quests in which they do the work, even if they think they are doing the work for us. The hypnotherapist Milton Erickson frequently gave clients tasks to complete before they came back to see him. Traditional healers also do this frequently, and it happens in traditional stories such as this one.

> *Badger completed his quest, but only returned with clay from the lower world instead of rocks. At first, Wisakedjak was angry, but then considered that clay could work after all. But he didn't actually know how to make a mountain out of clay, or anything for that matter. He knew that powerful medicine had been blown onto the tops of mountains to cause them to grow tall, and then something else had been blown on the two sides so they would stretch along the edges of the land, but Wisakedjak had no clue what these medicines were, and he was too proud to ask.*

"We often find ourselves in Wisakedjak's position," John said. "We know what we want to do, and we know that others have done it, but we don't have a clue how to proceed. Wisakedjak inspires us to go ahead and figure it out as we go. No one besides tricksters can start without a plan and improvise as they go. Wisakedjak did just that. He teaches us how to be flexible and creative. So, without showing that he didn't know what medicine to use, Wisakedjak asked Badger to go ask Buffalo for the medicine that would make the mountains grow. He found a way to persuade Badger to go do another task."

John did the same with Henry on his repeated visits. When he got there, John would send Henry to get some sturgeon from the lake or haul firewood or find new stones. Always one of John's children or grandchildren was there to help him so he didn't feel frustrated.

> *Wisakedjak's constructions are never perfect, nor even close to perfect. His mountains turned into three large hills, a small hill, and a huge canyon where he let the medicine spill and trickle down into the ground. He didn't even think*

to build a doorway into his hills, which had turned hard as rock. So he had to convince his digging friends—Mole, Skunk, Gopher, and Badger—to build him four doors. When they were done, he threw them out to find their own homes.

Finally Badger realized he knew enough to build his own home. Lucky for him, he had kept enough of the sacred dirt and clay from the underworld to have the raw material. He knew where to gather the growing medicine, and when all this was done, he set about making his home, which is now called Badger Mountain. So Badger had learned enough from his trials and tribulations to do a remarkable piece of work for himself, and this was Wisakedjak's gift.

"You can do the same, Henry," John told him. "You're just as clever as that Badger." John's point in telling this story was that Henry knew within himself what he needed to know to survive. I think he was also telling Henry that he (John) could see things that Henry couldn't and could help him to figure things out. That's certainly what I meant to imply to April in telling the same story. Even though John could and did help, by identifying Henry with Badger, John was telling him that he had enough capacity to do well on his own. He didn't really need me or John, just as Badger did not really need Wisakedjak. He had enough inner resources to rebuild his own world whether we helped or not.

This story was just a seed. Many more stories came. Each one reinforced the idea that Henry knew enough to figure things out for himself. The context of those stories, however, was the inclusion of Henry in a community of people orbiting around John (his healing circle) who cared about Henry.

We shared the sweatlodge ceremony the afternoon of our first visit. In this lovely ceremony, we sat near the fire while rocks roasted. In John's style of leadership, the opening to a canvas-covered oval is to the south. John sits in the north surrounded by helpers who will sing for him and provide emotional support. Those of us who wish prayers give him tobacco and cloth before the ceremony starts, telling him our concerns. He brings the tobacco and cloth into the lodge to pray over it. We enter the lodge, and each person tells John again what prayers they wish him to offer. When we are done, hot stones are brought in. When enough stones have entered, a bucket of water is brought inside, and the door is closed. We begin with songs, initially for the four directions. All are sung in Cree.

That day, when the songs were over, John asked specific people to pray. When they were done, he sang a final song, said a concluding prayer, and called for the door to open. When John felt we were ready, he called for more stones to be brought inside. Another bucket of water entered, and the door closed. This happened twice more. At the end of the fourth round, berries, salmon, and corn entered to be passed around for everyone to eat. In between rounds, people talked about their lives and their situations. John had words to share, but mostly he absorbed the words and sentiments of others.

After the formal conclusion of the ceremony, we shared a feast in John's small house next to the lake, with baked sturgeon and a buffalo stew. Henry's appetite had returned. He ate with gusto. The ceremony and the participation in community had reminded him about what was good in his childhood. As we were leaving, Henry mentioned he was ready to do another lodge, just as soon as John would have one. John laughed and told him to be back the next Sunday, and to come early so he could get doctored again. Henry was ready to return. He was "infected" with John's new stories, which united the traditional stories about being Cree with a modern presence in the world. John had stories of healing and stories of community. Henry could participate in a world in which being employed was unimportant. He was a good person regardless of his external circumstances.

Becoming Muskrat

Another time, I brought John a woman whose husband had been murdered by a gang. She was distraught. She wanted to die. "Terri" had cut her wrists, but the cuts had not been deep enough to cause much damage. When her sister brought her to me she was contemplating hanging herself. I sat with her and heard her story for several hours.

Terri's story was not so different from many that I have heard. Her mother and father had been alcoholic during her childhood but had sobered up during their later years. Nevertheless, that didn't help Terri's memories of childhood, which largely consisted of staying away from home as much as possible and knowing where to hide when her parents were really drunk. Terri had done everything she could to get away from her family, though she still loved them and felt conflicted about her reactions to them.

Terri's husband, Jeremy, had been her ticket off the reserve, though he had his own unsavory attributes. Jeremy was a hustler. He dallied with the Indian Posse, a local gang. He dabbled with drugs. He eked out a living by dealing, fencing stolen property, gambling, and other quasi-legal activities. Nevertheless, he could be quite charming, and Terri loved him. In the stories she told about him, he sounded simultaneously rakish, generous, compassionate, dangerous, and exciting.

Without Jeremy, Terri was lost, hopeless. I realized a traditional healer would be most helpful for her since she had grown up on one of the reserves just north of Saskatoon. I asked Terri if she would be willing to see an elder. She was. This is the beauty of aboriginal culture; most people are willing to see an elder if asked. We went to see John, who sat with Terri in his living room and let her talk on and on about her childhood, her parents, and her escape from the reserve.

Then John took her into her the small room that he used for his doctoring. He sat Terri down and began to sing. After several songs, he made a formal request to the spirits to help him understand. He announced that Jeremy's spirit had appeared. Jeremy was sorry to have left Terri. He wished things could have been different, but he lived a lifestyle that was associated with death. He was sorry.

John then began to doctor Terri. He fanned her with his eagle wing. He sang songs. He burned sage and cedar. He prayed. When he was done, he invited Terri to stay for his sweatlodge ceremony, which she did. When all was done he told her a story that she could take with her, a story about Wibasa.

Wibasa was the grandson of the Moon and the son of the West Wind. His mother had died in childbirth, but he was born fully developed and with all knowledge, so that he did not have to be raised. Wibasa made the earth, invented fishing nets, water, fish, and deer. He lived where the sun rises. After the great flood had covered the earth, Wibasa told Raven to bring him a lump of clay from which to remake earth, but Raven couldn't find any. Wibasa then

sent Otter to dive for clay, but Otter brought nothing back. Then Wibasa sent
Muskrat, who returned with some soil that was used to remake the earth.

John told Terri that he understood that her entire world had just been wiped out, just like what had happened in the great flood. Nevertheless, if she would dive deep into her soul, she could bring forth a life for herself out of what was left of the old. Like Muskrat, she was the one who could dive deep into the ocean and bring back what was needed for rebuilding. I felt inspired too. I also wanted to be like Muskrat. I wanted to bring back the dirt that would reestablish the earth. I wanted to be that helpful.

Then we assembled for the sweatlodge. Every lodge ceremony is transformative in its own way. Terri sat within a community of women and found hope again. Sensing her plight, the women there told stories of grief and loss—of having lost a child, a husband, parents, and a sister. They talked about the presence of those departed spirits and how close they seemed in ceremony. The prayers acknowledged those who had left and requested strength for those who were left behind. Again, everyone including John made sure Terri knew that each person was available for her to call or visit when the sadness overtook her. What a change for her to feel this community of concern!

In a later meeting, John told another story (among many) to Terri.

After the Creator made all the animals and the people, he asked Wisakedjak
to take good care of the people and teach them how to live. He asked him to
show the people all the bad roots that would hurt and kill them. He was asked
to keep the people and the animals from quarreling with each other.

"Obviously Wisakedjak didn't do a good job because people still quarrel, as you know. If he'd done his job, we wouldn't have any gangs like we do today. You probably told Jeremy much the same. You asked him to straighten up and stop dealing, and he didn't listen either." Terri was nodding her head in agreement. Bare branches danced in the winter winds outside. We had passed the time for the arrival of spring, but no one had seen it. The sky was overcast, and the air had the odor of snow coming.

Wisakedjak did not listen. He let the people and the animals do whatever they wished. Soon they were quarreling and fighting and shedding blood. The Creator was unhappy with Wisakedjak and threatened to take everything away from him and make him miserable if he didn't keep better order among the animals and the people.

"Creator does give us lots of warning before calamity befalls."

Wisakedjak didn't believe the Creator and didn't change his ways. He got even more careless and disobedient, tricking the animals and the people and making them angry with each other. They quarreled and fought so much that the earth became red with blood. Maybe that's why the people have been so miserable. Finally the Creator got really angry, threatening again to take everything away from Wisakedjak and wash the ground clean.

Wisakedjak didn't believe Creator until the rains came and the streams began to swell. The rains continued day after day and night after night. The water in the rivers and the lakes rose higher and higher until they overflowed their banks and washed the ground clean. The sea came onto the land and drowned everyone except for Wisakedjak, Otter, Beaver, and Muskrat.

"That's probably about where we are now. You can be Muskrat because she's going to save the day in this story. That's your role. Madrona can be Otter since they're smaller than beavers. I'll be Beaver because I work harder than he does. You're going to have to dive deep down inside yourself to pull out what Creator originally put there so we can rebuild your life. You'll see that neither Madrona nor I can do it for you."

Wisakedjak tried to stop the sea, but it was too strong for him. He sat down on the water and wept. Otter, Beaver, and Muskrat sat beside him and rested their heads on one of his thighs. In time the rain stopped, and they were left bobbing on the sea. Wisakedjak still didn't dare to speak to the Creator.

Taking pity on him, the Creator said, "I will give you the power to re-make everything if you will use the old materials buried under the water."

"That was me telling you that your life wasn't over yet. That's what I told you to do, to dive down deep inside and bring back something useful. And you did."

Wisakedjak didn't have the power to create anything, but he did have the power to expand what had already been created. As he could not dive and did not know how far it was to the old earth, he did not know what to do. Still floating on the flood, Wisakedjak said to the three animals beside him, "We shall starve unless one of you can bring me a bit of the old ground beneath the water. If you will get it for me, I will make an island for us." Then he turned to Otter: "You are brave and strong and active. If you will dive into the water and bring me a bit of earth, I will see that you will have plenty of fish to eat."

"I guess I didn't make you such a good offer, though we did have fish after the ceremony."

Otter dived, but came up without reaching the ground. A second time and a third time Wisakedjak praised Otter and persuaded him to dive. After the third time, he was too weary to dive again. "You are a coward!" exclaimed Wisakedjak. "I am surprised by your weak heart. Beaver, I know, can dive to the bottom of the flood. He will put you to shame."

Then Wisakedjak turned to Beaver. "You are brave and strong and wise. If you will dive into the water and bring me a bit of the old earth, I will make a good house for you on the new island I shall make. There you will be warm in the winter. Dive straight down as a brave Beaver does." Twice Beaver dived, and twice he returned without earth. After the second time he was so tired that Wisakedjak had to let him rest.

Wisakedjak begged Beaver to dive once more. "If you will bring me a bit of earth, I will make a wife for you."

"Too bad I didn't offer you a husband."

To obtain a wife Beaver dove a third time. He stayed so long that he was almost lifeless on his return, still with no earth in his paws. Wisakedjak was now very sad. If Otter and Beaver could not reach the bottom of the water, surely Muskrat would also fail. But he must try, as he was their last chance.

Wisakedjak told Muskrat how brave and strong and quick he was, even if he was small. He promised Muskrat plenty of roots to eat if he would dive into the water and bring back a bit of the old earth at the bottom. He promised to create rushes so that Muskrat could make a nice house with rushes and dirt.

Wisakedjak said that Otter and Beaver were fools. They had gotten lost. He told Muskrat that he would find the ground if he dove straight down. Muskrat jumped headfirst into the water. Down he went but brought back nothing. The second time he dived, he stayed a long time. When he returned Wisakedjak looked at his forepaws and sniffed.

"I smell the smell of earth," he said. "Go again. If you bring me even a small piece, I will make a wife for you, Muskrat. She will bear you a great many children. Have a strong heart now. Go straight down, as far as you can go."

This time Muskrat stayed down so long that Wisakedjak feared he had drowned. At last bubbles appeared in the water. Wisakedjak reached down his long arm, seized Muskrat, and pulled him up. The little creature was almost dead, but his forepaws held a piece of the old earth. Joyously, Wisakedjak seized it. In a short time he had expanded that bit of earth into an island. There he, Muskrat, Otter, and Beaver rested and rejoiced that they had not drowned in the flood.

What John offered Terri was love and the power of prayer. Implicit within his story was the story of hope—that anything is possible. Terri continued to visit John each weekend and made progressively greater strides to health. Eventually she got over the death of her husband and began to find meaning and purpose in the culture on her own reserve. She began to spend more time there with her elders and eventually moved back to work for the local tribal government.

Trickster Healers

I have been drawn to the trickster motif—seen in Wisakedjak, Coyote, Rabbit, Nanabush, and others—as a model for healing, since the trickster characters help us to see what we cannot see on our own. Trickster characters might have been the first healers/psychotherapists. Like psychotherapists, tricksters can be smart, cunning, and employ many ruses to overcome difficulties. Trickster stories also contain immense wisdom about change and transformation. Tricksters serve as cultural heroes who transform the world to be more habitable for humans by ridding it of dangerous monsters or by providing us with the means to live or live well (such as fire, ways of capturing animals, inventing of rain, and so on).

Trickster qualities tend to get assigned to those species—such as Coyote, Raven, Crow, and Rabbit—that are most adaptable, a highly valued trait in indigenous cultures. Coyote brought fire to the southern Dene people as well as to the California coastal Indians. Crow brought light to the far north for his people. The Norse god Odin was informed about the world by his two ravens, Hugin and Munin (Thought and Memory). Among the Haida people of the Queen Charlotte Islands, Raven stole light from an old grandfather who was hiding it under boxes. It was only through his trickery and inventiveness that Raven could succeed in this quest of gathering and sharing the light, thereby allowing the world to emerge from perpetual darkness. As a side effect, he invented birth and reincarnation.

Trickster shows us our contradictions;[2] many trickster tales relate to foolish, mischievous, and occasionally disastrous activities. They describe encounters with other animals and beings, attempts to trick them, to become like them, or to outwit them, attempts that inevitably rebound. In such stories the typical trickster figure is greedy, vain, foolish, cunning, and occasionally capable of displaying a high degree of power.

In the Pacific Northwest, Raven is always getting into trouble. In one Haida story, Raven assumes the form of a woman's husband and succeeds in getting into bed with her. When her husband returns early from his fishing trip and sees himself in bed with his wife, he knows something is wrong, and this something can only be Raven. He cuts Raven into little pieces, ties the pieces into a bundle, and throws them deep into the sea with weights attached. In this story, Raven's deceit was entirely for his own pleasure, and the result offers an instructive lesson to the hearer.

In the next cycle of that story, Raven gets tired of being tied into a bundle at the bottom of the ocean. He puts himself back together and rises toward the surface, but then Whale swallows him. Raven thinks nothing of inflicting a mortal wound in Whale as he digs out of Whale's stomach into the external world.

Trickster makes us laugh by doing all the wrong things, but in service to helping us understand how things actually work. Whenever a trickster tries to cruelly satisfy his desires, it backfires. Wile E. Coyote of cartoon fame never actually gets Road Runner. When Coyote gives Rabbit his penis to hold so that he can sneak into the women's sweatlodge, Rabbit runs off with it and establishes his reputation for sexual prowess. The next morning Coyote finds that Rabbit put his penis to good use all night long. No one suspected that a small animal could have such a large organ. Coyote's desires were thwarted, though he forgave his friend, Rabbit, for even he could appreciate a good joke when he saw one.

Trickster sometimes forces us to evolve, grow, and change, for our own good (as in the Dene stories from Arizona in which Coyote steals fire, only to set the mountain ablaze, thereby forcing First Woman to invent rain). Similarly, Coyote's theft of Water Monster's coat (with her babies in the pockets) was what precipitated the rage that led to the flood that forced the people to flee the Fourth World into the Fifth World in which we live today.

Trickster stories also allow us to share ideas with others that we could never directly approach. They are historically and across cultures the best stories for broaching taboo subjects. A Dene story about Coyote loaning his eyes allows people to indirectly talk about blindness, which would otherwise be taboo lest you lose your vision by talking about it (which is that culture's viewpoint). The taboo-breaking aspect of trickster stories helps us to look at aspects of ourselves and the stories we live that are not so savory as we might wish. We can talk about the trickster's antics, while we cannot talk about our own.

Coyote is sometimes associated with meanness and uncontrollable sexual passion. He can be pictured as rude, interfering, and restless, yet also vital to creation. In Dene stories, Coyote causes the flood that leads the people to emerge into this world, originates death, helps to place the stars, and generally pokes his nose into everyone's business. He was, however, also accorded knowledge above that of other beings. When there was uncertainty over the desirability of death, for example, when "no one knew what to do . . . they asked Coyote."[3] Also implied in the trickster is the indigenous cultural value of learning from animals. In an Arizona Dene story, people learn how to build houses by observing animal behavior. In that story, First Woman and the people went to the animals, one by one, to learn how they built their houses, then used all that information to settle on the hogan structure still in use today. On the way, they also learned how to weave blankets from spiders and make baskets from the birds.

Coyote represents the original knowledge on which the world rests and functions. Through his astuteness and manifestations in animal form, he gives omens and signs to the Dene people and provides warnings to travelers. Coyote stories are similar to other trickster tales found elsewhere in North America[4] "in the sense that the situations in which they may be related are much less ritually bound than for ceremonial and Creation myths."[5]

Coyote makes many appearances and has elaborate roles in the creation myths relating to the very important blessingway ceremony.[6] The blessingway ceremony is done to restore a state of harmony or beauty (*hozho*) and to exclude evil. Coyote wanders off by himself, only to turn up and offer advice and instruction when needed. He gives names to Talking God and Calling God, suggests the twelve hogan songs, insists on the mountains being given life, is enlisted by Changing Woman to steal dreams from people to give to the Holy People, so that they would receive forewarning that a blessingway ceremony was needed. He sanctified the sun, moon, corn, and plants and was responsible for ordering proper and necessary life patterns, including crop growing, to ensure the people's survival. From pieces of his fur and bone come all coyotes (for both the Dene and the Pima of Central Arizona) and the colors of the four different directions.

Trickster tales are amusing and entertaining and are frequently told to children, as they convey moral messages in an entertaining (and therefore memorable) way, as well as demonstrate possibilities and limitations in the world.[7] For the Dene people, for example, Coyote challenges and thereby authenticates and legitimizes the order established in the universe. "Coyote both extends the area of activities that have been and may be attempted and correspondingly demonstrates the limitations and/or consequences of such actions."[8] Coyote is a unique being who, in folklorist J. Barre Toelken's words, "experiences everything: he is, in brief, the exponent of all possibilities."[9]

In the Navajo story "Homes for Coyote and Badger,"[10] (which is remarkably similar to the Cree stories told earlier in this chapter) Badger is looking for a hill or mesa large enough to burrow into and build himself a house. "You will find nothing but hummocks here," Coyote says, making it clear that they will have to build their own mountain to have warm and safe homes. Badger had never thought of building a mountain, but Coyote had watched First Man when the four sacred mountains were made and had been with Fire Man when he started his mountain, so now he thought that he could easily build a mountain for himself. By mimicking the spirits, gods, and sacred people, Coyote conveys to humans and other animals the sense that we can do anything. Coyote observes and imitates, not always successfully, but in a way that stimulates and incites thoughtfulness not previously present.

We often find ourselves in Coyote's position. We know what we want to do, and we know that others have done it, but we don't have a clue how to proceed. The trickster inspires us to go ahead and improvise as we go. In this story, Coyote does just that. He asks Badger to go ask Hosteen Seal for the medicine that will make the mountains grow. Again, Coyote finds a rationale to persuade Badger why he must go instead of Coyote. Coyote is always looking to get others to work instead of himself. We helping professionals would sometimes do well to be so lazy, so that others can work and help themselves. If I can find someone else to lead ceremony or who wants to do the healing work, let them proceed. I step forward, like Coyote, when no one else is available, or all the others have given up. Then the task is clear, and we know what hasn't worked.

Fire Tales

I'm impressed with the number of cultures in which Coyote or another trickster figure steals fire. Coyote boldly sauntered up Fire Mountain, offering the Do'tsoh the gift of beautiful, multicolored shells, which were "magic" and able to bring moisture to the air and turn rocks to soft sand. Coyote employs deception to gain the fire. He gets permission to "warm up" by standing with his back to the interior of the mountain from which the fire rises. But he slips in a faggot to catch fire. When the Do'tsoh suspect what he is doing, he throws salt in their lidless eyes and grabs the burning faggot. Coyote then runs down the mountainside and sets most of the bushes on fire, creating a new problem for the people to resolve.

The Ojibway have a similar character known as Nanabush or Nanabozho, who also steals fire for the people. He is a vaguely human character except when he turns into an animal, which is most often a hare.[11] The Menominee name for Nanabush is derived from two Menominee words that mean "Great Rabbit." Chamberlain reports that Nanabush is one of several brothers born at the same time.[12] One of these brothers, Wabassa, who fled north almost immediately after his birth, was transformed into a rabbit and became a great manitou (spirit). In another story, Nanabush's grandmother puts him under a wooden bowl for his protection. She forgets him, so to avoid starvation, he changes into an animal that can eat the grass under the bowl—a rabbit, which is what his grandmother eventually finds when she remembers Nanabush and turns the bowl over.[13]

> *An old man has two daughters and is carefully guarding fire, an important commodity in an often frozen world. Nanabush wants fire for the people and for himself. By hiding he observes the habits and routines of the family who holds fire and decides he can trick them. He turns himself into a rabbit and hops into the lodge. The daughters find him so cuddly they cannot resist him. The father suspects trickery or magic, but the daughters will not listen. When all are asleep, Nanabush resumes his usual shape and runs away with some of their sacred fire.*

These stories are important sources of inspiration for us, because we always have to steal something from the gods—fire, independence, wisdom, and so on. It never comes easy. We must work to get what we want.

PART IV

Examples of Narrative Psychiatry in Action

14

Narratives for Anxiety and Depression

We must rely on the capacity people have for the narrative construction of their life and we must redefine therapy as a skill in participating in that process.

HARRY GOOLISHIAN, PLENARY ADDRESS
FOR THE HOUSTON-GALVESTON INSTITUTE'S
1991 DIS-DISEASING CONFERENCE

Through collaborative interaction, we can transform the narrative that is called depression into a narrative with a new name: health. The job of psychiatrists becomes facilitating the change from people believing they are defective to restoring dignity and purpose to lives. Then the various maladies of suffering, crime, and substance misuse can disappear. We can discard a series of labels that focus on dangerousness, hopelessness about change, and deserving punishment for people suffering from life burdens, to find respectful narratives that lead to new meanings, new understandings, and new relational social actions. Resolution is inherent in client-driven discourses and client-driven codirectorship with the therapist or doctor within the journey of burden and pain.

Gergen wrote, "Constructionist dialogues consistently underscore the significance of relationship as the matrix from which meaning is derived.

It is from the generation of coordination—of actions, words, objects—that human meaning is born. In this sense meaning does not originate in individual minds but in relationships among persons."[1] From this perspective, whether we use herbs, drugs, or meditation, psychiatry becomes a mediation of meaning among people. It becomes a return to what our forefathers were trying to create before the biological detour.

University of New Hampshire professor John Shotter wrote, "Relational knowing, which, while hard to learn from others, helps one to find a position in relation to the other(s) such that the relationship becomes more useful for those who take part in it."[2] From a social constructionist perspective, psychiatry becomes primarily the science of relationship as the catalyst for the transformation of suffering into health.

In any context involving doctor and patient, both bring positions, values, preconceptions, and ideas to any situation and both actually do poorly at disguising their subtle reactions to what the other person says. Their biases and values interact, and what emerges from a session is contextualized by the nature of the conversation and their preconversational assumptions. Collaborative work teases out those assumptions and allows new information to emerge. New meaning is born through fresh combinations and sharing of each individual's unique and context-bound contributions to the conversation. This kind of work has resulted in remarkable changes from anxiety and depression to psychological and spiritual wholeness.

Pilgrim's Progress

One example of narrative healing of an anxiety disorder comes from John Bunyan's story of transformation in *The Pilgrim's Progress from This World to That Which Is to Come,* a Christian allegory. In Bunyan's case, the "conversation" was more internal and with scripture, but in the story he created, there are many helpful dialogues. The first part was published in February 1678, and the second part in 1684; since then it has never been out of print. It is regarded as one of the most significant works of English literature and has been translated into more than two hundred languages. "Bunyan began the work while in the Bedfordshire county jail [1660–1672] for violations of the Conventicle Act, which prohibited the holding of religious services outside the auspices of the established Church of England."[3] *Pilgrim's Progress* represents one of the great epic hero's journeys, the seventeenth-century version of Luke Skywalker in *Star Wars*.

For those unfamiliar with *Pilgrim's Progress,* the following summary provides a helpful outline.

> Christian, an everyman character, is journeying from his hometown to the "Celestial City" atop Mt. Zion. The burden of his sins, which would cause him to sink into hell, impels him to seek deliverance. Christian leaves his home, his wife, and children to save himself when his attempt to persuade them to go with him fails.
>
> Christian is diverted by Mr. Worldly Wiseman into seeking deliverance from his burden through the Law, supposedly with the help of a Mr. Legality and his son Civility in the village of Morality, rather than through Christ, who stands at the Wicket Gate. The character, Evangelist, meets the wayward Christian where he has stopped before a life-threatening mountain on the way to Legality's home. Evangelist shows Christian that he had sinned by turning out of his way, but he assures him that he will be welcomed at the Wicket Gate if he should turn around and go there, which Christian does.
>
> At the Wicket Gate Christian is directed onto the "straight and narrow" King's Highway by the gatekeeper, Good Will. In the Second Part, Good Will is shown to be Jesus himself. Christian makes his way from there to the House of the Interpreter, where he is shown pictures and tableaux that portray or dramatize aspects of the Christian faith and life. From the House of the Interpreter, Christian finally reaches the "place of deliverance," where the "straps" that bound Christian's burden to him break. After Christian is relieved of his burden, he is greeted by three shining beings, who give him the greeting of peace, new garments, and a scroll as passport into the Celestial City.

As night falls Christian enters the Valley of the Shadow of Death. When he is in the middle of the valley amidst the gloom and terror he imagines the voice of his friend Faithful, with whom he grew up, speaking the words of the Twenty-third Psalm: *Yea, though I walk through the valley of the shadow of death, I will fear no evil: for thou art with me; thy rod and thy staff they comfort me* (Psalms 23:4). As he leaves this valley the sun rises on a new day.

Just outside the Valley of the Shadow of Death he encounters Faithful, who accompanies him to Vanity Fair where both are arrested and detained because of their disdain for the wares and business of the fair. Faithful is put on trial, and executed as a martyr. Hopeful, a resident of Vanity, takes Faithful's place to be Christian's companion for the rest of the way.

Along a rough stretch of road, Christian and Hopeful leave the highway to travel on the easier By-Path Meadow, where a rainstorm forces them to spend the night. In the morning they are captured by Giant Despair, who takes them to his Doubting Castle, where they are imprisoned, beaten, and starved. The giant wants them to commit suicide, but they endure the ordeal until Christian realizes that a key he has, called Promise, will open all the doors and gates of Doubting Castle. Using the key, they escape.

Christian and Hopeful make it through the dangerous Enchanted Ground into the Land of Beulah, where they ready themselves to cross the River of Death on foot to Mount Zion and the Celestial City. Christian has a rough time of it, but Hopeful helps him over; and they are welcomed into the Celestial City.

The Second Part of *The Pilgrim's Progress* presents the pilgrimage of Christian's wife, Christiana; their sons; and the maiden, Mercy. They visit the same stopping places that Christian visited, with the addition of Gaius' Inn between the Valley of the Shadow of Death and Vanity Fair; but they take a longer time in order to accommodate marriage and childbirth for the four sons and their wives. The hero of the story is Greatheart, the servant of the Interpreter, who is a pilgrim's guide to the Celestial City. He kills four giants and participates in the slaying of a monster that terrorizes the city of Vanity.

The passage of years in this second pilgrimage better allegorizes the journey of the Christian life. By using heroines, Bunyan, in the Second Part, illustrates the idea that women as well as men can be brave pilgrims.[4]

From my reading of *The Pilgrim's Progress* and Bunyan's autobiography, *Grace Abounding to the Chief of Sinners,* I believe Christian was created by Bunyan as an allegorical characterization of himself. Bunyan provides us with an early example of what today would be called an obsessive-compulsive disorder.[5] Bunyan's obsessive fear of "selling" his Savior (a fear of giving way to the temptation to blaspheme God and reject salvation) and his consequent compulsive, repetitious, and torturous examination of the "Esau text" (Hebrews 12:16–17) drove him to what Bunyan self-described as a kind of "madness," but also eventually toward healing. Bunyan heals through the help of hope, envisioned as Hopeful, the empathetic listener and provider of wise advice. Hope, according to John Calvin,[6] is applied faith, or faith in action. Calvin refers to hope as "the nourishment and strength of faith." Hopeful exhorts Christian (Bunyan's character) to put his faith in action, to hope in the promises.

At the outset Bunyan's irrational and obsessive fears and his desperately compulsive readings of scripture contribute to his dark despair. But his gradually developing proficiencies as a reader and his practice of faith in hope eventually bring him and his Christian pilgrim to a place of sustained health by way of Easter at Doubting Castle. No longer are his perceptions clouded and his thoughts paralyzed with doubts. Bunyan's progress toward a clear understanding and acceptance of God's grace, like Christian's, opens his mind to real hope and thus to spiritual and psychological health.

Stories like *Pilgrim's Progress* guide every aspect of our lives. When the themes of those stories are predominantly supportive of suffering, psychiatric disorders are diagnosed. When trauma has preceded these stories of suffering, posttraumatic stress disorder is diagnosed, which includes anxiety and depression. Excesses of sadness have been called depression or grief, excesses of fear and worry have been called anxiety disorders of various kinds, and excesses of joy and irritability have been called bipolar disorder. The breakdown in the ability to talk story with other people has been called psychosis.

Psychological disturbance can make God seem awfully far away. His grace seems unavailable. In this, hope is lost and despair sets in. However, as Bunyan's life attests, hope, conveyed to a sufferer in the context of a caring, loving relationship, is a primary ingredient in psychological therapy that can make a world of difference between deepening despair and healing. When Bunyan's reading of scripture finally provided comfort and hope, his anxieties and despair concerning his salvation quieted. His faith then promoted an obedient and faithful response (hope in action), and he experienced a transformation toward wholeness, or at least toward a remission of his obsessive thoughts and compulsive rituals.

Creating the Future

In the narrative view, patients become participants in a collaborative process, part of an emerging new relationship. Without directing the conversation, the role of the psychiatrist is to create "space in which dialogical conversation can occur" and to continually guide the conversation in a dialogical direction.[7] This dialogical conversation is nonhierarchical and collaborative, involving mutual sharing about the concerns of the participant, and not predefined by researchers, scientific truths, or theories. Patients become partners in contributing their expertise to the change process. Genuine collaboration involves working together on a mutually agreed-upon creative exploration or goal.

These elements are all present in my first story about healing anxiety and depression at a rural and remote Cree reserve in northwestern Saskatchewan. During my four years in Canada, I would fly into small villages to ply the trade of psychiatry. Mostly I tried to motivate people to solve their own problems, because conventional psychiatric solutions had not helped them in the past and probably weren't going to help them in the future. I would often visit people in their homes, since that was easier than expecting them to show up at the clinic. Life has a timeless quality in the north, which is neither good nor bad, but makes it difficult for people to keep track of appointments. There is a quality of "sameness" to people's days. One of my family doctor colleagues said that the north was like a still photograph, while life elsewhere was a movie.

"Gerty" was one of those people I visited at home. Gerty was still grieving the death of her son, who had been stabbed months earlier in the house across the street. Apparently the families on either side of that street had been feuding for as long as anyone could remember. In the dimly lit historical past, after treaty was taken and the people had been placed on reserves, the Indian agent had the bright idea to house these families across the street from each other. That had never changed. Tragedy happened in every generation, sometimes on alternating sides of the street. One side died, and the other side went to prison; both were tragedies.

I had been asked to see Gerty because her daughter "Louise," who worked at the clinic, thought her mother's grief had lasted too long. "We buried him six months ago," she had said about her brother. "I know the Cree way is to grieve for a year, but I think my mom has taken it too far." I had asked Louise to drive me to the house and introduce me to her mom and to stay with us for that first visit. Louise had taken her mother to see a new family doctor at the health clinic, who had just come to Saskatchewan from India. He had diagnosed her as having major depression and had given her an antidepressant medication (sertraline, brand name Zoloft), which she hadn't taken because she "wasn't no nut case."

We bumped over the frozen snow in Louise's Dodge Ram four-wheel-drive pickup. It was December, and the temperature outside was −43 degrees. I remember that well because it's the temperature at which the Fahrenheit and Celsius scales collide into the same number. It's also terribly cold. Smoke hung in the air above the chimneys. Many of the homes were heated by wood, and it was a great effort to lay in enough for the entire winter. People trudged along the frozen road, perhaps going to the clinic or going to the Northern Store, the area's only grocery, which had very little actual food in it, or at least very little of what I called food. It was full of soda, chips, dip, powdered drinks, dry cereal, and other food items that were light to ship, heavily processed, and full of fat and sugar.

How can I describe Gerty's house? Imagine snow everywhere. The front steps are missing so we must enter through the side door, through the mud room and into the kitchen. Probably no one ever thought to enter any other way. Wood is piled in great heaping stacks all around the house. A smoke house stands off to one side and back in the pine trees.

We climbed the rickety steps into the mud room, stamped the snow off our boots, and entered the kitchen. We could smell coffee and cigarettes. Pictures of "Tom," the lost son, were everywhere. Gerty was Anglican with a smattering of traditional Cree. She had created an altar of sorts in the living room with pictures of Tom under a statue of Jesus on the cross and surrounded by sage, tobacco, and cedar. Various small items of Tom's ringed the base of the cross. A Christmas tree, sparsely decorated, stood in the corner of the room. The house was clean and warm.

"Ma," Louise said. "I brought that doctor I been telling you about. He came to talk to you."

"I don't need to talk to no damn doctor," she said. "No offense," she added quickly, looking at me.

"No problem," I answered. "But since we're here anyway, and I gotta show some justification for them flying me all the way up here, maybe we could sit for some coffee and Louise and I could chat."

"That would be okay," Gerty answered. "So long as I'm not being psychoanalyzed."

"Wouldn't dream of it," I said.

"All right," Gerty said, getting off her sofa and going to get coffee for me and her daughter. Just like in my childhood home, nobody ever turned off the blaring television or even thought to do so. *Days of Our Lives* or something very similar was playing.

"What do you think of my younger brother?" Louise asked, stirring her coffee. Louise had studied nursing in Prince Albert, graduated with her B.S.N., and now worked in the health clinic. Even though she was only twenty-five or so, she was very quick, and I could see she knew exactly what she was doing.

"He was a handsome fellow," I replied.

"He sure was," she said.

"What a shame, his death," I added. We both held our breaths, expecting Gerty to jump into the discussion. We didn't have to wait long. Before the coffee was half gone, Gerty had launched into a long story about her son.

Before too long, however, she had changed subjects and was talking about the family of the young man who had killed Tom and how they were always looking over their fence at her. She had put up a higher fence after the murder, so she couldn't see their house from anywhere inside her house, nor could they see her. Her expression changed from how she had greeted her daughter to one of pursed lips, rigid shoulders, and clenched fists.

"I want to kill all of them," she said, shaking her fist. "Then I'd kill myself. The only thing that stops me is my grandbabies. I have to help my girls take care of my grandbabies."

"You sure do, Mom," Louise added. "We need you." Louise didn't have any children yet, but was rumored to be flirting with one of the new single doctors. Her four sisters, however, had four children each, and two of them lived in the village. Her two brothers also had two children each, but they lived with their mothers, who had different sets of grandparents to look after their children, so Gerty didn't see her sons' children very often.

Before long, Gerty was sobbing. "I just want to die," she was saying. "I just want to go to heaven and be with my little Tommy and my Roy." Gerty's husband "Roy" had died six years previously of a heart attack. "I'm just a burden on folks," she said. "I'm just a useless old woman. See, I can't even take care of my grandchildren I'm so broken up." Then, almost without warning, Gerty got angry again and launched into another diatribe against the family across the street. The third time she did this, I suspected that anger arose when tears were not far away.

"What have you done to commemorate Tom's life?" I asked Gerty.

"What do you mean?"

"Have you written down the stories of his life?" Gerty still looked confused. "You still don't know what I mean, do you?" I said.

"No," Gerty said, shaking her head.

"I'm proposing that you and Louise and your entire family get together and write down or make a video tape of all the stories you can remember about Tom. Put together all the photographs of Tom. Make a book of photos and stories about him. That'll help you focus on Tom." We spent the rest of our meeting discussing how to do this. We agreed that I would visit Gerty the next month when I came to their community.

My January drive with Louise to visit Gerty was a duplicate of December's visit. The day was cold and bright, the temperature slightly warmer at −39 degrees. We went into the house the same way. Dogs ran free outside in the snow, appearing to thrive with thick, healthy coats despite the temperature. This second visit resulted in more coffee and tears after tears after tears as Gerty showed us the photographs that the family had been assembling and shared with us some of the stories that had been written down. A toddler stumbled through the living room dressed only in a diaper. The Christmas tree stood in the corner amid wreaths and other decorations. I didn't hear any talk of the family across the street. Louise agreed that she would continue to shepherd her mother through the completion of the Tom memorial project.

For my February visit, the temperature had risen to −22 degrees. Louise was feeling better about her mother. For this visit the entire family was present—at least, all the family still living on or around the reserve. The living room was packed when Louise and I walked into the house. I counted two young men, three young women, and two women around Gerty's age. A gaggle of toddlers and young children were running helter-skelter around the house. An unrecognizable children's TV program blared from the corner of the room.

Louise made introductions. The men were Gerty's sons; the younger women, daughters. Two of Gerty's sisters had come. The children remained nameless and in constant motion. I began to get a sense of which children belonged to which adults by watching who they bounced up against the most often.

We talked for three hours about Tom, the family across the street, the feud, Gerty's sadness and anger, and how to move forward beyond Tom's death. The children and sisters had marvelous ideas. We brainstormed about how the feud could end and how this family could perhaps reach out to the family across the street and offer forgiveness. I suggested that the Anglican priest who visited the community periodically might be able to help broker a meeting for the purpose of forgiveness and reconciliation. That was agreed on. We continued to brainstorm, and plans were made to finish the Tom memorial project and to support Gerty in letting out all of her sadness and anger.

When I visited in March during a driving snow, everyone was feeling better. This time there was one son, two daughters, and one sister, plus Louise and Gerty present. The priest had scheduled a meeting with the family across the street. Gerty was uncertain about how she would react to those people, but she had committed to go through with the meeting. Everyone was happy with Gerty's progress. She was back to her "old self" of being vivacious and active and "in charge" of all of her children's and grandchildren's lives. We decided that my work was done, though I looked forward to hearing about the meeting with the family across the street.

I saw Gerty several more times when I visited her community. Her DSM diagnosis would have been "complicated bereavement" or "major depression." But she quickly overthrew these diagnoses through the involvement of her family and friends. We transformed her suffering into health through everyone's contributing to a story about the son she had lost. Through engaging her in a memorial project, she was able to channel her grief and create meaning from her son's life. The family and the priest generated a kind of healing circle around her. This work was much more effective than giving her medication, which she had refused on principles (her own story about people who take medication and what that means about them). Activating her social network through providing them with a project on which to work together started the healing process.

The Wolf's Advice

Here's another story of transforming anxiety and depression. I met "Petra" as part of a social services case in which Petra's daughter "Shawna" had reported Petra's boyfriend for molesting her. The report took place at school. The boyfriend was charged, but so was Petra, and her daughter was placed with a relative. Petra was forbidden to visit her daughter Shawna. I was asked to evaluate Petra's psychiatric status. Her attorney was looking for a defense. Petra was distraught. She had no idea that her boyfriend had done anything to her daughter. She alternately refused to believe that he had molested anyone and blamed herself that it had happened.

As I reviewed the situation, it seemed problematic. The reported abuse came after a school presentation on abuse. No physical evidence existed. It was possible that the abuse had happened; it was possible that it had not. The accusation was that the boyfriend had asked Shawna to "touch his pee-pee." These were the exact words used in a vignette at the school presentation. Shawna reported having touched it, then having a "yuck" response and running out of the bathroom.

Petra had been coping marginally before the arrest. After the arrest she fell into a deep well of despair. She could no longer see her boyfriend if she wanted to be able to eventually visit her daughter (by court order). Petra believed that her boyfriend had been the glue that held her life together. But without her daughter, she was lost. One weekend she drank continually and was eventually arrested for possession of alcohol on the reserve, which made her case to regain her daughter even more difficult.

Here is where I rail against the retribution system. (I fail to see how it is a justice system.) Petra had not done anything overtly wrong. Could she have failed to notice telltale signs for fear of losing her boyfriend and his financial and emotional support? That was possible, but is it reasonable to punish a mother for missing clues that are subtle anyway? And what if there were no clues? Or had there been no abuse? That was also possible, for Shawna was known to resent the boyfriend's moving into the house. Shawna's recitations of her story seemed rote and memorized and without much emotion, though she had a lot of feeling and anger about not being able to see her mother. She thought that was terribly unfair.

If we weren't so keen on punishing people, we could have worked with this family without any charges being filed. Social services could have mandated family counseling to sort through these accusations, rather than jump to recommending arrests. If actual abuse has occurred, it usually emerges in family talking circles. As it was, Petra's life had been devastated by accusations.

Petra's attorney recommended that she see me during my monthly visits to her reserve in order to show the court that she deserved to have Shawna back. The paradox was that Shawna lived just a few houses down from Petra and the family still had to go through the pretense that Petra never saw Shawna. The police, of course, had their eye on Petra and would have jumped to jail her if they saw the least hint of any contact between mother and daughter. I suspected, however, that the family was facilitating a modicum of contact in safe ways. The matriarch of the family was very unhappy with Petra's being charged. Petra's mother was a strong, controlling, iron-fisted woman, tight with the Roman Catholic Church.

By the time of the initial hearing, which happened nine months after the arrest, Petra was a lost soul. She had lost all will to live. She dreamed of being united with Shawna and, if that didn't happen, planned to slip off into the snow and die. She thought she'd just drive her brother's snowmobile into the bush until it ran out of gas and then lie down and go to sleep in the snow. Her mother had taken her to the health clinic, and the doctor there had given her fluoxetine (Prozac), but Petra rarely took it, and no one else paid attention either. She guessed she took a pill maybe once per week. We had to do something to jumpstart Petra.

In my first meeting alone with Petra that didn't involve evaluation and preparation of court documents, I asked her how religious she was. "I'm a good Catholic," she said.

"How's that," I asked, "when you're thinking about killing yourself?"

"That's different," she said.

"Oh, okay. So do you think God has a plan for you and your life?" I asked.

"Of course," she answered.

"So what is that plan?" I countered.

"I don't know," she said. "Only God knows why I'm being tortured like this. It's maybe like the Book of Job."

"So maybe God's torturing you to prove to the Devil that you are too strong to break?"

"Yes," Petra said.

"So shouldn't we be trying to learn God's purpose for all this?" I asked.

"I guess so," she answered, somewhat hesitantly. I think she saw where I was taking this and wasn't sure if she wanted to go there.

"Then let's have a meeting of everyone who knows you," I said. "Today perhaps we could do some guided imagery together and just see what happens."

"What's guided imagery?" she responded.

"It's just me talking and telling you stories and asking you to let images form in your mind's eye, kind of like you are having a dream, but you're awake. It's kind of fun, I think, and we might learn something."

"But isn't that some kind of devil stuff?" she asked, suspicious now that I was in league with Satan.

"No, good Catholics do it all the time—priests like Thomas Merton. They call it contemplative or reflective prayer."

"I don't know about that," Petra said.

"Well, I'll tell you what. If we do this, and you don't like it, we'll stop it," I said, trying not to be too eager or threatening.

"Okay, I guess," she said. I asked her to rearrange herself in the chair so she could be more relaxed, although that wasn't too likely. I proceeded with my somewhat standard induction with Petra, using images from the north—falling snow, the stillness after a winter storm, the moon's reflection on the snow, her sadness at missing her daughter. Then I told her a story about someone who had lost everything and found a way back.

After the story, I asked Petra to imagine that she was out in the woods. She'd driven out onto the frozen lake in her snowmobile and was thinking about dying, just like she had told me. Probably she was hoping that she would fall through the ice. Imagine if an angel appeared at that very moment to tell her about God's plan for her. (I was drawing my material from the television show *Touched by an Angel,* about the Irish angel who keeps appearing to desperate people to convince them to change the course of their lives.) How would an angel look? What would an angel say? What would the angel's message be?

"It looks like a wolf," she said. "The angel is a wolf who's come for me, to take me home. It's such an honor to be addressed by a wolf. It's such an honor to be led home by a wolf. It's going to walk with me until I get back to the house. It won't let me freeze."

"So God wants you to live?" I asked.

"I guess so," Petra answered.

"Ask the angel why you're supposed to live," I directed.

"Okay," she said. Silence ensued and then she answered. "It says I'm supposed to learn to be a fighter. I'm supposed to learn how to take on the system and fight for people who can't fight for themselves. How can that be? I can't even fight for myself. How can I fight for anyone else?"

"I guess the wolf thinks you can learn," I said.

During my next month's visit to the community, we met with Petra's entire family and several family friends to form a healing circle. We used the talking stick and talking circle format. I began the discussion by asking everyone to offer whatever thoughts they had about how Petra could change her situation. For three hours, the stick passed from person to person, each of them expressing their love for Petra and offering their suggestions.

Our consensus at the end of the day was that Petra and her older sister, who worked with Services Canada, should start a healing circle for women at the church. Then women who were afraid of losing their children or had lost children or had been beaten by boyfriends or girlfriends or had been raped or otherwise felt lost would have a place to go for healing. I volunteered to talk to the part-time priest about his sanctioning and encouraging this activity. He and I had a meeting scheduled for the next day anyway.

During the next day's meeting, the priest and his student intern were more than excited about the women's circle. He pledged to support it at the highest possible levels and even to provide refreshments. "Perhaps we could pay one of the high school students to provide child care," he said. "This is too important for anyone to have to stay home." (Many women had large families and had husbands who worked in the mines, one week or two weeks at work, then one or two weeks at home. Childcare was sometimes difficult to find.) "This gives me an opportunity to keep an eye on Petra," he said. "I'll try to help her and in doing that, stay aware of how she's doing."

"That would be wonderful," I said. "We have to keep finding reasons for her not to ride that snowmobile off into the bush for good."

"Definitely," he agreed.

Petra and her sister did start the women's circle. Perhaps women could relate to it better with Petra as one of the leaders because they knew she was suffering. That was better than a professional leader with the usual shielding of personal life from visibility.

The day of the hearing finally came. Charges against Petra's boyfriend were dropped because of insufficient evidence. Charges against Petra were continued because of her additional charge of drinking on the reserve. The priest and I wrote impassioned letters to the presiding judge, urging him to also drop all charges against Petra for the sake of her mental health, but also for the sake of the child. The boyfriend was now allowed to visit the child, but not Petra. (This is typical "justice system" logic as I have seen it enacted.)

I continued to see Petra every month. The priest joined one of our guided imagery sessions to pronounce it "Catholic friendly." Petra slowly forged a new story. She went from "helpless and unable to cope without a man" to "strong in a community of women." Slowly but surely drumming was introduced into the healing circle. Women drummed to Christian hymns with the priest's blessings.

Three months later, Petra's charges were reduced to a lesser offense to which she pleaded guilty in order to end her legal nightmare. She was sentenced to probation for child endangerment (despite no crime having been officially committed) and allowed supervised visitation with her child, who was now in the custody of her boyfriend and his new girlfriend (who was Petra's cousin).

Though her legal status never changed, Petra's daughter began living most of the time with her when Petra's cousin became pregnant and didn't want an extra child hanging around. Petra proceeded to claim her power and become a powerful community member. She overthrew her label of depression. Clearly engagement in her life did matter and did make a difference.

Moving Mountains

"Noreen" provides us with another example of healing anxiety and depression. She was referred to me by her family doctor for severe depression, unresponsive to medication. She had tried a variety of pharmaceuticals, but none had worked. Being a consultant in a rural and remote village, I had the luxury of spending as much time as I wished with patients (unless a crisis was happening in the community). I got to hear people's stories.

Noreen's story had begun two years earlier when she had called the police after her common-law husband, "Bill," had beaten her up. He had cracked a bone in her face and broken her nose. Apparently there was blood everywhere when it happened. Bill was charged with domestic assault, and Noreen was charged with possession of alcohol on the reserve. She had been kept in a cell for twenty-four hours before anyone thought of seeking medical attention for her. In fact, her husband was released from jail hours before she was. Nothing else happened for one year while Bill waited to go to court, except that she could not pay her fine to the court and thus was sentenced to some jail time, which she served.

Bill didn't go to jail during that year. He did take the incident as a wake-up call to give up alcohol. He sought community support and stopped drinking. He and Noreen lived together in relative happiness. Then came Bill's hearing in court. Noreen attended Bill's court appearance and urged the judge to drop the charges since Bill had stopped drinking and had been sober for the past year. Despite their having lived together peacefully without incident for the past year, the judge issued a restraining order that Bill could not come within a hundred yards of his partner. This meant that Noreen had to leave the family home, since Bill owned it, was the breadwinner, and it was their children's home. Logic dictated that Noreen leave alone instead of with all the children, which would have made them all homeless.

Initially Noreen went to her parents' house, but that was a nightmare since they regularly drank themselves into oblivion, but not before torturing Noreen. Noreen began couch surfing among all the people she knew in the community. Noreen had no money to go anywhere, and housing was so scarce on the reserve that she wasn't likely to get a house for years, if ever. It takes ages for a new house to be built, and when it is, there is a long waiting list to occupy it. Families take first precedent. Realistically, a single mother almost never qualifies.

Noreen and Bill would occasionally meet in secret. They knew that the police officers were watching them closely with the ardent goal of catching them together. Then the police could throw Bill back into jail for violating his order. Noreen didn't want that because Bill was the only support for the family. He was the breadwinner for their children. On one of their clandestine encounters, Noreen conceived.

When I met Noreen, she was six months pregnant and absolutely miserable. She had been homeless for almost a year. She couldn't tell the judge she was pregnant because then she would have to name Bill as the father, and he would be thrown into jail for violating the restraining order. She couldn't see or spend time with her kids because she couldn't come to the house, and they didn't want to go to her friends' homes or to their alcoholic grandparents' house. Noreen was beside herself. She had not even told her doctor that she was pregnant, and somehow he hadn't noticed. She hadn't taken any of the medications he had prescribed because of the pregnancy (the doctor had diagnosed an anxiety disorder).

Noreen had survived a year of homelessness. I began by celebrating her fortitude and her loyalty for not naming Bill and mentioning her pregnancy. Noreen exemplified some very important aboriginal values in refusing to hurt Bill despite great personal harm. I complimented Noreen on living traditional values above all else. She hadn't realized she was doing this, so the compliment worked. She felt better. She smiled. She relaxed.

"Now," I asked, "what are we going to do?" No wonder Noreen could be labeled as depressed. She felt useless, hopeless, weak, a pawn at the mercy of others. She had been able to continue only through the strength of her faith in God. Again I wrote a letter to the presiding judge urging him to drop the restraining order. I outlined how it was only making

Noreen suffer. She wouldn't allow me to mention the pregnancy. Per her wishes, I could only discuss her year of homelessness. I wasn't allowed to mention her parents' alcoholism or her limited number of places to go. I didn't even know if anyone at the court read my letters. Court never seemed to happen when I was in the community, or I would have gone on behalf of my clients. The judge didn't revoke the restraining order.

On my next visit to the community, Noreen was one month more pregnant. She did not want to take her baby to her parents' home after giving birth. She couldn't go home. Where could she go? Throughout this time I continued to emphasize her nobility (which I truly felt) and her selflessness in sacrificing for the benefit of her children and her husband. I told her the story of Joan of Arc, which she had never heard. I found stories of saints to tell her since she was Catholic. At the same time, I was talking to her priest, wondering if it wasn't possible for the Church to intervene. The priest and I had a good time one evening, brainstorming into the wee hours about how ancient saints or Saint Francis of Assisi would have handled Noreen's situation.

"Saint Francis would have her deliver her child in the church surrounded by the animals of the forest," I said. In true Benedictine fashion, we had been sipping some red wine.

"By George," the priest said, "you've got it. We'll create a media event by announcing that she'll have the baby in the church because she has no where else to go, thanks to the provincial court."

"That's great," I enthused. "How about some hay and a manger?"

Father Frank looked at me askance. "Don't you think that's taking it a bit too far?" His glasses fell down on his nose.

"Sorry," I said. "Just an idea. No offense meant."

"None taken," he said. "Church is enough. We don't need any more virgin births."

"You mean one is enough," I said.

"For all time," he said.

"We'll have to get Noreen's permission to talk about the pregnancy," I said. "She hasn't been willing to let me mention it."

"We'll do it," he said. "Count on me."

Father Frank had his discussion with Noreen, and she agreed. We crafted a letter to the media about how Noreen would be delivering her baby in the church since she had no home. We had arrived at a Noreen-approved version of her story. Father Frank agreed he would drop by the hotel where the judge was staying before the next court. He happened to mention the judge was Catholic.

"Thanks be to the saints," I said.

We never released the letter. A mysterious reversal of the restraining order occurred, and Noreen went home. This incident reminded me that we should never underestimate the power of the Church to move mountains where psychiatry cannot budge an anthill.

Noreen went home a much stronger woman than when she had left. I continued to see her for several months, reinforcing my incredible admiration for her strength, sacrifice, and moral convictions. In the biomedical model, she was just "an anxiety disorder." In a narrative perspective, she is the rich, complex story that I have just told. In the biomedical story, a medication is prescribed to treat the anxiety. In the narrative approach, the story is transformed.

Within a narrative model of psychiatry, all stories of anxiety and depression are unique. I had the opportunity to read the medical charts for the clients I have described. The charts read in the standard, checklist manner without any of the interesting detail of their stories. The DSM criteria were reviewed and, when met, were indicated as present. The diagnosis was made, and a medication prescribed. The richness of the life situation was unimportant. But that is exactly what matters in narrative psychiatry: we work within the richness of peoples' lives, helping to empower and to transform them. We continue to work together to transform stories, which changes lives.

15

Narratives and Bipolar Disorder

The distinction between the mental and the physical is false. Everything we know, whether it is about the physical or the mental world, comes to us through our brain. But our brain's connection with the physical world of objects is no more direct than our brain's connection with the mental world of ideas. . . . Our brain creates the illusion that we have direct contact with objects in the physical world. And at the same time our brain creates the illusion that our own mental world is isolated and private. Through these two illusions we experience ourselves as agents, acting independently upon the world.

CHRISTOPHER FRITH, *MAKING UP THE MIND: HOW THE BRAIN CREATES OUR MENTAL WORLD*

At the Tree of Life

The broad expanse of lake seemed to stretch forever like a prairie of water rolling toward the lighter blue horizon, broken only by the occasional tree-covered island and lined by the dense forest of the shore. While eagles circled overhead, it was not hard to imagine the game that roamed through the forest, though no moose would appear today. We had come to Nick Standing Bear's reserve for sun dance. One year ago I had brought "Daniel" to see Nick to be doctored at the tree of life that forms the center of the sun dance. Like others I have known, Daniel found traditional healing to his liking and jumped into working with Nick as an alternative to what he had been experiencing with conventional psychiatry. I looked forward to seeing him again, having kept in touch by e-mail and having seen him twice during the year at other ceremonies.

I had first met Daniel when I was taking psychiatric emergency calls. Our meeting was clear serendipity, for no other psychiatrist in the call schedule could have related to his culture and beliefs. Daniel had just crashed from a short spell of elation and was severely down, considering suicide. He came from a small reserve in Manitoba near Lake Winnipeg. His parents had attended residential schools and had been abusive alcoholics. Daniel had lived a traumatic childhood, dodging beatings from his parents and run-ins with the law. He had long periods of struggle with alcohol and mood swings. He had been hospitalized every two years for as long as he could remember. Conventional psychiatry had not served him well. The medications had given him serious side effects, limiting their use. He had preferred the misery off drugs to the misery on drugs. The day we met he was considering ending all the misery.

Daniel had been diagnosed as having bipolar disorder and, like most people who are given this label, spent 85 percent of his time depressed. Unfortunately, the few times he had become elatedly happy and expansive, he had behaved so bizarrely as to be jailed. Daniel's elation had spiritual themes in which he would feel powerful historic ancestors speaking through him. Not everyone around him liked the messages they delivered. He felt pressured to talk for these spirits and would inevitably say more to people than they wanted to hear, making everyone uncomfortable. At the extremes of his elation, he would try to help political figures, which invariably got him arrested. The prime minister of the province did not want to receive a lecture channeled from the famous Cree leader Big Bear, who had fought against taking treaty. Generally, the prime minister had a cadre of police to prevent such historical lessons, and that was when Daniel went to jail.

Daniel bitterly described his trauma of being tied up and secluded, both in jails and in hospitals. The mental health care system was brutal to him. I suggested to Daniel that he needed to see an elder. "What would Big Bear say for you to do if he was speaking through your lips right now?" Daniel agreed that Big Bear would want him to get to an elder. I didn't know any on his reserve, but I knew Nick on the nearby reserve. It was almost time for sun dance. Nick would be doctoring people throughout the dance, so I suggested that Daniel go. I would introduce him to Nick before it was time to get into costume and dance.

The sun dance is a four-day ceremony in which the dancers eschew food and water. The dance is focused around a tree of life, which is cut down and placed in the middle of the dance arbor the day before the dance begins. The dancers are there so that the people in the community can be healed and so that they can acquire powers to help with healing. A constant stream of people show up to be doctored by the leaders at the tree of life while the dancers proceed. Piercing ceremonies are usually included, as described earlier. The purpose is to sacrifice so those who are coming for healing can be healed. I have sun danced for ten years now and plan to continue as long as I can.

The year before, when I had first brought Daniel, he made his way to the tree of life during one of the dances, joining the line of people coming to the tree, some in wheelchairs, some using crutches or canes, and children being carried in the arms of their parents. Nick doctored Daniel for a long time at the tree, assisted by other elders. After the dance, Daniel announced that he was moving back to his reserve to complete his healing and to be closer to Nick. That way he could attend ceremonies regularly, helping Nick whenever he could and becoming a part of Nick's hocokah, or healing community.

Now, a year later, Daniel was much better. He was content in a way he had never been. His moods were tolerable, and he was avoiding all drugs. Daniel had changed his stories about his identity. He had absorbed the traditional stories that were intrinsically healing. They competed with the stories he had absorbed while growing up and the stories he had heard about himself in the psychiatric hospital. Daniel no longer believed in the inevitability of collapse and descent into the abyss. He had seen the abyss, and spirits had carried him out. He believed in the perpetual possibility of human life to be healed. He believed he could carry power tools and sharp tools again. He no longer subscribed to the inevitability of suicide.

Daniel had new knowledge, illustrating an important narrative principle often spoken by indigenous knowledge keepers—that knowledge is the outcome of interactions and relationships between the inquirers and participants. Daniel didn't know what he was going to learn and experience until it happened. The knowledge of how to help Daniel came from the relationships he created with healers on the reserve and with his friends and family members. It didn't exist in textbooks on mental disorders. Here is the radical difference in views—that there is no a priori, pre-set way to "treat" bipolar disorder, but rather a conversation among specific people that generates knowledge about how things work for those people. The biomedical paradigm diagnoses bipolar disorder through applying a set of criteria in cookbook fashion. Then it generates a list of medications to be applied, also in cookbook fashion. Narrative approaches, on the other hand, generate action plans unique to the people creating them.

Biomedicine takes the DSM-IV-TR (*Diagnostic and Statistical Manual of Mental Disorders,* 4th edition, text revised) as real and essential. Within a narrative approach we do not avoid it, but rather, recognize DSM as one way of specifying similarities and differences among people, somewhat arbitrary, and replaceable by equally valid other ways. Applying DSM is a process like applying any other categorization system. I personally prefer three-dimensional SPECT (single photon emissions computed tomography) scans—which show how blood is flowing through various regions of the brain—as generating a more reliable story about what is happening in a person's brain.

It is within my repertoire of stories to recognize that the social environment can radically change the brain and that patterns of neuronal activity, even as found on a SPECT scan, are socially constructed. Without relationship, we would have a largely useless brain, for it would not have matured. Our social relationships can change dendritic connections within the nervous system, can change regional blood flow and metabolism, and can transform the story we tell about who we think we are.

DSM is not necessary to prescribe medications, which are given based on predominant symptoms and not diagnosis. Of interest is that almost all psychiatric drugs can treat all psychiatric diagnoses. SSRIs, for example, though usually classified as antidepressants, reduce anxiety, reduce obsessions and compulsions, and treat psychosis. So-called antipsychotics reduce mania and improve depression, reduce anxiety, reduce obsessions and compulsions, and so on. Anticonvulsants have equally widespread therapeutic properties. Apparently the brain doesn't correspond to our DSM in its response to drugs. Thus, picking these neat diagnostic categories doesn't improve our success in prescribing drugs either.

Daniel found a better story—the same story we have seen for others, the story of what can happen in community, especially when that community is living traditional values. Daniel discovered a story of healing that was cocreated through all of his interactions with others in the community. He began to believe in possibility instead of inevitable destruction. This made all the difference.

Elsewhere, I have written more narratives of people who earn the label of bipolar disorder and who recover.[1] I have made the point that DSM diagnoses (the standard psychiatric labels) are arbitrary taxonomies, arbitrary characterizations of human suffering, arbitrary divisions that often fail to acknowledge that each of the traits with which we measure are distributed from a little to very much. The distributions of traits, moods, and emotions within individuals may poorly correspond to the categories of DSM. These diagnoses are, therefore, social constructions. People have created them and can uncreate them.

I am not against DSM; rather, I object to its being regarded as the only valid classification system for human suffering and pain. As a classification system, it has taken descriptive categories and inappropriately reified them. I am opposed to labels being used to convince people to follow a particular, specific story that mitigates against recovery and healing.

The Meaning of Madness

The meaning of "madness" cannot be found in chemicals or diagnostic nomenclature. No two mental illnesses are the same, despite DSM. Each madness has its own unique meaning that can only unfold within the context of the person's life who lives that madness and only becomes understandable by seeing the person against the backdrop of his family and community. Just as each woman gives birth in her own style, each individual recovers from insanity in her own manner.

This can be seen in the story of "Fran," who was a thirty-five-year-old woman who had lived a fairly ordinary life (with the exception of what was called a manic episode that resolved in her twenties). Then, two years before I started working with her, she had abruptly ended a ten-year relationship to be with a man she had met on the Internet, who turned out to be married and have two children. The family's story about Fran was that she realized too late that this man was unavailable and broke down over the pain of the simultaneous loss of her past relationship and anticipated future relationship. She had been hospitalized and diagnosed with bipolar disorder. She had been started on medications meant to "treat" this disorder, and none had worked. Fran's psychiatrist sent her to me when she took maternity leave, but I gathered from subtle hints in her notes (between the lines, so to speak) that she was glad to pass Fran along, since Fran wasn't responding to her ministrations.

At first, I liked the family's interpretation of Fran's story, but I slowly became aware that Fran detested this interpretation. She felt it trivialized her struggles and her pain. She believed that she had been meant to be the vampire queen, to ascend to sit at the right hand of God as his queen. When the time came to be called, she had been too selfish and had been tossed aside. She had been punished by being made to live among the undead (the rest of us). She was waiting for an angel to come to take her to her rightful place in the cosmos, which involved dying to eternal life. I thought of Jukka Aaltonen at first and how he would work so hard to bring this story around to one that was more ordinary. I tried that approach, but Fran was insulted by it and accused me of conspiring with her family to torture her. That was when I realized that we had to respect and work within her story.

A colleague suggested that we begin with the notion of time. Perhaps Fran's sense of time was off. Perhaps sitting by the front window, watching through the glass for the angel, was unrealistic. Perhaps she would have to busy herself to make her prison better since angels might not come for twenty years. Since she didn't want to have an accidental death (to choke or drown or otherwise die through nonascension), she would have to give some care to her physical world for a while. This was a better strategy. It also revealed the family conflict. Everyone (including me at first) was trying to deny the reality of the "otherness" of Fran. We wanted to bring her down from her Wagnerian operatic world into our ordinary world of high school-ish dramas. She refused to be dislodged.

When we acknowledged Fran's otherness, what emerged was the exhaustion of family members from the work of trying to change her. Within the consultation group in which this family presented itself, the recommendation was to surrender, to stop trying to change Fran, to leave her alone unless she became imminently dangerous to herself; then the proper course of action would be to call the police to intervene. Otherwise, we were to accept her edict—that she was the queen and therefore in control of her destiny. Members of the consultation group offered to pray for Fran and for the family. A suggestion was made for everyone to write letters to God, that they could be given to Fran as origami hangings, like Sodaka's thousand cranes for world peace in Hiroshima, Japan. A member of the group told about praying for her daughter for twenty years before her daughter found a way out of alcohol and drug problems. "God works slowly," she said. "Maybe twenty years is not long to God," she added, reinforcing what we had told Fran—that she might need to revise her time frame for angelic ascension.

We encouraged the family to get their lives back and to acknowledge Fran's fundamental differentness from them. She was not speaking in metaphor or parable. She was telling her story as she experienced it. This approach opened the door to change, which had hitherto been closed.

Crow: Bipolar Trickster

Narrative psychiatry recognizes that "bipolar disorder" is only a metaphor, a story, and that there are sometimes better stories. Within traditional North American healing, a very helpful concept is that of the spirit behind an illness, or the spirit that drives or fuels the illness. Again, though indigenous people take spirit literally, its interpretation as metaphor will not weaken this argument. I call the spirit that drives the symptoms we call "bipolar disorder" Bipolar Trickster; I think the concept of trickster is useful for understanding what this entity does as it drives the bipolar symptoms, pushing people outside the range of good judgment and often into the realms of psychosis.

Bipolar disorder, like trickster, forced "Cameron" to change even when he didn't want to. In the state called bipolar disorder, he was tricked to venture out onto the ledge of judgment so far that he crashed through the thin snow and tumbled far down into the valley below. He should have been dead, but he wasn't. It just felt that way. Bipolar Trickster knew how much Cameron wanted to lose control, to blast out of the orbit of social accountability, to soar above the confines of normalcy. Bipolar Trickster practiced severe cruelties, taking him to bars to proposition women in ways that would never succeed, which he would have known had he not been intoxicated with the elixirs of Bipolar Trickster.

Driven by that trickster, Cameron obsessed over satisfying his hungers—sexual, spiritual, experiential. He wanted to screw more than any human being had ever done. He wanted to fly with the eagles and sit at the right hand of God. Cameron's sexual desires were never satisfied. When trickster fell asleep and Cameron returned to sanity, Cameron sobered in the realization of his frustrations. Bipolar Trickster drove Cameron in gruesome manners, causing him to break taboos of every kind.

Bipolar Trickster is not to be admired in every situation and can be an example of what not to do. Sometimes it led him to revel in his role as cultural hero to transform the world to be more inhabitable for humans by ridding it of dangerous monsters or by providing the means to live or live well. Like Coyote, Cameron saw himself stealing fire for the people, inventing rain, and heroically defeating human-eating monsters. Nevertheless, Bipolar Trickster's amoral nature and lack of positive restraint often made him appear villainous even in his heroic triumphs. At the height of his successes and triumphant moments, Cameron would get carted away to the hospital or to jail, depending on the whim of the policemen at hand.

Bipolar Trickster can exemplify the cleverness of the Crow or Raven trickster, noted by the Reverend Henry Ward Beecher when he wrote, "If men had wings and bore black feathers, few of them would be clever enough to be crows."[2] Just as the legends say that Raven brought light to the far north for his people, Bipolar Trickster did indeed deliver great wisdom to Cameron. Some of the spiritual insights he delivered following a run of mania were amazing and profound. Raven succeeded in bringing the light only through his trickery and inventiveness, but there are side effects to the seduction by Bipolar Trickster. Cameron's was the fall into the depths of darkness. "I have been to hell," he said, "and it is dark. Hell is cold and lonely. There are no kindred suffering souls burning together. That would have been infinitely preferable."

We solved Cameron's bipolar disorder by admiring and appreciating his trickster. Using guided imagery techniques, we started a dialogue with Bipolar Trickster. To Cameron I said, "Once upon a time, we appreciated the gifts and wisdom of Bipolar Trickster. Today is different. Just as when humans became largely agrarian, and crows became our competitors—stealing food and raiding crops—and had to be scared off with 'scarecrows,' so did we lose track of the gifts of Bipolar Trickster. He became an evil being to be eradicated with drugs. His wisdom was dismissed. Similarly, just as crows even later came to be associated with disease and death as they scavenged the corpses of the victims of plague or war, and are still used to represent evil and death in horror literature and films, so did Bipolar Trickster come to be seen as evil and only worthy of elimination and suppression.

"Instead, let's invite Bipolar Trickster to come forward and teach us. We could definitely learn survival from Bipolar Trickster. Just as we needed to learn cooperation and group living to defend our kills against scavenging crows and other predators, Bipolar Trickster pushed us to bind together to defend our moods against extremes."

Being able to dialogue with Bipolar Trickster made a big difference for Cameron. We used techniques in which we identified the voices within his head who spoke to him. Bipolar Trickster was one of these characters. Bipolar Trickster said that its job was to shake up things and prevent stagnation. Its job was to force fun where there is none. Its job was to prevent boredom. We found another character, which Cameron called Moody, who suffered the consequences of Bipolar Trickster. After Bipolar Trickster wrecked havoc in Cameron's life, Moody appeared to clean up the pieces. Moody suffered deeply and plunged Cameron into the abyss of deep depression. Other voices complicated the mix. Cameron had the voices of his parents, who criticized him continually, but differently. He had the voices of his first several psychiatrists, who told him he was hopeless except if he took their medications.

We created images for the bodies of these voices. We carried out conversations between them. We introduced new voices (characters). Cameron found spirit helpers. One of these was the spirit of the land on which he was born, which he called Land and which was a voice of healing. He identified the spirit of Big Bear, who could moderate the other voices. Over time Big Bear and Land, in the context of a community healing circle in which Cameron regularly participated in ceremony, got control of Bipolar Trickster and prevented him from taking over. Once Bipolar Trickster was under control, then Moody did not appear, since she appeared in reaction and as a consequence of Bipolar Trickster. Big Bear and Land were able to manage the voices of the parents and psychiatrists. A new voice appeared—the medicine man whom Cameron had incorporated. Cameron could hear him telling stories and teaching moderation. Cameron was able to learn how to regulate Bipolar Trickster and Moody to his best advantage.

Rabbit: Bipolar Trickster

Here's another story of someone who was diagnosed as bipolar. His medical chart is as equally unrevealing about him as a person as each of the other examples I have given. In all three cases, the hundreds of pages of their medical records did not reveal as much as the few pages written here. Rather, their medical records were a repetitious documentation of signs and symptoms without need for explanation.

This young man was named "Jason." He lived at home with his mother. He mostly felt too depressed to do anything and used marijuana to make the day go faster. Sometimes, however, when he got some energy, he would go out in the world and play tricks on people. He fancied himself a bit like a successful Wile E. Coyote or Daffy Duck or Alvin the Chipmunk as he let air out of tires, rewired alarms to ring the opposite of how they were supposed to work, opened telephone router boxes to change the wires so neighbors received each others' calls, and more.

My work with Jason involved telling him stories to inspire him to venture out into the world. We had to catch him on the upswing, yet before he was out of control. Our work resembled the work with Cameron; we needed to identify the various voices in his head. We needed to give them substance so he could dialogue with them. We needed to create a community to surround Jason and to perform ceremony with him.

As part of all this effort, I told Jason a Rabbit story as a template to help us catch a glimpse of the bipolar spirit—that being behind his tricks who left him crumpled in a depressive heap when it departed.

Rabbit trickster folktales reflect social satire and social morality while revealing the binary nature of tricksters who embody the struggle between the needs of the individual and the needs of the group. Thus, they are perfect Bipolar Tricksters. One of the great lessons of trickster stories may be in the portrayal of the disasters that happen when the needs of the individual are put ahead of the group and the value of self-sacrifice. People who receive the bipolar label enact this dichotomy. Jason was in this situation. He was so absorbed with his own needs that he ignored the distress he was creating in his parents and his siblings as he sat alone in his room, day after day, doing nothing but smoking weed.

I told Jason a Cambodian rabbit story collected by Chanthyda called *Subhā Dansāy Jā Bāky Rāy*, or *The Story of Subhā Dansāy in Prose:*

There was a rabbit who came out from a well and was relaxing near a village. While relaxing, the rabbit saw an old lady who was selling bananas.

"This rabbit is like your Bipolar Trickster," I said. "He's not going to let this lady off easy, just as you wouldn't have at the height of those times when you're possessed." Jason appeared to like this entrance into the story and seemed to be identifying with the rabbit right away.

"I am very exhausted," thought the rabbit. "What can I do to get those bananas? I will pretend that I am dead," he thought. Thinking that, he ran to pretend that he was asleep on the path. When the lady passed the path, she saw the rabbit lying on the ground.

"How lucky I am!" she thought. "I have never tasted rabbit before. Today, I will cook it for the first time." After that she took the rabbit into her basket and continued on her way to sell bananas. Along the way, the rabbit ate all the bananas in the basket. When a passerby asked the lady to buy bananas, she noticed that all the bananas were gone and that the rabbit had run away. "Oh! That rabbit was still alive. I thought it was dead. Damn it!" yelled the lady.

Jason chuckled. "That's what I do," he said. "I eat all your goodies and then I run away." Jason could really relate to this metaphor for the ways in which he caught people up into his web of excitement and crash. He metaphorically lay down on their path, and they picked him up and put him in their basket.

After escaping from the lady, the rabbit reached a pond in the forest and really wanted to drink water from it. There was a shellfish in the pond, and he stopped the rabbit from drinking.

"Hey, why do you drink my water?" asked the shellfish.

"If I drink, what does it matter to you?" replied the rabbit.

"Of course, this pond is mine," the shellfish continued.

"So, let's have a race around the pond. If I win, I will drink water from this pond, and if you win, I will never drink water from any pond anymore," said the rabbit proudly.

The shellfish then discussed with his fellow shellfish how to defeat the rabbit. They wanted the rabbit to leave them alone. They thought of a trick that required a shellfish to hide under the water every two or three yards around the pond. Each shellfish would jump up just ahead of the rabbit to trick him into thinking that he was always behind.

The rabbit thought that the shellfish ran fast, so the rabbit tried to run faster. Every time the rabbit thought he was winning, another shellfish popped up ahead of him. When he reached the goal point, a shellfish was already there. The rabbit, without thinking clearly, thought that he had lost, so he ran away. From that day on, the rabbit never drinks water from any ponds; he just drinks dew.

"That's how I feel about my life," Jason said. "That's my story. I'm always racing as hard as I can and always losing. It feels rigged just like the rabbit racing those shellfish. That's why I never succeed."

"We'll skip over much of this story where much the same plot continues but with different characters and turn to the ending, where the rabbit gets caught while eating rice in an old man's field."

An old man brought the rabbit home and put him in a trap. He had also caught a fish and placed it next to the rabbit. Then the old man thought about a monk in a pagoda that was near his house. He had heard that this monk was good at telling fortunes. So he went to see him to get his fortune told.

Before leaving the house, the old man told his wife, "You should look after the rabbit and the fish so they don't get away." Then he went to the pagoda. He bowed respectfully to the monk and politely said, "I have heard that you have the best reputation for telling horoscopes."

"I can tell them, but I don't claim that they're completely right," said the monk.

"Please, just guess what I will have to eat this morning?" asked the man.

"I am afraid that I can't guess for you," replied the monk.

The man begged. "Please, please, I want to know," he begged.

"I am afraid that you will be upset," answered the monk.

The man thought to himself, "If this monk guesses correctly, I will give him meat and fish to eat. However, if he guesses wrongly, I will give him nothing. I will eat the rabbit and the fish with my wife only." Then he said, "I won't be upset actually. Please tell me!"

"Today, you get nothing delicious to eat!" said the monk. After that, the man went back home. He thought, "That monk was good at guessing, but he guessed completely wrong. I have the rabbit and the fish!" Then when he arrived home, he asked his wife to cook the rice.

However, the rabbit and the fish had found a way to escape. The rabbit told the fish, "Brother Fish, you should pretend to be dead, float with your stomach up. When they catch you, they will put you nearby the water; you can jump into the water and slowly swim away. When they run to catch you, you do the same as before until they take the trap from me to put over you. Then you can go to the deep place in the river."

As soon as the old man's wife had boiled the rice, he took the fish to scrape its skin and clean it near the edge of the pond. The fish pretended to be dead according to the rabbit's advice. Then he jumped in the water. Seeing that the man tried to catch him, just like the rabbit predicted, the fish acted like this again and again until the man called out to his wife to bring him the trap. That woman forgot that the rabbit was caught in the trap. When the wife lifted up the trap, the rabbit ran away quickly into the forest. Then the fish swam to a deep place in the river. The couple felt angry, and went back to their house. They were so cold they could barely stand. They sat in front of the fire and thought that what the monk had said was really right. They believed the monk's prophecies after that.[3]

Jason reflected that his exploits were so much like the rabbit's. It seemed as if guardian spirits had averted him from disaster, keeping him alive when he should have died or gone to jail by any reasonable estimation. Jason wanted to stop playing the rabbit role. "I think Rabbit eventually dies," he said.

"I fear you are right. Bipolar Trickster never lives forever. The rabbit survives against all odds through his wits. Nevertheless, wits usually give out. As entertaining as he is, the rabbit is doomed to destruction."

"Much as I love playing the rabbit, I'm ready to give him up," said Jason. "I think I'd like to be a more sedate character who runs less risk of sudden death and certainly less trauma. Better to be occasionally tricked than to die tricking."

I thought that perhaps I was the monk in the story, there to give wise advice to whomever would listen. The old man wouldn't listen. He's another character in the trickster story. Someone has to play the role of always being tricked by the rabbit, usually another family member.

I now had Jason's attention. Through the story of the rabbit, Jason realized that I understood his Bipolar Trickster. Now we were ready for genuine dialogue. Jason was fun when he was manic. His exploits were exciting. Unfortunately they were sufficiently over the top that they got him in trouble. Once we had characterized Bipolar Trickster, we could work on Jason's other characters and voices. Later I told Jason the story about Wisakedjak, the Cree trickster, which I shared in chapter 13. Jason also felt like he was at the end of his rope just like Wisakedjak. He had to dig deep to transform his inner voices, just as Muskrat did. This dialogue led to a more detailed discussion of all of Jason's internal voices and characters, including the voices he heard when he was really manic or really depressed.

We were able to construct a story to explain his extremes—that he had been born into a family of extremes. His parents were radical hippies in a generation of conformists, forever in conflict with their parents and grandparents. He was raised in a counterculture environment in which the opposite of what most people believed was true for his parents. Jason told the story of pleasing his parents by acting bizarre; it almost seemed the more bizarre, the more they approved.

But the cuteness of acting bizarre ends at a certain age. No matter what the values of our parents, at a certain age, they expect conformity to the norms of earning money and being self-supporting and respecting them. Perhaps this is a cultural invariant—I'm not sure—but it was true for Jason. Being home schooled, he had no peers. So he found an exit in extreme survival camp. He convinced his parents to let him go to summer survival school and progressively immersed himself deeper and deeper into that movement. Then he discovered marijuana. Jason believed (and perhaps he is right) that he would never have fallen off the deep end of the pool without marijuana, which seemed to loosen the corners and borders of his brain in such a way that anything seemed possible. Marijuana opened the door for Bipolar Trickster.

Then, puzzlingly, like other clients I have had, Jason believed he could defeat evil once and for all in the world. He credited marijuana for making him believe so. Like others with whom I have worked, Jason defied evil, claiming that he could destroy it. The Hawai'ian demigod, Maui, did the same to death and was consumed. Jason called out evil, and it overtook him and possessed him, leading him into a career of ineluctable highs and lows. Now we could reverse this and give him back a story of balance and harmony.

We used guided imagery to see Evil as a character, whom we denied access to the Round Table of Jason's inner voices. Song and ceremony and drama helped to drive Evil away. Over time Jason was able to realign the configuration of his inner world and drive out Evil and Bipolar Trickster. He transformed into being able to regulate his moods. Madness had allowed Jason's unbearable emotions to leak out and be expressed even if cryptically and in gibberish. Our narrative work helped him to reconstruct a sense of worth and meaning for his life within a saner context. Over the course of the next year, we struggled with and negotiated with these voices to arrive at a compromise in which Jason could be occasionally outrageous and still not fall over the edge.

16
Narrative Approaches to Psychosis

Inside my head there is an amazing labor-saving device. Better even than a dishwasher or a calculator, my brain releases me from the dull, repetitive task of recognizing the things in the world around me, and even saves me from needing to think about how to control my movements. I can concentrate on the important things in life: making friends and sharing ideas. But, of course, my brain doesn't just save me from tedious chores. My brain creates the "me" that is released into the social world. Moreover, it is my brain that enables me to share my mental life with my friends and thereby allows us to create something bigger than any of us are capable of on our own.

CHRISTOPHER FRITH, *MAKING UP THE MIND:*
HOW THE BRAIN CREATES OUR MENTAL WORLD

Psychosis is a disorder of storytelling, especially in its primary form of disrupting our narrative embeddedness as characters in a plot with other characters, moving toward an end, sequentially in time, and with a purpose or value that will be demonstrated. Psychotic individuals are poor at storytelling. Their social relationships suffer; they are isolated and alone. If they do not learn to become storied, their stories eventually evaporate and disappear. At its worst, psychosis becomes a wasteland of what are called negative symptoms—no words, no voice, nothing, extreme passivity, a complete shutdown.

I believe that psychotic people can become restoried, given a suitable context and sufficient relationships. The deficits in storying can be offset and perhaps even corrected. The recovery from psychosis can be a unique time in which a person, having shattered, can put together the pieces, learning how to be an entirely different self. Psychosis often occurs at times of shifts in social status, such as the adolescent transition to adulthood or the child's transition to adolescence. Aiding a person through such a transition is like taking them through labor, in which you are more like a midwife or a shepherdess of the energy of healing, keeping the process moving, than the one deciding where it shall go. At the same time, like a shepherdess, you have a responsibility to make sure the flock arrives at a destination and does not fall off the cliff on the way. These are the Native American metaphors of working with insanity: the idea of leading the sheep to greener, higher mountain pastures in the summer and bringing them down from the high country before the first snows of winter.

I have been struggling to keep people out of hospitals ever since I began my training. It is curious, because hospitals are meant to be compassionate, healing places. But the praxis of psychiatric institutions for the psychotic is to make them, in general, worse, meaning more hopeless, despondent, and demoralized. Foucault would have probably said that the institutions of power and those who hold positions of power within them cannot accept solutions that they cannot control, and healing is clearly outside of anyone's control. Drug therapy can be controlled. It does not apparently cure or heal, although it can reduce suffering temporarily, though sometimes offset by its side effects.

We noted previously Loren Mosher's questioning of the emerging psychopharmacological domination of the treatment of very disturbed and disturbing people. He noted that those people seemed to appreciate his sometimes clumsy attempts to understand them and their lives, which duplicates my observation that even the most hopeless recognize when someone is actually listening. He worried "about what went on in the one hundred and sixty-four hours a week when my patients were not with me; was the rest of their world trying to understand and relate meaning-fully to them?"[1] He wrote that he "never became a true believer in the 'magic bullet' attribution" of psychotropic medication, having "somehow never found a Lazarus among those I treated with the major tranquil-izers."[2] Nonetheless, our culture has cast aside wisdom in its search for these magic bullets. This is like in the Japanese story of Abandonment Canyon, recorded by Norma Livo in her book, *Story Medicine*.[3]

> *A warlord took control of a village and was much feared by the people. He ordered them to take all those over age sixty to a canyon high in the mountains and leave them there to die. He had decided that those over age sixty could not possibly work at full efficiency and were therefore useless to him and the society he wished to create. One man, however, rebelled on the road to Abandonment Canyon. This son simply could not leave his father on the high slopes to starve. He brought his father back home and created a hiding place under his porch.*
>
> *As luck would have it, the warlord found another way to torment the people—to give them impossible tasks and torture them for not succeeding. The warlord demanded a rope woven from ashes. The distraught son came to his father's hiding place to discuss his inability to give the warlord what he wanted. "Easy," said the father. "Weave a rope and then carefully burn it so that it turns to ashes." The son did so and the warlord was pleased.*
>
> *But next, the warlord demanded a conch shell with a silk string passed completely through it. Again the son consulted his father, as he was perplexed about how to accomplish this task. Again, his father knew what to do. He told the son to get a conch shell and point the tip toward the sun. He told the son to find a silken thread and attach it to a grain of rice, then show the rice to a hungry ant, put the thread and the ant into the mouth of the shell, and watch for the ant to work its way through the shell with the rice grain attached to the string. The son did this and the project was accomplished. The next morning the warlord was again impressed and asked the son how he had managed to become so clever.*
>
> *The son fell to his knees before the warlord and told him how he could not take his father to certain death and had hidden him under the porch. He told the warlord how his father had the wisdom to solve both of the tasks when he did not. Then the warlord realized that elders had their usefulness*

beyond what they could physically produce and should be allowed to live, so he
rescinded his former proclamation.

In the same manner, cultures of storytelling have wisdom for the healing of psychosis that modern psychopharmacologically dominated culture has ignored. We need to access the wisdom of our ancestors to learn how to help people who are in the midst of breakdown.

Kiss of Coherence

My work with people who are psychotic is very similar to my work with people diagnosed with cancer. Both tend to involve long time periods. I suspect that cancer and psychosis are bookends in some strange topology. Cancer is psychosis of the body. Cells are running amok, out of control, reproducing faster than they should, losing their ability to differentiate. In short, they lose their ability to tell a coherent story through coordinated function with neighbor cells and the body as a whole. Psychosis of the mind is similar. Thoughts and feelings run amok, out of control, reproducing faster than they should, losing their ability to communicate with the outer world—again, losing their ability to render a coherent narrative.

To illustrate this, I will tell a story about "Chris," a nineteen-year-old man who had been hospitalized after he entered the office of a local software company and announced that he was now in charge; he was the new CEO. Chris had taken the "Joel Test" for software engineers, an online spoof, and had determined that it meant he needed to be in charge of all software production on the planet, or at least in Saskatchewan.

Chris had recently returned from Malta, where he had been obsessed with cathedrals. He had decided to become an architect to design them. He described wandering about the streets, basking in the rain, the darkness, the sunshine. Sometimes he would take things from stores, but he would usually leave something in its place—like a modern-day packrat. His time in Malta had ended when he had taken a shirt from a rack in a store. He believed that Jesus had told him to take the shirt, but the shopkeeper disagreed. The police were called and quickly arrested him.

His mother flew to Malta to get him and brought him back to Saskatoon, where she taught French at the university.

I met Chris after his second discharge from the hospital—after the software takeover incident. Chris remained silent throughout our first meeting, with his mother doing all the talking. When asked why he was so quiet, he said he was dead and made a reference to the Grateful Dead rock band. For our second meeting, both of his parents came. They had been divorced since Chris had been five years old. They related how, two years earlier, they had sought psychiatric care for Chris because he had become so tense that he could not do his homework. He would shake if he got even close to his desk. Without completing his homework, he was doing poorly in school, but couldn't see that as related to him. He believed that the teachers had a conspiracy to ignore his good works.

After his most recent hospitalization, Chris had been put on risperidone (brand name Risperdal). He had been diagnosed as having bipolar disorder with psychotic features. The medication made him look calmer to others, he said, but inside, he felt just as weird. He didn't want to continue taking it, which led to fighting with his parents, who objected to this decision. He said it wasn't fair that he should have to take a medicine that just made him look good on the outside but feel no better on the inside. He said his dreams were becoming true and that worms would eat him alive if he didn't get something to do. He wanted to spend his days at the university library searching for websites that gave money to charity based on the number of hits they got (a common activity these days among my younger psychotic patients). He said he could save his little part of the world by visiting these websites all day long. He believed this was his job. Meanwhile, he was living with his mother, and his parents were reluctantly supporting him. But his father resented paying "child support" now that Chris was over eighteen.

I asked Chris if he had a dream that hadn't yet come true. He smiled sheepishly. He wanted a girlfriend who would kiss him. I pursued the question of what stopped him from dating and finding a girlfriend. The answers became more and more vague. Here was the unstoried territory of Chris's life. He couldn't really tell a story about himself and girls. I wondered aloud if he wanted to work together on the project of getting a girlfriend. He most certainly did, though his father promptly rejected the idea because that was not why they had brought Chris to see me. I held my ground, asserting that we had to start where Chris was at, and what concerned him was more important than what concerned his father, and that all roads eventually led back to the same place. The father reluctantly agreed.

I learned from Chris that he had been largely isolated most of his life and tended to avoid people. He had not yet dated, thinking himself ugly and undesirable. I learned that he saw one of his purposes in life as keeping his mom's child support coming to her. He viewed his mother as helpless and pathetic in the face of his father's rage and sought to protect her. He was afraid to grow up and leave her for fear she would no longer receive his father's financial support. He saw himself as an ally for his mother, her friend and confidante against his father, whom he perceived as Zeus, Saturn, or all of the gods rolled into one.

I suggested Chris join a healing circle. There we would periodically talk around the circle about his efforts to find a girlfriend, along with any other concerns he had. He did not dominate the group and was initially shy, but slowly began to seek feedback from the women in the group about his efforts at dating. It was through these meetings and my separate sessions with him that change occurred.

Part of my work with Chris involved putting stories to the experiences of his life that he hadn't been able to explain and helping him build a repertoire of stories for how to be in the world effectively. We built a series of stories for how to behave around women, how to date, how to avoid getting hospitalized, and eventually, how to finish school and get a job without appearing to be too strange. After two years, no further signs or symptoms of psychosis existed for Chris, and he was taking no medication.

In three years Chris even found the girlfriend he was seeking. Granted, she's not the girl that you'd bring home to conservative parents, with her piercings and tattoos and streaked purple hair. But the two fit together, and when I met her it seemed that they complemented each other and helped each other and appreciated each other's foibles. (For example, Chris still froze with fear when he tried to cross a busy city street. "Libby" told him to close his eyes and guided him across. She found this endearing.)

It reminded me of studies showing that when people with schizophrenia marry, both people do amazingly better than they had done before the relationship. Chris's girlfriend does not have a schizophrenia diagnosis, but she's sufficiently different from conventional mainstream expectations, and sufficiently complementary to Chris, that they can help each other.

Nurturing Real Boy

Here's another story to illustrate the narrative psychiatry of psychosis. "Nathan" was quite intelligent but disadvantaged. (Some people believe it is not possible to be psychotic without being smart—that only with intelligence does reality become unbearable.) He was the youngest of four sons, all from different fathers. His mother, "Natalie," was also brilliant, but erratic. She managed to function as a professor at a nearby university, teaching sociology, but she suffered from alternating over- and under-involvement in her work and in her children's lives. She was passionate in everything she said or did, which sometimes annoyed her colleagues.

Nathan similarly annoyed his peers. He was exceptionally smart, easily bored, often irritating and obnoxious, arrogant, and therefore easy to reject. Arrogance breeds its own punishment. Nathan didn't seem to be able to learn from his rejections, which were frequent and included ejection from virtually every campus club.

Nathan rarely talked to his father, who was a plumber and couldn't relate to any of Nathan's extravagant stories. When Nathan wasn't being disdainful of his father, he bragged about being descended from the working class.

Nathan's mother brought him to me when he stopped going to classes. His grades plummeted, though he was close to graduating. His future plans alternated between touring Uganda with a rock band to chasing the secrets of the universe through the campus computer center. He was aware of a conspiracy into which he could tap. This conspiracy was controlling the world through the manipulation of currencies (maybe he was correct!).

When I spoke to Nathan alone, I could feel the desperation in his voice. When he was with his mother, his derision and mockery hid it. Nathan wanted to destroy everything. His theory was that anything worthwhile would rise again, like the phoenix from its ashes, and the rest would perish as it should. He loved the slogan, "Burn, baby, burn."

Nathan was not willing to take any medication, as is true with many people who are labeled psychotic (and few of whom are sufficiently dangerous to warrant going to court to get an order for their taking medication). We needed to pursue another course.

"Aren't you being a little too obvious for this conspiracy?" I asked.

"What do you mean?" Nathan asked.

"Don't you think that the way you live is making you more and more obvious? Can't you blend better? Isn't that what you secret agents are taught—how to blend?"

"I'm not a secret agent," he said.

"Then you responded correctly," I said, "because I'm not looking for a secret agent. I need someone who can watch and observe, protecting themselves only when necessary."

"What do you need me to do?" Nathan asked.

"I want you to write down at least one dream every night," I said, "so we can examine them to make sure that no one has tampered with your mind."

"That's ridiculous," he said. "They haven't done that."

"I won't know unless I can examine your dreams," I said. "Plus I want you to keep a diary of what happens during the day: what you're thinking and what you're feeling. That way we can also look for subtle signs of takeover."

"Are you crazy?" he asked.

"Are you?" I countered.

"No," he responded, indignantly.

"Well, neither am I," I said.

Nathan agreed to the record keeping. Nathan depended on his mother to make appointments. I saw him as often as she would bring him. He brought dreams and journals. We poured over his dreams and journals and began to construct a theory about the conspiracy in which he was enmeshed. At first this conspiracy was fantastic, with gods and aliens and other supernatural beings manipulating him and his mother like puppeteers. Slowly but surely, the conspiratorial maze began to more closely resemble a social network. We began to construct a story about Nathan being controlled by people instead of gods and aliens. That was my goal with Nathan: to help him become aware that he was a human being enmeshed in human social networks under human control and that he had some choice over how they controlled him. Nathan slowly built a sense of human agency, of ability to push back and change the ways in which he was controlled. This awareness took six months to evolve.

Along the way, Nathan had a strange dream about killing his parents. I wondered if this was a kind of declaration of independence in metaphorical form, one that every child has to accomplish. (I had no fear of Nathan actually killing his parents; if I had, I would have handled the situation very differently.) I decided to tell Nathan a classic Choctaw story about how Real Boy, with the help of Spirit Boy, overthrew the gods/parents and created a new freedom on the earth (but with much more uncertainty). I told Nathan this story to assist us in identifying the voices inside his head.

"Nathan," I said. "I want to tell you a story about a man named Lucky Hunter and his wife, Maize, their child, and a strange spirit boy who just showed up and started living with them. Maybe these characters will remind you of some you know. Lucky Hunter and Maize were holy people with special powers. I know you have had thoughts about having your own special powers. I know you have wanted to overthrow the gods just like Real Boy and Spirit Boy will eventually want to do in this story. These youngsters were not happy being children of the gods; they wanted to be in charge. You can probably relate to that. But, by the same token, it can be pretty lonely when the gods disappear, and apparently, they're pretty hard to kill off. They always keep returning in one form or another, like the voices inside your head.

Lucky Hunter always lived up to his name and never failed to catch game. The child of Lucky Hunter and Maize liked to play in the river where Maize cleaned her husband's catch every day. This child, named Real Boy because he was the first human, began playing with a creature that sprang from the river, proclaiming himself the boy's elder brother. He said their mother had thrown him into the river. Lucky Hunter and Maize, however, knew he had come from the blood of the animals that had been released into the river. He was a spirit boy.

At first, no one could see Spirit Boy very clearly. Lucky Hunter told his son to wrestle Spirit Boy and pin him down so that he could be seen. Real Boy did as he was told. Once Spirit Boy was pinned down he became material and everyone could see him, so Lucky Hunter and Maize took Spirit Boy home with them. He was a disobedient and wild child, who quickly developed skills in magic. He was also called Wild Boy.

"Perhaps you can relate to that. Probably you have some disobedient and wild characters and voices inside of you, also."

Spirit Boy and Real Boy followed Lucky Hunter on a hunting trip one day, because Spirit Boy wanted to find out where Lucky Hunter caught all his game. Spirit Boy turned himself into a bit of down and floated onto Lucky Hunter's shoulder without his knowledge. He watched Lucky Hunter make arrows from the reeds of a swamp. Then he came back to tell Real Boy what he had seen. Neither was certain of the purpose of an arrow.

"Maybe there are parts of you that are similarly confused about how things work and what things are for," I said to Nathan.

The boys followed Lucky Hunter farther and watched him go into a cave. They crept behind him. Inside the cave they saw many deer. They saw Lucky Hunter shoot one of those deer with his arrows, and then they understood what arrows did. Then they made arrows of their own, trying to imitate Lucky Hunter as best as they could. When they were done, they went into that cave and tried to shoot a deer. They only succeeded in scaring the deer, who ran out of the cave. As the cave emptied, the boys were so surprised that they killed nothing, though Spirit Boy did shoot a deer in the tail, pushing its tail upward. The boys decided shooting the deer's tails was fun, and did it to all the deer (this is why deer tails go up, instead of down, like most animals, when they are frightened). After the deer, raccoons, rabbits, and all the other four-footed creatures fled from the cave, followed by the birds.

I noted to Nathan, "These boys were challenging the way things were. They wanted to know how things worked. They wanted to do things themselves. Of course, Spirit Boy inspired Real Boy. In any case, they weren't content with the status quo. Maybe you're like that, Nathan. Maybe you're tired of your parents providing everything for you. Maybe you want to know more about how to do things yourself."

The flapping of the birds' wings made so much noise that Lucky Hunter heard what was happening and rushed to the scene. He was furious at what he saw. When he came to the place where he kept the game, only the two boys were left standing by the rock that marked the entrance to the cave. All the birds and animals were gone. Without saying a word he went down into the cave and kicked the covers off four jars in one corner. They contained bedbugs, lice, gnats, and fleas, which swarmed all over the boys. When Lucky Hunter felt that the boys had been sufficiently punished, he knocked the insects off the boys, who had nearly been bitten to death.

"Ever since then, humankind has had to hunt to find the animals instead of snaring them in a cave. And we have been bothered and hampered in those efforts by the bug nations, who bite us and sting us."

Maize was an excellent cook and kept the food that she cooked in a storeroom. The boys wondered what she did in the storeroom, and they spied on her through a small hole. She leaned over a basket in the middle of the room and rubbed her stomach counterclockwise. When she did that, the basket filled with corn. The boys decided Maize was a witch and that she would have to be killed.

"Now what you need to know, Nathan, is that they can't really kill her, because she's a god, and this is a symbolic story. No one really dies."

Maize read their minds and knew they would kill her. She asked the boys to drag her body around a circle drawn on a cleared spot in front of the house, and watch the circle all night so that they would have food the next day. They killed her with a club and put her head on the roof of the house facing west.

They didn't follow her directions exactly, clearing only seven small spots instead of the one large circle as she said; this is why corn does not grow everywhere, but only in the places where her blood fell as they dragged. The next morning (after they watched all night) the corn was full grown.

When Lucky Hunter came back, he saw Maize's head and was furious. He went to stay with the wolf-people. Once again Spirit Boy changed himself into duck down and accompanied Lucky Hunter. The wolf-people were meeting in council, and Lucky Hunter asked them to challenge his boys to a ballgame and then kill them. They agreed.

Spirit Boy and his brother made a wide circle all around the house, making a trail all around except in the direction from which the wolf-people would be coming. They made themselves arrows and waited. As soon as the wolf-people passed through the break in the trail, it magically transformed into a high fence, locking them in. Spirit Boy and Real Boy had trapped the wolf-people, who agreed to leave through the swamp and bother the boys no more. The wolf-people who survived became our modern wolves.

A series of dramas followed in which the boys tried unsuccessfully to kill Lucky Hunter and he tried unsuccessfully to kill them. Finally, the boys made their way to the end of the world, where the sun rises, and found Lucky Hunter and Maize sitting there, waiting for them. They all stayed together for seven days and then returned to their homeland and were known as "the little men." The boys then oversaw the populating of the world with people. They sang seven songs, and deer came out from the woods for the people to eat. The people learned those songs, which the hunters always sang when hunting deer. Now the people had corn and deer and could survive.

"Who are your internal characters?" I asked Nathan. "Who are the characters who live within your mind? Do you have a wild boy like Spirit Boy? Do you have internal parents like Lucky Hunter and Maize whom you wish to overthrow? Are they like your parents? What do they say all day when you are talking to yourself?"

Through dialogue inspired by the story, we discovered that Nathan had several inner voices who were attached to internalized characters. He had his Wild Boy who tried to destroy everything and everyone in his path. Wild Boy was the spirit who fueled going crazy. He had his internalized parents who were like Lucky Hunter and Maize in some ways. His inner mother was always sacrificing herself to take care of him. His inner father was a solid worker though not particularly inspired and not very creative. He loved and hated them simultaneously. He loved them because they were his parents, but he hated them because he detested their lives. He detested the very idea that he would be like them. Real Boy represented the inner part of Nathan who could negotiate among these other parts.

We had hours of interesting and provocative conversations between these inner parts of Nathan. In the throes of his psychosis, they behaved like the characters in the story, trying to kill each other and behaving erratically. Through our negotiations they learned to coexist. Real Boy placed Wild Boy on notice that he could no longer destroy everything he touched. A truce was declared among the inner parents, Wild Boy, and Real Boy. Once the truce existed, life could move forward.

Nathan and I also talked about "hunting deer" as meaning he had to leave home and make it on his own. He had to make it in the world of ordinary people. "But you don't have to do that in an ordinary way," I said. "Let's figure out how you can follow your passion without going overboard. How can you support yourself doing music or something else that means a lot to you? How can you play the music you love and maybe tour Saskatchewan before touring Uganda?"

As part of the guided imagery we did in conjunction with the above story, Nathan had constructed a story that he was so terrified of being like his parents that he had rebelled too far and gone off the deep end. He didn't want to live from mortgage to mortgage, a quiet conventional life with a bohemian flare like his mother. He wanted excitement. He wanted passion. He wanted to live, but he had gone too far. Once over the deep end, as many of my friends who have been there will tell you, it's hard to get back, and one lives in the constant fear of going there again. It's very frightening to be psychotic because the world is out of control.

I believe the world is always out of control, but we maintain a sense of control and order through the stories or narratives that we impose on it. These stories filter out evil spirits, bad energies, ghosts, aliens, and everything else that would disturb our comfort zone; they create a seamless narrative for us. I have a friend whose experience nicely illustrates this concept of the creation of a seamless reality. He had a pituitary tumor that was surgically removed. Because he has no pituitary, he has to take artificial hormones. When the hormones get out of balance, sometimes he gets swelling that affects his optic nerve. When this happens, he loses a quarter of his vision. What amazes me is that his brain still creates a full visual field even when a quarter of its perception has been eliminated. My friend only knows that he's missing part of the world because he knows that he has a right arm and that he's moving it and that it's missing from his vision. Otherwise he would never know that he's not seeing the world as it is.

Psychosis allows us to see the naked, unstoried raw material of existence and the world, and it's terrifying. We need stories (contexts) to prevent us from going crazy from the overwhelming sensory data of perception. Stories organize our perception into comprehensible wholes. Helping Nathan to make stories allowed him to structure his world into manageable chunks that no longer seemed overwhelming.

Nathan decided he would start playing music in coffeehouses and other venues for free. "It's not too hard to find gigs that pay nothing," he said, "and it's good practice." I reminded him that the Beatles had played together about ten thousand hours before they made it big, mostly in strip clubs in Hamburg, Germany. Nathan began to play guitar all over his town as we continued our dialogue and storytelling for the next eighteen months, after which time he felt completely recovered. For three of his worst months I had given him low doses of risperidone (Risperdal), since I didn't have a social network to surround him and heal him.

By the time we parted ways, Nathan was getting paid for gigs and was doing studio musician work. He was living on his own, though not yet fully supporting himself. His parents were still paying his rent and utilities. His parents were thrilled to pay this small cost to reap the benefit of how his life had changed. Luckily for Nathan, in his world of music, you can be a bit strange and still be accepted. Completing his financial independence was the intended project for the next year or two. Patience is needed with more severe disturbances, as progress is slower, but it is still significant, since most people in today's modern world make no progress at all.

Saying Goodbye to Satan

"Beth" was a forty-three-year-old woman who believed she was possessed by the devil. She believed that angels and demons followed her around, laughing at her and trying to poison her food. They made ongoing, running, derogatory comments on her activities, thoughts, feelings, and behavior. The worst of the voices (the most negative) came from the devil himself. Beth felt so cursed that not even the church could save her. She had been diagnosed as having paranoid schizophrenia seventeen years previously and had been "channeling" the devil for the past fifteen years.

Sometimes Beth saw monsters and demons on the street, and then she would go inside stores or shops until the visions passed. This sometimes got her in trouble with the police, since she didn't look like the typical consumer in those shops and I suppose the merchants thought she would scare away other customers.

Beth believed the devil routinely broke into her house and rearranged objects and pictures. She could sometimes see his eyes peering out at her. I came into contact with Beth when I was on psychiatry emergency call. She came to the hospital because she couldn't go home. The devil was occupying her living room, and she was too terrified to open her apartment door. Beth needed a place to sleep. When the resident called me, I agreed that we could give her some lorazepam (Ativan, an antianxiety drug) and just let her sleep the night in the emergency room, as long as we didn't need the room (we had two designated psychiatry rooms at the hospital). Then I'd see her in the morning in my office or at the emergency room if she couldn't get to the office. In the morning, the ER nurses were ecstatically glad to be able to send Beth by taxi to my office.

Beth was an interesting-looking character. She had tattoos up and down her arms, although I couldn't tell whether they were patterns like Maori tattoos or poorly drawn pictures. She wore multiple layers of purple, red, and orange clothing, which was actually refreshing against the background of solid white snow that Saskatoon saw for months. Beth was aboriginal—Cree from Manitoba—and had been in Saskatoon for as long as she remembered. I didn't intend to interfere with her treating psychiatrist, who only saw her for medication, but I thought we could do some interesting work together (in Canada, I had that option; I was on salary).

I began by asking Beth to tell me about the time the devil had first appeared in her life. It seemed logical to return to that time to hear about what was happening in her life.

"I was watching my mom die of cancer," Beth said.

"Wow," I said. "That must have been awful."

"No," she said. "The devil was worse."

"So tell me what happened."

"Well, my mom always took care of all twelve of us kids. My mom was a really strong woman. We lived on the reserve, and we had a small house. My dad had died when I was twelve. He went out fishing and never came back. They never found his body, but the boat was found capsized and wedged up against some trees. So we figured he had drowned. He had been drinking, and there were beer cans floating near the boat, so maybe the boat turned over and he was too drunk to swim or whatever, and so we had a funeral for him even though no one ever found his body, though lots of people looked when the weather turned warm."

"Did you ever see his spirit?" I asked. Beth smiled.

"I did. Many times. But the doctors told me that was just a hallucination."

"But we know differently, don't we?" I said. Now Beth was truly relaxing. "You really are an Indian doctor," she said. "I didn't know Indians could become psychiatrists."

"Well, I come from the U.S.," I said. "We had a different kind of Indian Act. It sort of read, 'kill them all,' but anyone who survived wasn't prohibited from getting an education and going to college. My grandmother only made it through Grade 3," I said, "but my mother, to her credit, got through college and blazed the trail for me to follow. She went to this cool college that was free except that she had to work, so she quilted her way through college."

"That's awesome," Beth said. "My mother quilted, too."

"I'll bet your mom was an amazing woman, just like mine," I said.

"She sure was. I was so devastated when she died. It was like a big part of me died with her. And I had all my younger brothers and sisters to look after. And I was number four so there was help, but the older ones were busy with their own families, and I just couldn't do it. I tried so hard to help the younger ones, but I broke down."

"Is that when you first met the devil?" I asked.

"Yes, he was the one that gave my mother cancer and killed her," Beth said.

"How did you know?"

"I could see him inside of her as she was dying. He was eating her alive. He finally ate her heart, and then she died."

"That's terrible. Were you ever afraid that he would eat you?"

"All the time," Beth confessed. "I fear for my life—that he'll take me just like he took my mother."

"What do you do to prevent that?" I asked.

"I pray to Jesus and Mary. I pray to God. I smudge. I sacrifice." Beth showed me scars all along her arm where she had cut herself as a sacrifice so the devil could not possess her.

"Like a flesh offering," I said.

"Exactly," she responded. She was obviously relieved that I understood this custom.

"So, here's my question," I said. "It's been seventeen years that Satan has been stalking you, and he hasn't gotten you. You must have some incredibly strong protection. Who is it?"

"What?" she asked. I guess no one had ever posed this question to her before.

"Who protects you?" I asked again.

"What do you mean?"

"If you didn't have protection, you'd be dead. So I'm wondering who protects you?"

"Wow," she said. "I never thought of that."

"I'm guessing Jesus and Mary must like you, or maybe it's the spirit of your mother, or maybe it's another ancestor, or maybe an animal out in the bush took a hankering to you and wards off evil for you."

"Maybe," she said slowly. "I never thought of that." I had her attention.

"It's worth thinking about," I said, "'cause maybe you're scared for nothing. You know, it's been seventeen years, and if Satan were going to kill you, I think you'd be dead by now." Beth had no way to dispute my unassailable logic. "Of course," I added, "don't stop doing what you're doing. I'll bet you tie prayer flags in trees also."

"Sure do," she said.

"Well, don't stop," I said. "But maybe we could stop worrying. I'm guessing that even if Satan is sitting in the middle of your living room, that your protectors will chase him out before you even unlock the apartment door."

"Wow," Beth said. "Maybe so."

"Let's do an experiment," I said. "Let's see if you can relax a bit and still be safe. I'm betting you can. I'm also betting that Satan will protest. His voice will get louder and louder inside your head when he finds out he's powerless to hurt you. It might feel like he's powerful when that happens, but it's really because he's powerless, and the only way he can hurt you is to get you to hurt yourself. You see, the death of your mother may have given you a powerful medicine against Satan that not even he can counteract. So let's relax and be less fearful and see if the voice gets stronger and if, even then, nothing bad happens." Beth agreed.

We spent more time talking, and before she left I told her a story to take with her. "If you get scared," I said, "just remember this story and tell it back to yourself and then my spirit and the spirit of the story will be with you." I was able to use our shared aboriginal beliefs for her benefit, an example of why therapists from the same spiritual perspective or culture or worldview as the client can be more effective.

For the next three months, I continued to see Beth at intervals of about every seven to fourteen days. My predictions had come true. When Beth relaxed, Satan's voice had gotten louder, but nothing bad happened. She proudly reported to me at the next visit that she had told Satan the story I told her, and it had quieted him down. She had redoubled her efforts at prayer and at smudging, and was still alive. After one month, she was really starting to relax. "You know," she said. "Satan can't kill me."

"No," I said. "He can't." This is when I introduced her to the idea of speaking to an aboriginal elder. I had in mind John C., a man who had first been an Anglican priest before he became a traditional healer and used both Christian and Cree traditions freely, mingling them at will. Over the next month, Beth fretted about whether she could see a healer. She was scared. After about six weeks, she was ready to go. It turned out that I was going to a sweat and a doctoring ceremony that John was having, so I offered to take her. She was glad because she had no transportation and no money to pay her way. All she had to offer John was a few cigarettes, but I knew that would be fine with him, because it came from her heart and cigarettes were really valuable to her. (Research has shown that the nicotine in cigarettes counteracts the adverse effects that antipsychotic drugs have on thinking. This may be why so many people on these medications smoke.)

I drove Beth and a couple of friends to see John the very next Saturday morning. John was so glad to see Beth. He told her that he'd been dreaming for weeks that she would be coming. "My girl," he said, "we are going to remove these demons once and for all. And then, you keep coming by here, and we'll be sure that they never return."

Beth was doctored by John, who gave her protection (a pouch of herbs and tobacco, tied with silk ribbons of many colors and fastened to an eagle feather) to put on her door so Satan could never get in.

The next part of my "treatment" of Beth involved making sure she got to the ceremonies at John's. After that first contact, she wanted to be a regular. After three months, Beth decided to move nearer to John so she wouldn't have so much trouble getting there on a regular basis. We figured out how she could do that and worked out the details. I stopped seeing her so often except at ceremonies at John's place.

Later I heard that she and John had chased out the devil. They had silenced that voice. Of course, we all participated. When I left Canada, Beth was slowly decreasing her medications. She hadn't found a psychiatrist who would help her, but we did find a cooperative and friendly family doctor, and we laid out a regimen that involved a 10 percent decrease in medications across the board every three months. If symptoms worsened, the plan was for her to go back upward and stay at the level that prevented symptoms from returning for another three months and then try again. Since Beth had been on drugs for eighteen years by then, it was important for her to taper off slowly. The last I heard, she was down to 50 percent of her former medication level and still decreasing. She is happy in her community and even has a boyfriend whom she met at one of John's sweats and doctoring. Her boyfriend had been labeled bipolar psychotic, so they have a lot to talk about, and they look after each other nicely, which is very sweet.

The Promise

The symptoms of all of my patients who have been labeled with psychotic disorders have a sort of logic, a meaning within the context of their lives. That enables me or the other healers who work with them to construct a narrative from their symptoms even if they can't. We create a zone of proximate development to make stories together when the person cannot make stories on his or her own. Within that zone of proximate development, he or she learns from us and by example how to structure experience into a quality narrative. It is like putting up a temporary scaffolding, then slowly removing it while helping to build a new narrative. When the scaffolding is gone, the new story stands on its own. The healing comes when the person constructs his or her own narrative.

The healing process involves realizing that many of the truths we hold about ourselves are merely stories, learned through our experiences in a social network, and changeable. As we begin to find better stories for life, our old stories gradually drop away. Through finding healthier social networks—often with the aid of spirituality and traditional culture or other immersion in longstanding teaching tales that communicate good values for life—we mature and solidify our changes. We gain control over the voices and internal characters of our mind, finding ways for them to negotiate and live well together. Slowly our suffering and pain melts away, and we find more happiness and well-being. This is the power of story for healing the mind and the promise of narrative psychiatry.

Notes

Preface

1. Lewis Mehl-Madrona, *Narrative Medicine: The Use of History and Story in the Healing Process* (Rochester, Vt.: Bear & Company, 2007).

Introduction: There's Nothing But Story

1. Karl-Erik Sveiby and Tex Skuthorpe, *Treading Lightly: The Hidden Wisdom of the World's Oldest People* (Crows Nest, Australia: Allen & Unwin, 2006), 45.

2. *Layla and Majnun,* quoted in Patrick Colm Hogan, *The Mind and Its Stories: Narrative Universals and Human Emotion* (Cambridge: Cambridge University Press, 2003), 147.

3. Brian Boyd, *On the Origins of Stories: Evolution, Cognition, and Fiction* (Cambridge, Mass.: Belknap Press of Harvard University Press, 2009), 197.

4. Ibid., 198.

5. M. M. Merzenich, P. Tallal, B. Peterson, S. Miller, and W. M. Jenkins, "Some Neurological Principles Relevant to the Origins of—and the Cortical Based Remediation of—Language Learning Impairments," in *Neuroplasticity: Building a Bridge from the Laboratory to the Clinic,* ed. J. Grafman and Y. Christen (Amsterdam: Elsevier, 1998), 169–87.

6. Boyd, *Origins of Stories.*

7. J. Liepert, W. H. R. Miltner, H. Bauder, M. Sommer, C. Dettmers, E. Taub, and C. Weiller, "Motor Cortex Plasticity during Constraint-induced Movement Therapy in Stroke Patients," *Neuroscience Letters* 250 (1998): 5–8; B. Kopp, A. Kunkel, W. Muehlnickel, K. Villringer, E. Taub, and H. Flor, "Plasticity in the Nervous System Related to Therapy Induced Improvement of Movement after Stroke," *NeuroReport* 10, no. 4 (1999): 807–10.

8. Norman Doidge, *The Brain That Changes Itself: Stories of Personal Triumph from the Frontiers of Brain Science* (New York: Penguin, 2007), 55.

9. M. M. Merzenich, "Cortical Plasticity Contributing to Childhood Development," in *Mechanisms of Cognitive Development: Behavioral and Neural Perspectives,* ed. J. L. McClelland and R. S. Siegler (Mahway, N.J.: Lawrence Erlbaum Associates, 2001), 64–73.

10. T. N. Wiesel, "Early Explorations of the Development and Plasticity of the Visual Cortex: A Personal View," *Journal of Neurobiology* 41, no. 1 (1999): 7–9.

Chapter 1. Conventional Mental Health Today

1. C. J. Murray and A. D. Lopez, "Global Mortality, Disability, and the Contribution of Risk Factors: Global Burden of Disease Study," *Lancet* 349, no. 9063 (1997): 1436–42.

2. Norman Sartorius and Hugh Schulze, *Reducing the Stigma of Mental Illness: A Report from a Global Association* [World Psychiatric Association Global Programme against Stigma and Discrimination because of Schizophrenia] (New York: Cambridge University Press, 2005); Kim Hopper, Glynn Harrison, Aleksandar Janca, and Norman Sartorius, eds., *Recovery from Schizophrenia: An International Perspective: A Report from the WHO Collaborative Project, the International Study of Schizophrenia* (New York: Oxford University Press, 2007).

3. Irving Kirsch, Brett J. Deacon, Tania B. Huedo-Medina, Alan Scoboria, Thomas J. Moore, and Blair T. Johnson, "Initial Severity and Antidepressant Benefits: A Meta-Analysis of Data Submitted to the Food and Drug Administration," *PLoS Medicine* 5, no. 2 (2008), www.plosmedicine.org/article/info:doi/10.1371/journal.pmed.0050045 (accessed August 18, 2009).

4. L. L. Altshuler, M. J. Gitlin, J. Mintz, K. L. Leight, and M. A. Frye, "Subsyndromal Depression Is Associated with Functional Impairment in Patients with Bipolar Disorder," *Journal of Clinical Psychiatry* 63 (2002): 807–11.

5. Leonardo Tondo, Göran Isacsson, and Ross Baldessarini, "Suicidal Behaviour in Bipolar Disorder: Risk and Prevention," *CNS Drugs* 17, no. 7 (2003): 491–511.

6. David Kaiser, "Commentary: Against Biologic Psychiatry," *Psychiatric Times* XIII, no. 12 (1996): 1.

7. Ibid., 2.

8. Ibid., 5.

9. Ibid., 6.

10. Phillip Sinaikin, "Categorical Diagnosis and a Poetics of Obligation: An Ethical Commentary on Psychiatric Diagnosis and Treatment," *Ethical Human Sciences and Services* 5, no. 2 (2003): 141–48.

Chapter 2. Good Stories and Mental Health

1. Rita Charon, "Narrative Medicine: A Model for Empathy, Reflection, Profession, and Trust," *JAMA* 286 (2001): 1897–1902.

2. Mehl-Madrona, *Narrative Medicine*.

3. Roger C. Schank and Robert P. Abelson, "Knowledge and Memory: The Real Story," in *Knowledge and Memory: The Real Story,* ed. Robert S. Wyer Jr. (Hillsdale, N.J.: Lawrence Erlbaum Associates), 1–85.

4. Gerald Prince, *A Dictionary of Narratology,* rev. ed. (Lincoln: University of Nebraska Press, 2003).

5. Victor Erlich, *Russian Formalism* (New Haven, Conn.: Yale University Press, 1981).

6. Vladimir Propp, *Morphology of the Folktale* (Austin: University of Texas Press, 1968).

7. Raymond A. Mar, "The Neuropsychology of Narrative: Story Comprehension, Story Production and Their Interrelation," *Neuropsychologia* 42 (2004): 1414–34.

8. M. F. Mason, M. I. Norton, J. D. Van Horn, D. M. Wegner, S. T. Grafton, and C. N. Macrae, "Wandering Minds: The Default Network and Stimulus-independent Thought," *Science* 315 (2007): 393–95.

9. D. A. Gusnard, E. Akbudak, G. L. Shulman, and M. E. Raichle, "Medial Prefrontal Cortex and Self-referential Mental Activity: Relation to a Default Mode of Brain Functioning," *Proceedings of the National Academy of Sciences of the United States* 98 (2001): 4259–64; M. E. Raichle, A. M. MacLeod, A. Z. Snyder, W. J. Powers, D. A. Gusnard, and G. L. Schulman, "A Default Mode of Brain Function," *Proceedings of the National Academy of Sciences of the United States* 98 (2001): 676–82.

10. Norman A. S. Farb, Zindel V. Segal, Helen Mayberg, Jim Bean, Deborah McKeon, Zainab Fatima, and Adam K. Anderson, "Attending to the Present: Mindfulness Meditation Reveals Distinct Neural Modes of Self-reference," *Social Cognitive and Affective Neuroscience,* advance access published August 13, 2007, Oxford University Press, http://scan.oxfordjournals.org/cgi/reprint/nsm030v1 (accessed November 7, 2009).

11. E. Waitkins and J. D. Teasdale, "Rumination and Overgeneral Memory in Depression: Effects of Self-focus and Analytic Thinking," *Journal of Abnormal Psychology* 110 (2001): 353–57.

12. Mason et al., "Wandering Minds."

13. Yale University, "Brain's 'Default Mode' Awry In Schizophrenia," *Science Daily,* March 14, 2007, www.sciencedaily.com/releases/2007/03/070313172329.htm (accessed November 7, 2009).

14. Schank and Abelson, "Knowledge and Memory."

15. Lewis Mehl-Madrona, *Coyote Medicine: Lessons from Native American Healing* (New York: Fireside/Simon & Schuster, 1998.)

16. Boyd, *Origins of Stories,* 154.

17. Jerome Bruner, *Acts of Meaning* (Cambridge, Mass.: Harvard University Press, 1990).

18. L. S. Vygotsky, *Mind in Society: Development of Higher Psychological Processes,* ed. Michael Cole, Vera John-Steiner, Sylvia Scribner, and Ellen Souberman, 14th ed. (Cambridge, Mass.: Harvard University Press, 1978).

19. National Institute of Mental Health, "Questions and Answers about the NIMH Clinical Antipsychotic Trials of Intervention Effectiveness Study (CATIE)," April 1, 2006, www.nimh.nih.gov/health/trials/practical/catie/phase2results.shtml (accessed January 29, 2010).

20. Robert A. Rosenheck, Marvin S. Swartz, and Jeffery A. Lieberman, "Practical

Clinical Trials in Psychiatry: Studies of Schizophrenia from the CATIE Network," *Psychiatric Services* 57, no. 8 (2006): 1093, http://psychservices.psychiatryonline .org/cgi/reprint/57/8/1093 (accessed August 18, 2009); "CATIE Studies Cite Need for Tailored Treatment Plans, Community Supports" (Clinical Antipsychotic Trials for Intervention Effectiveness), *Mental Health Weekly,* March 5, 2007, www .accessmylibrary.com/coms2/summary_0286-32769659_ITM (accessed August 18, 2009).

21. L. L. Altshuler, M. J. Gitlin, J. Mintz, K. L. Leight, and M. A. Frye, "Subsyndromal Depression Is Associated with Functional Impairment in Patients with Bipolar Disorder," *Journal of Clinical Psychiatry* 63 (2002): 807–11; F. Goodwin and Kay Jamison, *Manic-Depressive Illness,* 2nd ed. (New York: Oxford University Press, 2007).

22. Richard C. Schwartz, *Internal Family Systems Therapy* (Westport, Conn.: Guilford Press, 1996).

23. Vernon Hamilton, Gordon H. Bower, and Nico H. Frijda, eds., *Cognitive Perspectives on Emotion and Motivation,* NATO Science Series D (New York: Springer, 1988).

24. Schwartz, *Internal Family Systems Therapy.*

25. Boyd, *Origins of Stories,* 154.

26. John W. Perry, *The Far Side of Madness* (Dallas, Texas: Spring Publications, 1974), 139.

27. D. L. Rennie, "Qualitative Analysis of the Client Experience of Psychotherapy: The Unfolding of Reflexivity," in *Psychotherapy Process Research: Paradigmatic and Narrative Approaches,* ed. S. G. Toukmanian and D. L. Rennie (London: Sage Publications, 1992), 211–33.

28. M. R. Henriques, B. C. Machado, and Ó. F. Gonçalves, "Anorexia Nervosa: Validação Divergente de uma Narrativa Protótipo: Revista Internacional de Psicología Clínica y de la Salud," *International Journal of Clinical and Health Psychology* 2, no. 1 (2002): 91–109.

29. Rudolf Botha and Chris Knight, *The Prehistory of Language* (New York: Oxford University Press, 2009); C. Whitehead, "Work Versus Play: What Recent Brain Research Can Tell Us about Play, Theatre, and the Arts, and Why It Is Taking Scientists Such an Unconscionably Long Time to Realize Their Importance," in *Consciousness, Theatre, Literature and the Arts 2007,* ed. D. Meyer-Dinkgräfe (Newcastle: Cambridge Scholars Publishing, 2007), 487–503; C. Whitehead, "Why Scientists Cannot Agree about Human Behavioural Universals, What Animal Cartoons Can Tell Us, and Some Suggestions as to When and Why Fundamental Human Differences Evolved" (lecture, "VI. Göttinger Freilandtage: Primate Behavior and Human Universals," Department of Behavioral Ecology and Sociobiology, Deutsches Primatenzentrum, Göttingen, Germany, December 11–14, 2007).

30. L. Luborsky, I. P. Barber, and L. Digver, "The Meaning of Narratives Told in Psychotherapy: The Fruit of a New Observation Unit," *Psychotherapy Research* 2 (1992): 277–90.

31. L. E. Angus and K. Hardtke, "Narrative Processes in Psychotherapy," *Canadian Psychology* 35 (1994): 190–203; L. E. Angus, K. Hardtke, and H. Levitt, *The Narrative Processes Coping System Manual,* rev. ed. (unpublished manuscript, North York, Ontario: York University, 1996); L. E. Angus, H. Levitt, and K. Hardtke, "The Narrative Processes Coding System: Research Applications and Implications for Psychotherapy Practice," *Journal of Clinical Psychology* 55, no. 10 (1999): 1255–70.

32. James W. Pennebaker and Janel D. Seagal, "Forming a Story: The Health Benefits of Narrative," *Journal of Clinical Psychology* 55, no. 10 (1999): 1243–54; M. E. Francis and J. W. Pennebaker, "Putting Stress into Words: The Impact of Writing on Physiological Function, and Self-Reported Emotional Well-Being Measures," *American Journal of Health Promotion* 6 (1992): 280–87.

33. J. W. Pennebaker, J. Kiecolt-Glasser, and R. Glaser, "Disclosure of Traumas and Immune Function: Health Implications for Psychotherapy," *Journal of Consulting and Clinical Psychology* 56 (1988): 239–45.

34. J. W. Pennebaker, M. Colder, and L. K. Sharp, "Accelerating the Coping Process," *Journal of Personality and Social Psychology* 58 (1990): 528–37.

35. Chad M. Burton and Laura A. King, "The Health Benefits of Writing about Intensely Positive Experiences," *Journal of Research in Personality* 38, no. 2 (April 2004): 150–63.

36. Joanne Frattaroli, "Experimental Disclosure and Its Moderators: A Meta-analysis," *Psychological Bulletin* 132, no. 6 (November 2006): 823–65.

37. Kenneth J. Gergen, "From Identity to Relational Politics," in *Social Construction in Context* (Thousand Oaks, Calif.: Sage Publications, 2001), 169–83.

Chapter 3. How Do We Learn to Be Who We Are?

1. Jerome S. Bruner, *Toward a Theory of Instruction,* rev. ed. (Cambridge, Mass.: Belknap Press of Harvard University Press, 1974).

2. Carl Ratner, "Vygotsky's Conception of Psychological Development," in *The Essential Vygotsky,* ed. Robert Rieber and David Robinson (New York: Kluwer Academic/Plenum Publishing, 2004).

3. Learning-Theories.com, "Social Developmental Theory (Vygotsky)," www.learning-theories.com/vygotskys-social-learning-theory.html (accessed June 24, 2009).

4. L. S. Vygotsky, *Mind in Society: Development of Higher Psychological Processes,* ed. Michael Cole, Vera John-Steiner, Sylvia Scribner, and Ellen Souberman, 14th ed. (Cambridge, Mass.: Harvard University Press, 1978), 57.

5. Lev Vygotsky, *Thought and Language,* ed. Alex Kozulin, rev. ed. (Cambridge, Mass.: Massachusetts Institute of Technology, 1986).

6. Ibid.

7. Lev Vygotsky, "Interaction between Learning and Development," in *Mind in Society,* www.comnet.ca/~pballan/Vygotsky(1978).htm (accessed June 24, 2009).

8. Lev Vygotsky, "Social Development Theory," http://tip.psychology.org/vygotsky .html (accessed June 24, 2009).

9. Nassim Nicholas Taleb, *The Black Swan: The Impact of the Highly Improbable* (New York: Random House, 2007).

10. Lev Vygotsky, *Collected Works,* vol. 5, *Child Psychology* (New York: Plenum Press, 1998), 168.

11. Ibid., 34.

12. Vygotsky, *Mind in Society,* 81.

13. S. Scribner, "Vygotsky's Uses of History," in *Mind and Social Practice: Selected Writings of Sylvia Scribner,* ed. Ethel Tobach, R. J. Falmagne, M. B. Parlee, L. M. W. Martin, and A. S. Kapelman (Cambridge: Cambridge University Press, 1997), 241–65 (reprinted from *Culture, Communication, and Cognition,* ed. J. V. Wertsch [New York: Cambridge University Press, 1985], 119–45).

14. Ibid., 259.

15. D. Purves, J. T. Voyvodic, L. Magrassi, and H. Yawo, "Nerve Terminal Remodeling Visualized in Living Mice by Repeated Examination of the Same Neuron," *Science* 238, no. 4830 (November 1987): 1122–26; Yuri Geinisman, John F. Disterhoft, Hans Jørgen, G. Gundersen, Matthew D. McEchron, Inna S. Persina, John M. Power, Eddy A. Van Der Zee, and Mark J. West, "Our Brain Changes Moment to Moment as We Learn: Remodeling of Hippocampal Synapses after Hippocampus-dependent Associative Learning," *The Journal of Comparative Neurology* 417, no. 1 (2000): 49–59.

16. John Shotter, "Vico, Moral Worlds, Accountability and Personhood," in *Indigenous Psychologies: The Anthropology of the Self,* ed. Paul Heelas and Andrew Lock (London: Academic Press, 1981), 265–84; John Shotter, *Conversational Realities Revisited: Life, Language, Body and World* (Chagrin Falls, Ohio: Taos Institute Publications, 2008).

17. Shotter, *Conversational Realities Revisited.*

18. Paul F. Ballantyne, "Psychology, Society, and Ability Testing (1859–2002): Transformative Alternatives to Mental Darwinism and Interactionism," 2002, www .comnet.ca/~pballan/Toc1.htm (accessed August 11, 2009).

19. Temple Grandin and Sean Barron, *Unwritten Rules of Social Relationships: Decoding Social Mysteries through the Unique Perspective of Autism* (Arlington, Texas: Future Horizons, 2005).

Chapter 4. How Do We Learn to Feel What We Feel?

1. Pyotr Bodor, *On Emotions: A Developmental, Social Constructionist Account* (London: L'Harmattan, 2004), 54.

2. Paul Ekman, *Emotion in the Human Face,* 2nd ed. (Cambridge: Cambridge University Press, 1977); R. Zajonc and H. Marcus, "Affect and Cognition: The Hard Interface," in *Emotion, Cognition, and Behavior,* ed. C. E. Izard, J. Kagan, and R. Zajonc (Cambridge: Cambridge University Press, 1984), 73–102.

3. Bodor, *On Emotions,* 54.

4. Joseph E. LeDoux, "Emotion, Memory and the Brain: The Hidden Mind," *Scientific American,* special editions, www.sciamdigital.com/index.cfm?fa=Products .ViewIssuePreview&ARTICLEID_CHAR=E2A4B18E-C338-4FCA-9384-A110917B5AD (accessed October 12, 2009); Joseph E. LeDoux, "The Emotional Brain, Fear, and the Amygdala," *Cellular and Molecular Neurobiology* 23, nos. 4–5 (October 2003): 727–38.

5. William James, "What Is Emotion?" in *Readings in the History of Psychology,* ed. Wayne Dennis (New York: Appleton-Century-Crofts, 1948), 291, 299.

6. E. Grastyan, "Emotion," in *Encyclopedia Britannica: Macropaedia III* (New York: Helen Hemingway Benton, 1974), 757–66.

7. S. Schachter and J. E. Singer, "Cognitive, Psychological, and Social Determinants of Emotional States," *Psychological Review* 69 (1962): 379–99.

8. Bodor, *On Emotions,* 56.

9. Carol Z. Stearns and Peter N. Stearns, "Introduction," in *Emotions and Social Change: Toward a New Psychohistory* (New York: Holmes and Meier Publishers, 1988), 1–23.

10. Stearns and Stearns, "Introduction"; Rom Harré and R. Finlay-Jones, "Emotion Talk across Cultures," in *The Social Construction of Emotions,* ed. Rom Harré (Oxford: Blackwell Publishers, 1989), 220–34.

11. J. M. Barbalet, *Emotion, Social Theory, and Social Structure: A Macrosociological Approach* (New York: Cambridge University Press, 1998), 29–61.

12. Carl Ratner, "A Social Constructionist Critique of Naturalistic Theories of Emotion," *Journal of Mind and Behavior* 10 (1989): 211–30.

13. Aaron Beck, *Love Is Never Enough* (New York: Harper & Row, 1988).

14. Ratner, "Social Constructionist Critique."

15. Beck, *Love Is Never Enough.*

16. James R. Averill, "Individual Differences in Emotional Creativity: Structure and Correlates," *Journal of Personality* 67, no. 2 (April 1999): 331–71.

17. Martha C. Nussbaum, "Emotion in the Language of Judging," *St. John's Law Review* 70 (1996): 23; Martha C. Nussbaum, *Upheavals of Thought: The Intelligence of Emotions* (Cambridge: Cambridge University Press, 2001).

18. Tom Lutz, *American Nervousness, 1903: An Anecdotal History* (Ithaca, N.Y.: Cornell University Press, 1991).

19. G. di Pellegrino, L. Fadiga, L. Fogassi, V. Gallese, and G. Rizzolatti, "Understanding Motor Events: A Neuropsychological Study," *Experimental Brain Research* 91 (1992): 176–80; G. Rizzolatti, L. Fadiga, L. Fogassi, and V. Gallese, "Premotor Cortex and the Recognition of Motor Events," *Cognitive Brain Research* 3 (1996): 131–41.

20. G. Buccino, A. Baumgaertner, L. Colle, C. Buechel, G. Rizzolatti, and F. Binkofski, "The Neural Basis for Understanding Non-intended Actions," *NeuroImage* 36, no. 2 (2007): 119–27; G. Buccino, F. Binkofski, G. R. Fink, L. Fadiga, L. Fogassi, V. Gallese, R. J. Seitz, K. Zilles, G. Rizzolatti, and H.-J. Freund, "Action Observation

Activates Premotor and Parietal Areas in a Somatotopic Manner: An fMRI Study," *European Journal of Neuroscience* 13 (2001): 400–4; J. Grèzes and J. Decety, "Functional Anatomy of Execution, Mental Simulation, Observation, and Verb Generation of Actions: A Meta-analysis," *Human Brain Mapping* 12 (2001): 1–19; G. Rizzolatti, L. Fogassi, and V. Gallese, "Mirrors in the Mind," *Scientific American* 295, no. 5 (2006): 54–61.

21. Rizzolatti et al., "Mirrors in the Mind." For more information about Rizzolatti, see www.unipr.it/arpa/mirror/english/staff/rizzolat.htm.

22. Rizzolatti et al., "Mirrors in the Mind," 59.

23. Charles Whitehead, ed., *The Origin of Consciousness in the Social World* (Exeter, UK: Imprint Academic, 2008), 43–57.

24. Brian Broom, *Meaning-full Disease* (London: Karnac Books, 2007), 42.

25. Colwyn Trevarthen, "The Psychobiology of Speech Development," in *Language and Brain: Developmental Aspects. Neurosciences Research Program Bulletin* 12 (1974): 570–85; Colwyn Trevarthen, "Communication and Cooperation in Early Infancy. A Description of Primary Intersubjectivity," in *Before Speech: The Beginning of Human Communication,* ed. M. Bullowa (Cambridge: Cambridge University Press, 1979), 321–47; Maya Gratier and Colwyn Trevarthen, "Musical Narratives and Motives for Culture in Mother-infant Vocal Interactions," in *The Origin of Consciousness*, ed. Whitehead.

26. Ekman, *Emotion in the Human Face.*

27. Michelle Rosaldo, *Knowledge and Passion: Ilongot Notions of Self and Social Life* (Cambridge: Cambridge University Press, 1980); Anna Wierzbicka, *Semantics, Culture, and Cognition: Universal Human Concepts in Culture-Specific Configurations* (New York: Oxford University Press, 1992).

28. R. W. Levenson, P. Ekman, K. Heider, and W. V. Friesen, "Emotion and Autonomic Nervous System Activity in the Miningkabau of Western Sumatra," *Journal of Personality and Social Psychology* 62, no. 6 (1992): 972–88.

29. Joan Y. Chiao, Zhang Li, and Tokiko Harada, "Cultural Neuroscience of Consciousness: From Visual Perception to Self-Awareness," in *The Origin of Consciousness,* ed. Whitehead, 58–69.

30. Paul Ekman, *Emotions Revealed: Recognizing Faces and Feelings to Improve Communication and Emotional Life,* rev. ed. (New York: Times Books, 2007). (first edition published 2004)

31. Carl Ratner, "A Cultural-Psychological Analysis of Emotions," *Culture and Psychology* 6 (2000): 5–39.

32. Jeff Coulter, *The Social Construction of Mind* (London: Macmillan; Totowa, N.J.: Rowman and Littlefield, 1979), 127; Hazel Rose Markus and Shinobu Kitayama, "The Cultural Construction of Self and Emotion: Implications for Social Behavior," in *Emotions in Social Psychology: Key Readings,* ed. W. Parrott, Key Readings in Social Psychology (New York: Psychology Press, 2000), 119–38.

33. Bodor, *On Emotions*, 63–64.

34. Rom Harré, "Toward an Emotionology of Local Moral Orders," *Common Knowledge* 2, no. 3 (1993): 12–14; Rom Harré and Grant Gillett, *The Discursive Mind* (London: Sage Publications, 1994).

35. cf. Émile Durkheim (1895–1938), *On Institutional Analysis* (Chicago: University of Chicago Press, 1978).

36. Lev Vygotsky, *Educational Psychology* (Boca Raton, Fla.: St. Lucie Press, 1997) (originally published 1926), 5, 53–54, 133.

37. Carl Ratner, *Cultural Psychology: A Perspective on Psychological Functioning and Social Reform* (New York: The Erlbaum Group, 2006).

38. Mavis Tsai, Robert J. Kohlenberg, Madelon Y. Bolling, and Christeine Terry, "Values in Therapy and Green FAP," in *A Guide to Functional Analytic Psychotherapy,* ed. Mavis Tsai (New York: Springer, 2009).

39. Ekman, *Emotions Revealed.*

40. Pierre Bleau, "On Emotions and Psychopharmacology" (lecture, Department of Psychiatry, University of Saskatchewan, Saskatoon City Hospital, 2005).

41. J. Dewey, *The Influence of Darwin on Philosophy and Other Essays on Contemporary Thought* (New York: Holt, 1910), 249–50; Lev Vygotsky, *Collected Works,* vol. 3, *Problems of the Theory and History of Psychology* (New York: Plenum Press, 1997): 272–73, 327.

Chapter 5. The Meaning of Pain and Depression

1. Peter Brown, *The Hypnotic Brain: Hypnotherapy and Social Communication* (New Haven, Conn.: Yale University Press, 1991).

2. Rom Harré, "Social Construction of Consciousness," in *Investigating Phenomenal Consciousness: New Methodologies and Maps,* ed. Max Velmans (Amsterdam: John Benjamins Publishing Company), 234–53.

3. Harré, "Social Construction of Consciousness," 234–53.

4. Ervin Laszlo, *The Connectivity Hypothesis: Foundations of an Integral Science of Quantum, Cosmos, Life, and Consciousness* (Albany: State University of New York Press, 2003).

5. D. C. Turk, R. H. Dworkin, R. R. Allen, N. Bellamy, N. Brandenburg, D. B. Carr, C. Cleeland, et al., "Core Outcome Domains for Chronic Pain Clinical Trials: IMMPACT Recommendations," *Pain* 106, no. 3 (2003): 337–45.

6. K. O. Anderson, S. P. Richman, J. Hurley, G. Palos, V. Valero, T. R. Mendoza, I. Gning, and C. S. Cleeland, "Cancer Pain Management among Under-served Minority Outpatients: Perceived Needs and Barriers to Optimal Control," *Cancer* 94, part 8 (April 15, 2002): 2295–2304.

7. Ibid.

8. Broom, *Meaning-full Disease,* 15.

9. cf., Jerome Bruner, *Acts of Meaning* (Cambridge, Mass.: Harvard University Press, 1990); Harré and Gillett, *Discursive Mind;* Charles C. Ragin and Howard Saul Becker, *What Is a Case? Exploring the Foundations of Social Inquiry* (Cambridge:

Cambridge University Press, 1992); D. Polkinghorne, *Narrative Knowing and the Human Sciences* (Albany: State University of New York Press, 1988); Theodore Sarbin, ed., *Narrative Psychology: The Storied Nature of Human Conduct* (New York: Praeger Publishers, 1986); Betty M. Bayer and John Shotter, eds., *Reconstructing the Psychological Subject: Bodies, Practice, and Technologies* (Thousand Oaks, Calif.: Sage Publications, 1998).

10. Óscar F. Gonçalves, "Constructivism and the Deconstruction of Clinical Practice," in *Constructivist Thinking in Counseling Practice, Research, and Training,* ed. Thomas Sexton and Barbara Griffin (New York: Teachers College Press, 1997).

11. Óscar F. Gonçalves and Paulo P. P. Machado, "Cognitive Narrative Psychotherapy: Research Foundations," *Journal of Clinical Psychology* 55 (1999): 1179–91.

12. N. L. Stein and M. T. Nezworski, "The Effects of Organization and Instructional Set on Story Memory," *Discourse Processes* 1 (1978): 177–93.

13. B. Sutton-Smith, "Children's Fiction Making," in *Narrative Psychology,* ed. Theodore Sarbin (New York: Praeger Publishers, 1986).

14. H. Waters, L. Rodrigues, and D. Ridgeway, "Cognitive Underpinnings of Narrative Attachment Assessment," *Journal of Experimental Child Psychology* 71 (1998): 211–34.

15. Jean M. Mandler, *Stories, Scripts, and Scenes: Aspects of Schema Theory* (Hillsdale, N.J.: Lawrence Erlbaum Associates, 1984).

16. Broom, *Meaning-full Disease,* 18.

17. Ibid., 22.

18. Kenneth Gergen, *Realities and Relationships: Soundings in Social Construction* (Cambridge, Mass.: Harvard University Press, 1995), 276.

Chapter 6. Story and the Shaping of Identity

1. Katerina Clark and Michael Holquist, *Mikhail Bakhtin* (Cambridge, Mass.: Harvard University Press, 1984), 2–3.

2. Joseph J. Tobin, David Y. H. Wu, and Dana H. Davidson, *Preschool in Three Cultures: Japan, China, and the United States* (New Haven, Conn.: Yale University Press, 1989).

3. Dan P. McAdams, "The Development of a Narrative Identity," in *Personality Psychology: Recent Trends and Emerging Directions,* ed. David M. Buss and Nancy Cantor (New York: Springer-Verlag, 1989), 161.

4. Ibid., 169; Polkinghorne, in Jerome Bruner, *Acts of Meaning* (Cambridge, Mass.: Harvard University Press, 1990), 115–16.

5. H. J. M. Hermans, H. J. C. Kempen, and R. J. P. van Loon, "The Dialogical Self: Beyond Individualism and Rationalism," *American Psychologist* 47 (1992): 23–33.

6. Bruner, *Acts of Meaning*; Robert Kegan, *The Evolving Self: Problem and Process in Human Development* (Cambridge, Mass.: Harvard University Press, 1982).

7. Nikolas Coupland and John F. Nussbaum, *Discourse and Lifespan Identity* (Newbury Park, Calif.: Sage Publications, 1993), xx.

8. Charles Taylor et al., *Multiculturalism: Examining the Politics of Recognition,* ed. Amy Gutmann, rev. ed. (Princeton, N.J.: Princeton University Press, 1994).

9. Ann Locke Davidson, *Making and Molding Identity in Schools: Student Narratives on Race, Gender, and Academic Achievement* (Albany: State University of New York Press, 1996), 4.

10. Ibid., 1.

11. Sheldon Stryker, "Identity Theory: Developments and Extensions," in *Self and Identity: Psychosocial Perspectives,* ed. Krysia Yardley and T. Honess (New York: John Wiley & Sons, 1987), 89–104.

12. Ibid., 90.

13. Kenneth J. Gergen, *The Saturated Self: Dilemmas of Identity in Contemporary Life* (New York: Basic Books, 1991).

14. Ibid., 139–40.

15. Evanthia Lyons, "Coping with Social Change: Processes of Social Memory in the Reconstruction of Identities," in *Changing European Identities: Social Psychological Analyses of Social Change,* ed. Glynis Breakwell and Evanita Lyons (Oxford: Butterworth-Heinemann, 1996), 34.

16. Ibid., 37.

17. Stephanie Coontz, *The Way We Never Were: American Families and the Nostalgia Trap* (New York: Basic Books, 2000).

18. Dora S. Dien, "Big Me and Little Me: A Chinese Perspective on Self," *Psychiatry: Journal for the Study of Interpersonal Processes* 46 (1983): 281–86.

19. Henri Tajfel, ed., *Differentiation between Social Groups: Studies in the Social Psychology of Intergroup Relations* (London: Academic Press, 1978); Henri Tajfel, *Human Groups and Social Categories: Studies in Social Psychology* (Cambridge: Cambridge University Press, 1981); Henri Tajfel, "Instrumentality, Identity and Social Comparisons," in *Social Identity in Intergroup Relations,* ed. Henri Tajfel (Cambridge: Cambridge University Press, 1982); Henri Tajfel and John C. Turner, "The Social Identity Theory of Intergroup Behavior," in *The Psychology of Intergroup Relations,* ed. Stephen Worchel and William G. Austin (Chicago: Nelson-Hall, 1985), 7–24.

20. Dora Dien, "The Evolving Nature of Self-Identity across Four Levels of History," *Human Development* 43 (2000): 1–18.

21. James Waldram, *Revenge of the Windigo: The Construction of the Mind and Mental Health of North American Aboriginal Peoples* (Toronto, ON: University of Toronto Press, 2004).

22. Shi-xu, "Cultural Perceptions: Exploiting the Unexpected of the Other," *Culture & Psychology* 1 (1995): 317.

23. William R. Penuel and James V. Wertsch, "Dynamics of Negation in the Identity Politics of Cultural Other and Cultural Self," *Culture & Psychology* 1 (1995): 343–59.

24. Ibid., 354; Waldram, *Revenge of the Windigo.*

Chapter 7. How Culture Changes Biology and Genetics

1. Fred Tyson, Ph.D., National Institute of Environmental Health Sciences, quoted in "'Epigenetics' Means What We Eat, How We Live and Love, Alters How Our Genes Behave," *Duke Medicine News,* October 26, 2005, http://dukehealth.org/HealthLibrary/News/9322?search_highlight=prental (accessed June 23, 2009).

2. M. F. Fraga et al., "Epigenetic Differences Arise during the Lifetime of Monozygotic Twins," *Proceedings of the National Academy of Sciences of the United States* 102 (July 26, 2005): 10604–9; G. M. Martin, "Epigenetic Drift in Aging Identical Twins," *Proceedings of the National Academy of Sciences of the United States* 102 (July 26, 2005): 10413–4.

3. Peter Roy-Byrne, M.D., et al., "Emerging Perspectives: Epigenesis—How Experience Sculpts Genes," *Journal Watch Psychiatry* 17 (August 2005), http://psychiatry.jwatch.org/cgi/content/full/2005/817/1 (accessed June 24, 2009).

4. L. D. Brown and M. F. Schneider, "Delayed Dedifferentiation and Retention of Properties in Dissociated Adult Skeletal Muscle Fibers In Vitro," *In Vitro Cellular & Developmental Biology—Animal* 38, no. 7: 411–22.

5. Andrea Mechelli et al., "Neurolinguistics: Structural Plasticity in the Bilingual Brain," *Nature* 431 (October 2004): 757.

Chapter 8. How Culture Is Context and Context Shapes Behavior

1. Christopher Frith, *Making Up the Mind: How the Brain Creates Our Mental World* (Malden, Mass.: Blackwell Publishing, 2007), 17.

2. Ibid., 16.

3. Lawrence W. Barsalou, "Grounded Cognition," *Annual Review of Psychology* 59 (2008): 617–45.

4. Boyd, *Origins of Stories,* 155.

5. Barsalou, "Grounded Cognition," 618–19.

6. Boyd, *Origins of Stories,* 156.

7. Boyd, *Origins of Stories,* 157.

8. Daniel L. Schachter and Donna Rose Addis, "The Cognitive Neuroscience of Constructive Memory: Remembering the Past and Imagining the Future," *Philosophical Transactions of the Royal Society* B 362 (2007): 773–86.

9. Randy L. Buckner, "Prospection and the Brain," *Behavior and Brain Sciences* 30 (2007): 318–19.

10. Antonio Damasio, *Descartes' Error: Emotion, Reason, and the Human Brain* (New York: Harper Perennial, 1995).

11. H. R. Markus and Shinobu Kitayama, "Culture and the Self: Implications for Cognition, Emotion, and Motivation," *Psychological Review* 98 (1991): 224–58; H. R. Markus, Shinobu Kitayama, and R. J. Heiman, "Culture and 'Basic' Psychological Principles," in *Social Psychology: Handbook of Basic Principles,* ed. E. T. Higgins and A. W. Kruglanski (New York: Guilford, 1996).

12. M. W. Morris and K. Peng, "Culture and Cause: American and Chinese Attributions for Social and Physical Events," *Journal of Personality and Social Psychology* 67 (1994): 949–71.

13. Shinobu Kitayama and D. Cohen, *Handbook of Cultural Psychology* (New York: Guilford, 2007); Shinobu Kitayama, S. Duffy, T. Kawamura, and J. T. Larsen, "Perceiving an Object and Its Context in Different Cultures: A Cultural Look at New Look," *Psychological Science* 14 (2003): 201–6; T. Masuda and R. E. Nesbitt, "Attending Holistically vs. Analytically: Comparing the Context Sensitivity of Japanese and Americans," *Journal of Personality and Social Psychology* 81 (2001): 922–34.

14. Hillary A. Elfenbein and Nalini Ambady, "On the Universality and Cultural Specificity of Emotion Recognition: A Meta-analysis," *Psychological Bulletin* 128 (2002): 203–35; K. C. H. Lam, K. Buehler, C. McFarland, M. Ross, and I. Cheung, "Cultural Differences in Affective Forecasting, the Role of Focalism," *Personality and Social Psychological Bulletin* 31: 1296–1309; Nico H. Frijda, *The Laws of Emotion* (Mahwah, N.J.: Lawrence Erlbaum Associates, 2007).

15. Joan Y. Chiao, T. Harada, H. Komeda, Z. Li, Y. Mano, D. N. Saito, N. Sadato, and T. Iidako, "Neural Basis of Individualistic and Collectivist Views of Self," *Cognitive Neuroscience Society Abstracts* (San Francisco, Calif.: Cognitive Neuroscience Society, 2008).

16. Joan Y. Chiao and Nalini Ambady, "Cultural Neuroscience: Parsing Universality and Diversity across Levels of Analysis," in *Handbook of Cultural Psychology,* ed. S. Kitayama and D. Cohen (New York: Guilford Press, 2007).

17. Joan Y. Chiao, Zhang Li, and Tokiko Harada, "Cultural Neuroscience of Consciousness: From Visual Perception to Self-Awareness," in *The Origin of Consciousness in the Social World,* ed. Charles Whitehead (Exeter, UK: Imprint Academic, 2008), 58–69.

18. Robert Turner, "Perfusion Studies and Fast Imaging," in *Cerebral Blood Flow: Mathematical Models, Instrumentation, and Imaging Techniques,* ed. A. Rescigno and A. Biocelli (L'Aquila, Italy: Proceedings of NATO ASI, 1988), 245–58.

19. Robert Turner, "Culture and the Human Brain," *Anthropology and Humanism* 26 (2002): 1–6.

20. Robert Turner and Charles Whitehead, "How Collective Representations Can Change the Structure of the Brain," in *The Origin of Consciousness in the Social World,* ed. Charles Whitehead (Exeter, UK: Imprint Academic, 2008), 43–57.

21. Norman Doidge, *The Brain That Changes Itself: Stories of Personal Triumph from the Frontiers of Brain Science* (New York: Penguin, 2007), 51.

22. Whitehead, "Editor's Introduction," *Origin of Consciousness.*

23. Ibid.

24. Charles Whitehead, "Social Mirrors and the Brain" (Ph.D. diss., Department of Anthropology, University College, London, 2003).

25. Doidge, *Brain That Changes Itself,* 265–66, 278–79.

26. Charles Whitehead, "Social Mirrors and Shared Experiential Worlds," *Journal of Consciousness Studies* 8, no. 4 (2001): 3–36.

27. R. M. Keesing, *Kwaio Religion: The Living and the Dead in a Solomon Island Society* (New York: Columbia University Press, 1982).

28. Chris Frith, *Making Up the Mind: How the Brain Creates Our Mental World* (London: Blackwell Publishing, 2007).

29. Chris D. Frith and Uta Frith, "Social Cognition in Humans," *Current Biology* 17, no. 16 (August 2007): R724–R732; Christof Koch, *The Quest for Consciousness: A Neurobiological Approach* (Greenwood Village, Colo.: Roberts & Company Publishers, 2004); cf. Émile Durkheim, *The Elementary Forms of Religious Life* (London: Allen & Unwin, 1912; reprint 1964).

30. Steven Pinker, *How the Mind Works* (New York: Norton, 1997), 207.

31. Colwyn Trevarthen, "First Things First: Infants Make Good Use of the Sympathetic Rhythm of Imitation, Without Reason or Language," *Journal of Child Psychotherapy* 31, no. 1 (2005): 91–113; Colwyn Trevarthen, "The Musical Art of Infant Conversation: Narrating in the Time of Sympathetic Experience, Without Rational Interpretation, Before Words," in *Musical Scientiae,* ed. M. Imberty and M. Gratin, special issue, Narrative in Music and Interaction (Liege: European Society for the Cognitive Sciences, 2008), 15–48.

32. Charles A. Nelson, "The Ontogeny of Human Memory: A Cognitive Neuroscience Perspective," in *Brain Development and Cognition: A Reader,* ed. Mark Henry Johnson, Yuko Munakata, and Rick O. Gilmore (New York: Wiley-Blackwell, 2002), 151–70; K. Nelson and G. Ross, "The Generalities and Specifics of Long-term Memory in Infants and Young Children," in *New Directions for Child Development—Memory,* ed. M. Perlmutter (San Francisco: Jossey-Bass, 1980), 87–101; Theodore J. Gaensbauer, "Representations of Trauma in Infancy: Clinical and Theoretical Implications for the Study of Early Memory," *Infant Mental Health Journal* 23, no. 3: 259–77.

33. Giacomo Rizzolatti and Corrado Sinigaglia, "Mirror Neurons and Motor Intentionality," *Functional Neurology* 22, no. 4 (2007): 205–10.

34. Max Weisbuch and Naline Ambady, "Non-conscious Routes to Building Culture: Nonverbal Components of Socialization," in Whitehead, *Origin of Consciousness.*

35. Max Weisbuch and Naline Ambady, "Unspoken Cultural Influence: Exposure to and Influence of Non-verbal Bias," *Journal of Personality and Social Psychology* 96, no. 6 (June 2009): 1104–19.

36. C. Trevarthen, "Instincts for Human Understanding and for Cultural Cooperation: Their Development in Infancy," in *Human Ethology,* ed. M. van Cronach, K. Foppa, W. Lepenies, and D. Ploog (Cambridge: Cambridge University Press, 1979).

37. Colwyn Trevarthen, "Conversations with a Two-month Old," *New Scientist* (May 1974): 230–35.

38. Boyd, *Origins of Stories,* 98.

39. Whitehead, "Social Mirrors."

40. Gratier and Trevarthen, "Musical Narratives."

41. Boyd, *Origins of Stories,* 51–53.

42. James E. King, Duane M. Rumbaugh, and E. Sue Savage-Rumbaugh, "Perception of Personality Traits and Semantic Learning in Evolving Hominids," in *The Descent of Mind: Psychological Perspectives on Hominid Evolution,* ed. Michael C. Corballis and Stephen E. G. Lea (New York: Oxford University Press, 1999), 98–116; Brothers, "The Social Brain: A Project for Integrating Primate Behavior and Neurophysiology in a New Domain," *Concepts in Neuroscience* 1 (1990): 27–51; L. Brothers, *Friday's Footprint: How Society Shapes the Human Mind* (New York: Oxford University Press, 1997); R. Adolphs, "Social Cognition and the Human Brain," *Trends in Cognitive Science* 3, no. 12 (1999): 469–79.

43. Boyd, *Origins of Stories,* 51–53.

44. Gratier and Trevarthen, "Musical Narratives."

45. Robert Turner, "Brain Images of Collective Representations," in *Brain, Mind, and Culture,* ed. A. Ioannides (London: Blackwell, 2005), 149–51.

46. Gratier and Trevarthen, "Musical Narratives."

47. Colwyn Trevarthen, "Intrinsic Motives for Companionship in Understanding: Their Origin, Development, and Significance for Infant Mental Health," in *Infant Mental Health Journal* 22, no. 1 (2001): 95–131.

48. Colwyn Trevarthen, "Infancy, Mind," in *Oxford Companion to the Mind,* 2nd ed., ed. R. L. Gregory (New York: Oxford University Press, 2004), 455–64.

49. Malcolm Gladwell, *Blink: The Power of Thinking without Thinking* (New York: Norton, 2005).

Chapter 9. Stories from Science: Change Is Always Possible

1. Louis Cozolino, *The Neuroscience of Human Relationships: Attachment and the Developing Social Brain* (New York: Norton, 2006).

2. Ernest Rossi, *The Psychobiology of Gene Expression* (New York: Norton, 2002).

3. Ibid., xv–xvi.

4. Eric F. Kandel, "A New Intellectual Framework for Psychiatry," *American Journal of Psychiatry* 155 (1998): 457–69.

5. J. F. Staiger, S. Bisler, A. Schleicher, P. Gass, J. H. Stehle, and K. Zilles, "Exploration of a Novel Environment Leads to the Expression of Inducible Transcription Factors in Barrel-related Columns," *Neuroscience* 99, no. 1 (July 26, 2000): 7–16.

6. Gerd Kempermann, "Why New Neurons? Possible Functions for Adult Hippocampal Neurogenesis," *The Journal of Neuroscience* 22, no. 3 (February 1, 2002): 635–38.

7. Boyd, *Origins of Stories,* 124.

8. Ibid.

9. Ibid., 95.

10. Rossi, *Psychobiology of Gene Expression,* 7.

11. Cynthia M. Kuhn and Saul Schanberg, "Responses to Maternal Separation: Mechanisms and Mediators," *International Journal of Developmental Neuroscience* 16 (1998): 261–270; Cynthia M. Kuhn, Saul Schanberg, Tiffany M. Field, R Symanski, E. Zimmermann, Frank Scafidi, and F. J. Roberts, "Tactile-Kinesthetic Stimulation Effects on Sympathetic and Adrenocortical Function in Preterm Infants," *Journal of Pediatrics* 119 (1991): 434–40.

12. J. V. Bartolomé, M. B. Bartolomé, S. Wang, and Saul Schanberg, "Involvement of c-myc and max in CNS Beta-endorphin Modulation of Hepatic Ornithine Decarboxylase Responsiveness to Insulin in Rat Pups," *Life Sciences* 64 (1999): 87–91; D. H. Russell, "Ornithine Decarboxylase: A Key Regulatory Enzyme in Normal and Neoplastic Growth," *Drug Metabolism Reviews* 16 (1985): 1–88; S. Wang, J. Bartolomé, and Saul Schanberg, "Neonatal Deprivation of Maternal Touch May Suppress Ornithine Decarboxylase via Downregulation of the Proto-oncogenes c-myc and max," *Journal of Neuroscience* 16, no. 2 (1996): 836–42.

13. G. Powell, C. Brasel, and C. Hansen, "Emotional Deprivation and Growth Retardation Simulating Idiopathic Hypopituitarism: I. Clinical Evaluation of the Syndrome," *New England Journal of Medicine* 276 (1967): 1271–78; G. Powell, N. Hopwood, and E. Baratt, "Growth Hormone Studies before and during Catch-up Growth in a Child with Emotional Deprivation and Short Stature," *Journal of Clinical Endocrinology and Metabolism* 37 (1973): 674–79.

14. Frances A. Champagne, Pablo Chretien, Carl W. Stevenson, Tie Yuan Zhang, Alain Gratton, and Michael J. Meaney, "Variations in Nucleus Accumbens Dopamine Associated with Individual Differences in Maternal Behavior in the Rat," *Journal of Neuroscience* 24, no. 17 (April 28, 2004): 4113–23; Frances A. Champagne, Darlene D. Francis, Adam Mar, and Michael J. Meaney, "Variations in Maternal Care in the Rat as a Mediating Influence for the Effects of Environment on Development," *Physiology & Behavior* 79 (2003): 359–71.

15. Christine M. Colvis, Jonathan D. Pollock, Richard H. Goodman, Soren Impey, John Dunn, Gail Mandel, Frances A. Champagne, et al., "Epigenetic Mechanisms and Gene Networks in the Nervous System," *Journal of Neuroscience* 25, no. 45 (2005): 10379–89.

16. Frances A. Champagne, Ian C. G. Weaver, Josie Diorio, Shakti Sharma, and Michael J. Meaney, "Natural Variations in Maternal Care Are Associated with Estrogen Receptor alpha Expression and Estrogen Sensitivity in the Medial Preoptic Area," *Endocrinology* 144, no. 11 (2003): 4720–24.

17. Ian C. G. Weaver, Frances A. Champagne, Shelley E. Brown, Sergiy Dymov, Shakti Sharma, Michael J. Meaney, and Moshe Szyf, "Reversal of Maternal Programming of Stress Responses in Adult Offspring through Methyl Supplementation: Altering Epigenetic Marking Later in Life," *Journal of Neuroscience* 25, no. 47 (2005): 11045–54.

18. Darren Sush, "A Final Solution with No End? The Transgenerational Effect of the Holocaust," http://judaism.about.com/od/holocaust/a/darrensash.htm (accessed January 12, 2010).

19. Sarah Thompson, Christine Kopperud, and Lewis Mehl-Madrona, "Healing Intergenerational Trauma in Aboriginal Communities," in *Mass Trauma and Emotional Healing around the World: Rituals and Practices for Resilience and Meaning-Making,* vol. 2, ed. Ani Kalayjian and Dominique Eugene (Santa Barbara, Calif.: Praeger, 2009), 343–60.

20. Frances A. Champagne, "Epigenetic Mechanisms and the Transgenerational Effects of Maternal Care," *Frontiers in Neuroendocrinology* 29, no. 3 (June 2008): 386–97.

21. Frances A. Champagne and Michael J. Meaney, "Transgenerational Effects of Social Environment on Variations in Maternal Care and Behavioral Response to Novelty," *Behavioral Neuroscience* 121, no. 6 (2007): 1353–63.

22. Avshalom Caspi, Ian Craig, Joseph McClay, Terri Moffitt, Jonathan Mill, Judy Martin, Alan Taylor, and Richie Poulton, "Role of Genotype in the Cycle of Violence of Maltreated Children," *Science* 297 (2002): 5592: 851–54.

23. H. G. Brunner, M. Nelen, X. O. Breakefield, H. H. Ropers, and B. A. van Oost, "Abnormal Behavior Associated with a Point Mutation in the Structural Gene for Monoamine Oxidase A," *Science* 262, no. 5133 (1993): 578–80; J. Kim-Cohen, A. Caspi, A. Taylor, B. Williams, R. Newcombe, I. W. Craig, and T. E. Moffitt, "MAOA, Maltreatment, and Gene-environment Interaction Predicting Children's Mental Health: New Evidence and a Meta-analysis," *Molecular Psychiatry* 11, no. 10 (October 2006): 903–13.

24. Alan Taylor and Julia Kim-Cohen, "Meta-analysis of Gene-environment Interactions in Developmental Psychopathology," *Development and Psychopathology* 16, no. 2 (2007): 271–83, vii.

25. Michael Rutter, "The Psychological Effects of Early Institutional Raising," in *The Development of Social Engagement: Neurobiological Perspectives,* ed. Peter J. Marshall and Nathan A. Fox (New York: Oxford University Press, 2005), 355–75.

26. Avshalom Caspi, Karen Sugden, Terrie E. Moffitt, Alan Taylor, Ian W. Craig, HonaLee Harrington, Joseph McClay, et al., "Influence of Life Stress on Depression: Moderation by a Polymorphism in the 5-HTT Gene," *Science* 301, no. 5631: 386–89.

27. Tracy Hampton, "Researchers Seek Roots of Resilience in Children," *Journal of the American Medical Association* 295, no. 15 (2006): 1756–60.

28. Caspi et al., "Influence of Life Stress."

29. Ronald Glaser and Janice K. Kiecolt-Glaser, "Science and Society: Stress-induced Immune Dysfunction: Implications for Health," *Nature Reviews Immunology* 5 (2005): 243–51.

30. For more information on theories about the relationship of schizophrenia to the immune system, see Rael D. Strousa and Yehuda Shoenfeld, "Schizophrenia, Autoimmunity and Immune System Dysregulation: A Comprehensive Model Updated and Revisited," *Journal of Autoimmunity* 27, no. 2 (2006): 71–80.

31. David Servan-Schreiber, *Anti-Cancer: A New Way of Life* (New York: Penguin, 2008).

32. John Shotter, "Dialogical Views of Mind and Self," in *The Plural Self: Multiplicity in Everyday Life,* ed. John Rowan and Mick Cooper (Thousand Oaks, Calif.: Sage Publications, 1999).

Chapter 10. The Power of Ceremony

1. See Andrew Weil and Anne-Marie Chiassaon, *Essentials of Energy Medicine* (Boulder, Colo.: Sounds True Productions, 2009).
2. Richard W. Voss, Victor Douville, Alex Little Soldier, and Gayla Twiss, "Tribal and Shamanic-based Social Work Practice: A Lakota Perspective," *Social Work* 44, no. 3 (1999): 228–41.
3. Ibid.
4. Malcolm Gladwell, *Outliers* (New York: Norton, 2008).
5. Voss et al., "Shamanic-based Social Work."
6. Kompare, 1980, quoted by Sandra Francis in "The Role of Dance in a Navajo Healing Ceremony," in *Handbook of Culture, Therapy, and Healing,* ed. Uwe Peter Gielen, Jefferson Fish, and Juris Draguns (Mahwah, N.J.: Lawrence Erlbaum Associates, 2004), 136. (Revised from book of same title by Uwe P. Gielen, 1980.)
7. James C. Faris, *The Nightway: A History and a History of Documentation of a Navajo Ceremonial,* 3rd ed. (Albuquerque, N.M.: University of New Mexico Press, 1995).
8. Francis, "Role of Dance," 135–150.
9. Ibid., 136–37.
10. D. Saleeby, *The Strengths Perspective in Social Work Practice* (New York: Longman, 1992), 11.
11. Doug Boyd, *Rolling Thunder* (New York: Harper and Row, 1982).

Chapter 11. How Communities Create Change

1. Joyce Vesper, "The Use of Healing Ceremonies in the Treatment of Multiple Personality Disorder," *Dissociation* 5, no. 2 (June 1991), 109–14.

Chapter 12. To Story or Not to Story

1. Edward Shorter, *A History of Psychiatry: From the Era of the Asylum to the Age of Prozac* (New York: John Wiley & Sons, 1997), 255.
2. Robert Whitaker, "The Case against Antipsychotic Drugs: A 50-year Record of Doing More Harm than Good," *Medical Hypotheses* 62 (2004): 5–13.
3. Ibid., 6–7.
4. Ibid.
5. Ann Braden Johnson, *Out of Bedlam* (New York: Basic Books, 1990; rev. ed., 1992).
6. Whitaker, "Case against Antipsychotic Drugs."
7. J. Cole, G. Klerman, and S. Goldberg, for the National Institute of Mental Health Psychopharmacology Service Center Collaborative Study Group, "Phenothiazine Treatment in Acute Schizophrenia," *Archives of General Psychiatry* 10

(1964): 246–61; P. Gilbert, M. Harris, L. McAdams, and D. Jeste, "Neuroleptic Withdrawal in Schizophrenic Patients," *Archives of General Psychiatry* 52 (1995): 173–88.

8. Jeffrey A. Lieberman, T. Scott Stroup, Joseph P. McEvoy, Marvin S. Swartz, Robert A. Rosenheck, Diana O. Perkins, Richard S. E. Keefe, et al., for the Clinical Antipsychotic Trials of Intervention Effectiveness (CATIE) Investigators, "Effectiveness of Antipsychotic Drugs in Patients with Chronic Schizophrenia," *New England Journal of Medicine* 353, no. 12 (2005): 1209–23; Elaine Zablocki, "Second-generation Antipsychotics Offer Mixed Results: Finding Most Effective Antipsychotic Drug Can Be Trial and Error Process," June 1, 2007, http://managedhealthcareexecutive .modernmedicine.com (accessed August 22, 2009); Richard P. Bentall, *Madness Explained: Psychosis and Human Nature* (New York: Penguin, 2004).

9. J. Hegarty, R. Baldessarini, M. Tohen, C. Waternaux, and G. Oepen, "One Hundred Years of Schizophrenia: A Meta-analysis of the Outcome Literature," *American Journal of Psychiatry* 151 (1994): 1409–16; C. Holden, "Deconstructing Schizophrenia," *Science* 299 (2003): 333–35; P. Weiden, R. Aquila, and J. Standard, "Atypical Antipsychotic Drugs and Long-term Outcome in Schizophrenia," *Journal of Clinical Psychiatry* 57, Suppl. no. 11 (1996): 53–60; P. Harvey, "Cognitive Impairment in Schizophrenia: Its Characteristics and Implications," *Psychiatric Annuals* 29 (1999): 657–60.

10. Emmanuel Stip, "Happy Birthday Neuroleptics! 50 Years Later: *La folie du doute*," *European Psychiatry* 17, no. 3 (May 2002): 115–19.

11. Robert Whitaker, *Mad in America: Bad Science, Bad Medicine, and the Enduring Mistreatment of the Mentally Ill* (New York: Perseus Books, 2002).

12. Raymond Mar, "The Neuropsychology of Narrative: Story Comprehension, Story Production and Their Interrelation," *Neuropsychologia* 42 (2004): 1414–34.

13. Maryanne Wolf, *Proust and the Squid: The Story and Science of the Reading Brain* (New York: Penguin Books, 2008), 215.

14. Jennifer C. Day, Richard P. Bentall, Chris Roberts, Fiona Randall, Anne Rogers, Dinah Cattell, David Healy, Pam Rae, and Cheryl Power, "Attitudes toward Antipsychotic Medication: The Impact of Clinical Variables and Relationships with Health Professionals," *Archives of General Psychiatry* 62 (2005): 717–24.

15. Ibid.

16. Ibid.

17. Boyd, *Origins of Stories,* 188.

18. Victor Robinson, *The Story of Medicine* (London: Kessinger Publishing, 2005), 190.

19. Ronald Havens, *The Wisdom of Milton H. Erickson: The Complete Volume* (Bethel, Conn.: Crown House Publishing, 2005).

20. James Hillman, *Healing Fiction* (New York: Continuum, 1994), 17.

21. Ibid.

22. Jacques Lacan, *The Four Fundamental Concepts of Psychoanalysis,* ed. Jacques-Alain

Miller, trans. Alan Sheridan, *The Seminar of Jacques Lacan,* book XI (New York: Norton, 1998).

23. Erving Goffman, *Asylums: Essays on the Social Situations of Mental Patients and Other Inmates* (New York: Anchor Books, 1961).

24. W. Fenton, L. Mosher, J. Herrell, and C. Blyler, "A Randomized Trial of General Hospital Versus Residential Alternative Care for Patients with Severe and Persistent Mental Illness," *American Journal of Psychiatry* 155 (1998): 516–22.

25. Loren Mosher, "Soteria and Other Alternatives to Acute Psychiatric Hospitalization: A Personal and Professional Review," *Journal of Nervous and Mental Disease* 187 (1999): 142–49.

26. See L. Mosher, A. Menn, R. Vallone, D. Fort, "Treatment at Soteria House: A Manual for the Practice of Interpersonal Phenomenology," published in German as *Dabeisein—Das Manual zur Praxis in der Soteria* (Bonn: Psychiatrie Verlag, 1994).

27. P. B. Braun, G. Kochansky, R. Shapiro, S. Greenberg, J. E. Gudeman, S. Johnson, and M. F. Shore, "Overview: Deinstitutionalization of Psychiatric Patients: A Critical Review of Outcome Studies," *American Journal of Psychiatry* 138 (1981): 736–49; S. M. Matthews, M. T. Roper, L. R. Mosher, and A. Z. Menn, "A Nonneuroleptic Treatment for Schizophrenia: Analysis of the Two-year Post-discharge Risk of Relapse," *Schizophrenia Bulletin* 5 (1979): 322–33; R. B. Straw, "Meta-analysis of Deinstitutionalization" (Ph.D. diss., Northwestern University, Ann Arbor, Mich., 1982); B. A. Stroul, *Crisis Residential Services in a Community Support System* (Rockville, Md.: NIMH Community Support Program, 1987); R. Warner, ed., *Alternatives to the Mental Hospital for Acute Psychiatric Treatment* (Washington, D.C.: American Psychiatric Press, 1995); R. J. Wendt, L. R. Mosher, S. M. Matthews, and A. Z. Menn, "A Comparison of Two Treatment Environments for Schizophrenia," in *The Principles and Practices of Milieu Therapy,* ed. J. G. Gunderson, O. A. Will, and L. R. Mosher (New York: Jason Aronson, 1983), 17–33.

28. Loren Mosher and A. Z. Menn, "Community Residential Treatment for Schizophrenia: Two-Year Follow-up," *Hospital Community Psychiatry* 29 (1978): 715–23; Loren Mosher, R. Vallone, and A. Z. Menn, "The Treatment of Acute Psychosis without Neuroleptics: Six-week Psychopathology Outcome Data from the Soteria Project," *International Journal of Social Psychiatry* 41 (1995): 157–73.

29. Rudolf H. Moos, *Evaluating Treatment Environments: A Social Ecological Approach* (New York: John Wiley, 1974); Rudolf H. Moos, *Evaluating Correctional and Community Settings* (New York: John Wiley, 1975).

30. Wendt et al., "Comparison of Two Treatment Environments."

31. Fenton et al., "Randomized Trial."

32. R. M. Hirschfeld, S. M. Matthews, Loren Mosher, and A. Z. Menn, "Being with Madness: Personality Characteristics of Three Treatment Staffs," *Hospital Community Psychiatry* 28 (1977): 267–73; Loren Mosher, Ann Reifman, and A. Menn, "Characteristics of Nonprofessionals Serving as Primary Therapists for Acute Schizophrenics," *Hospital Community Psychiatry* 24 (1973): 391–96.

33. M. Kresky-Wolff, S. Matthews, F. Kalibat, and Loren Mosher, "Crossing Place: A Residential Model for Crisis Intervention," *Hospital Community Psychiatry* 35, no. 1 (1984): 72–74.

34. Loren Mosher, M. Kresky-Wolff, S. Matthews, and A. Menn, "Milieu Therapy in the 1980s: A Comparison of Two Residential Alternatives to Hospitalization," *Bulletin of Menninger Clinic* 50 (1986): 262–64.

35. Ibid., 257–68.

36. Fenton et al., "Randomized Trial."

37. For more about Fountain House, see their website, www.fountainhouse.org/moxie/who/.

38. Paul Ricoeur, "Life in Quest of Narrative," in *On Paul Ricoeur: Narrative and Interpretation,* ed. David Wood (New York, London: Routledge, 1991), 20–33.

39. Juha Holma and Jukka Aaltonen, "The Self-Narrative and Acute Psychosis," *Contemporary Family Therapy* 17, no. 3 (September 1995): 307–16.

40. H. Anderson and H. Goolishian, "The Client Is the Expert: A Not-Knowing Approach to Therapy," in *Therapy as Social Construction,* ed. Sheila McNamee and Kenneth J. Gergen (London: Sage Publications, 1992), 23–39.

41. Y. O. Alanen, V. Räkköläinen, J. Laakso, R. Rasimus, and A. Kaljonen, "Towards Need-Specific Treatment of Schizophrenic Psychoses," *Monographien aus dem Gesamtgebiete der Psychiatrie = Psychiatry Series* 41 (1986): 1–295; Y. O. Alanen, K. Lehtinen, V. Räkköläinen, and J. Aaltonen, "Need-Adapted Treatment of New Schizophrenic Patients: Experiences and Results of the Turku Project," *Acta Psychiatrica Scandinavica* 83, no. 5 (1991): 363–72; V. Räkköläinen, K. Lehtinen, and Y. O. Alanen, "Need-Adapted Treatment of Schizophrenic Processes: The Essential Role of Family-Centered Therapy Meetings," *Contemporary Family Therapy* 13, no. 6: 573–82; J. Aaltonen, A. Vartiainen, M-L. Kalliokoski, and T. Riikonen, "Team Treatment of Acute Psychosis," *Journal of Family Psychotherapy* 5 (1994): 77–95.

42. Aaltonen et al., "Team Treatment."

43. Ibid.

44. V. Lehtinen, J. Aaltonen, T. Koffere, V. Räkköläinen, and E. Syvälahti, "Two-year Outcome in First-episode Psychosis Treated according to an Integrated Model: Is Immediate Neuroleptisation Always Needed?" *European Psychiatry* 15 (2000): 312–20.

Chapter 13. Indigenous Models for the Practice of Psychiatry and Mental Health

1. Sonam Rigzin, speaking on the radio in Australia (Australian Broadcasting Company, *The Road to Dharmasala,* Monday, June 7, 2004).

2. Paul Radin, *The Trickster: A Study in American Indian Mythology,* 2nd ed. (New York: Schocken Books, 1987), 165.

3. Yazzie, Ethelou, ed., *Navajo History,* vol. 1 (Chinle, Ariz.: Navajo Community College Press, 1971).

4. A. Hultkrantz, "Myths in Native North American Religion," in *Native Religious Traditions,* ed. Earle H. Waugh and K. Dad Prithipaul (Waterloo, Ontario: Wilfrid Laurier University Press, 1979), 77–96.

5. Guy H. Cooper, "Coyote in Navajo Religion and Cosmology," *The Canadian Journal of Native Studies* VII, no. 2 (1987): xx.

6. Leland Wyman, *Blessingway, with Three Versions of the Myth Recorded and Translated from the Navajo by Father Berard Haile* (Tucson: University of Arizona Press, 1970).

7. J. Barre Toelken, "The 'Pretty Language' of Yellowman: Genre, Mode, and Texture in Navajo Coyote Narratives," *Genre* 2 (1969): 211–35.

8. Cooper, "Coyote in Navajo Religion."

9. Toelken, "Pretty Language," 231.

10. F. J. Newcomb, *Navajo Folk Tales* (Albuquerque: University of New Mexico Press, 1990), 108–24.

11. Dorothy Reid, *Tales of Nanabozho,* 2nd ed. (London: Oxford University Press, 1979); Stith Thompson, *Tales of the North American Indians,* 2nd ed. (Bloomington: Indiana University Press, 2009), 53–59; *Indian Legends of Canada* (Toronto: McClelland and Stewart, 1977), 67; *Journal of American Folklore* 16: 229.

12. A. F. Chamberlain, "Nanabozho among the Otchipwe, Mississaugas, and Other Algonquin Tribes," *Journal of American Folklore* 4 (1891): 206–7.

13. W. J. Johnson, "Mythology of the Menominee Indians," *American Anthropologist* 3z (1890): 243–58; Chamberlain, "Nanabozho," 210–11; A. Skinner and J. V. Satterlee, "Folklore of the Menominee Indians," *Anthropological Papers of the American Museum of Natural History* 13, no. 3 (1915): 241.

Chapter 14. Narratives for Anxiety and Depression

1. Kenneth J. Gergen, *The Saturated Self,* 2nd ed. (New York: Basic Books, 2000), 211–12.

2. John Shotter, *Conversational Realities: Constructing Life through Language* (London: Sage Publications, 1993), 56.

3. This summary culled from Wikipedia, http://en.wikipedia.org/wiki/The _ Pilgrim%27s_Progress.

4. Ibid.

5. Vera Camden, "'That of Esau': The Place of Hebrews xii. 16, 17 in *Grace Abounding,*" in *John Bunyan: Reading Dissenting Writing,* ed. N. H. Keeble (Bern, Germany: Peter Lang, 2002).

6. J. T. McNeill, ed., *Calvin Institutes of the Christian Religion,* trans. F. L. Battles (Philadelphia: The Westminster Press, 1960).

7. Harlene Anderson and Harold Goolishian, "Human Systems as Linguistic Systems: Preliminary and Evolving Ideas about the Implications for Clinical Theory," *Family Process* 27 (1988): 371–93.

Chapter 15. Narratives and Bipolar Disorder

1. Lewis Mehl-Madrona, "Narrative Analysis: Alternative Constructions of Bipolar Disorder," *ADVANCES* 22, no. 2 (Fall 2007): 12–19.

2. John M. Marzluff and Tony Angell, *In the Company of Crows and Ravens* (New Haven, Conn.: Yale University Press, 2005), 80.

3. C. Chanthyda, "An Analysis of the Trickster Archetype as Represented by the Rabbit Character in Khmer Folktales" (master's thesis, Royal University of Phnom Penh, 2004).

Chapter 16. Narrative Approaches to Psychosis

1. Johnson, *Out of Bedlam.*

2. Ibid.

3. Norma Livo, "Abandonment Canyon," in *Story Medicine: Multicultural Tales of Healing and Transformation* (Englewood, Colo.: Greenwood Publishing Group, 2001), 177–78.

About the Author

A practicing physician since 1975 and an indigenous healer trained in Native American culture and ceremony, Lewis Mehl-Madrona, M.D., Ph.D., once more extends his new paradigm of healing approaches to "mental illness" and presents them to us in both a scientific and a practical manner. As a clinical assistant professor of family medicine at the University of Hawai'i School of Medicine and the director of training for the newly established Coyote Institute for Studies of Change and Transformation, where he directs its Center for Narrative and Indigenous Healing, he teaches courses on indigenous healing and narrative psychiatry and offers presentations, workshops, and healing sessions around the globe. He also teaches part-time at Johnson State College in Vermont and at Southwestern College in Santa Fe, New Mexico. He is a graduate of Stanford University School of Medicine, the Psychological Studies Institute in Palo Alto, and Massey University in Palmerston North, New Zealand, and is American board certified in family medicine and in psychiatry. His previous books include *Coyote Medicine: Lessons from Native American Healing* (1998), *Coyote Healing: Miracles in Native Medicine* (2003), *Coyote Wisdom: The Power of Story in Healing* (2005), and *Narrative Medicine: The Use of History and Story in the Healing Process* (2007). Visit his website at **www.mehl-madrona.com.**

Index

Books of Related Interest

Narrative Medicine
The Use of History and Story in the Healing Process
by Lewis Mehl-Madrona, M.D., Ph.D.

Coyote Healing
Miracles in Native Medicine
by Lewis Mehl-Madrona, M.D., Ph.D.

Coyote Wisdom
The Power of Story in Healing
by Lewis Mehl-Madrona, M.D., Ph.D.

Wheel of Initiation
Practices for Releasing Your Inner Light
by Julie Tallard Johnson

The Spiritual Anatomy of Emotion
How Feelings Link the Brain, the Body, and the Sixth Sense
by Michael A. Jawer with Marc S. Micozzi, M.D., Ph.D.

The Shamanic Wisdom of the Huichol
Medicine Teachings for Modern Times
by Tom Soloway Pinkson, Ph.D.

Shamanic Experience
A Practical Guide to Psychic Powers
by Kenneth Meadows

Shamanic Spirit
A Practical Guide to Personal Fulfillment
by Kenneth Meadows

INNER TRADITIONS • BEAR & COMPANY
P.O. Box 388
Rochester, VT 05767
1-800-246-8648
www.InnerTraditions.com

Or contact your local bookseller